2011
YEAR BOOK OF
ENDOCRINOLOGY®

The 2011 Year Book Series

Year Book of Anesthesiology and Pain Management™: Drs Chestnut, Abram, Black, Gravlee, Lien, Mathru, and Roizen

Year Book of Cardiology®: Drs Gersh, Cheitlin, Elliott, Gold, Graham, and Thourani

Year Book of Critical Care Medicine®: Drs Dellinger, Parrillo, Balk, Dorman, Dries, and Zanotti-Cavazzoni

Year Book of Dermatology and Dermatologic Surgery™: Dr Del Rosso

Year Book of Diagnostic Radiology®: Drs Osborn, Abbara, Elster, Manaster, Oestreich, Offiah, Rosado de Christenson, Stephens, and Walker

Year Book of Emergency Medicine®: Drs Hamilton, Bruno, Handly, Mullin, Quintana, and Ramoska

Year Book of Endocrinology®: Drs Schott, Apovian, Clarke, Eugster, Ludlam, Meikle, Schinner, Schteingart, and Toth

Year Book of Gastroenterology™: Drs Talley, DeVault, Harnois, Murray, Pearson, Philcox, Picco, and Smith

Year Book of Hand and Upper Limb Surgery®: Drs Yao and Steinmann

Year Book of Medicine®: Drs Barker, Garrick, Gersh, Khardori, LeRoith, Seo, Talley, and Thigpen

Year Book of Neonatal and Perinatal Medicine®: Drs Fanaroff, Benitz, Donn, Neu, Papile, Polin, and van Marter

Year Book of Neurology and Neurosurgery®: Drs Klimo and Rabinstein

Year Book of Obstetrics, Gynecology, and Women's Health®: Drs Dungan and Shulman

Year Book of Oncology®: Drs Arceci, Bauer, Chiorean, Gordon, Lawton, Murphy, Thigpen, and Tsao

Year Book of Ophthalmology®: Drs Rapuano, Cohen, Flanders, Fudemberg, Hammersmith, Milman, Myers, Nagra, Nelson, Penne, Pyfer, Sergott, Shields, Talekar, and Vander

Year Book of Orthopedics®: Drs Morrey, Beauchamp, Huddleston, Swiontkowski, and Trigg

Year Book of Otolaryngology-Head and Neck Surgery®: Drs Sindwani, Balough, Franco, Gapany, and Mitchell

Year Book of Pathology and Laboratory Medicine®: Drs Raab, Parwani, Bejarano, and Bissell

Year Book of Pediatrics®: Dr Stockman

Year Book of Plastic and Aesthetic Surgery™: Drs Miller, Gosain, Gurtner, Gutowski, Ruberg, Salisbury, and Smith

Year Book of Psychiatry and Applied Mental Health®: Drs Talbott, Ballenger, Buckley, Frances, Krupnick, and Mack

Year Book of Pulmonary Disease®: Drs Barker, Jones, Maurer, Raza, Tanoue, and Willsie

Year Book of Sports Medicine®: Drs Shephard, Cantu, Feldman, Jankowski, Khan, Lebrun, Nieman, Pierrynowski, and Rowland

Year Book of Surgery®: Drs Copeland, Behrns, Daly, Eberlein, Fahey, Huber, Klodell, Mozingo, and Pruett

Year Book of Urology®: Drs Andriole and Coplen

Year Book of Vascular Surgery®: Drs Moneta, Gillespie, Starnes, and Watkins

2011

The Year Book of ENDOCRINOLOGY®

Editor-in-Chief
Matthias Schott, MD, PhD

Associate Professor, Deputy Director of the Department of Endocrinology, Diabetology and Rheumatology, University Hospital of Düsseldorf, Düsseldorf, Germany

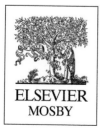

ELSEVIER
MOSBY

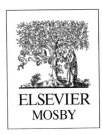

ELSEVIER
MOSBY

Vice President, Continuity: Kimberly Murphy
Developmental Editor: Patrick Manley
Production Supervisor, Electronic Year Books: Donna M. Skelton
Electronic Article Manager: Mike Sheets
Senior Illustrations and Permissions Coordinator: Dawn Vohsen

2011 EDITION

Composition by TNQ Books and Journals Pvt Ltd, India

Editorial Office:
Elsevier
Suite 1800
1600 John F. Kennedy Blvd
Philadelphia, PA 19103-2899

International Standard Serial Number: 0084-3741
International Standard Book Number: 978-0-323-08413-0

Printed and bound by CPI Group (UK) Ltd, Croydon, CR0 4YY

Transferred to digital print 2012

Associate Editors

Caroline M. Apovian, MD, FACP, FACN
Associate Professor of Medicine and Pediatrics, Boston University School of Medicine; Director, Center for Nutrition and Weight Management, Boston Medical Center, Boston, Massachusetts

Bart L. Clarke, MD
Associate Professor of Medicine, Mayo Clinic College of Medicine; Consultant, St. Mary's Hospital; Consultant, Rochester Methodist Hospital, Rochester, Minnesota

Erica Eugster, MD
Professor of Pediatrics, Director, Section of Pediatric Endocrinology/ Diabetology, Riley Hospital for Children, Indiana University School of Medicine, Indianapolis, Indiana

William H. Ludlam, MD, PhD
Director, Seattle Pituitary Center, Neuroscience Institute, Swedish Medical Center, Seattle, Washington

A. Wayne Meikle, MD
Professor of Medicine and Pathology, University of Utah School of Medicine; Director of Endocrine Testing, ARUP Laboratories, The University of Utah Hospitals, Salt Lake City, Utah

Sven Schinner, MD, PhD
Associate Professor of Medicine, Department of Endocrinology, Diabetes and Rheumatology, University Hospital of Düsseldorf, Düsseldorf, Germany

David E. Schteingart, MD
Professor, Department of Internal Medicine, Division of Metabolism, Endocrinology and Diabetes, University of Michigan Health System, Ann Arbor, Michigan

Peter P. Toth, MD, PhD, FAAFP, FICA, FAHA, FCCP, FACC
Director of Preventive Cardiology, Sterling Rock Falls Clinic, Ltd; Clinical Professor, University of Illinois College of Medicine, Peoria, Illinois; Southern Illinois University School of Medicine, Springfield, Illinois

Contributing Editors

Thomas Baehring, PhD
University Hospital of Düsseldorf, Düsseldorf, Germany

Rosane Ness-Abramof, MD
Meir Hospital, Kfar Saba, Israel, and Sackler School of Medicine, Tel Aviv, Israel

Megan Ruth, PhD
Post-doctoral Fellow, Endocrinology, Diabetes and Nutrition, Boston University School of Medicine, Boston, Massachusetts

Table of Contents

Journals Represented

Journals represented in this YEAR BOOK are listed below.

Acta Paediatrica
American Heart Journal
American Journal of Cardiology
American Journal of Clinical Nutrition
American Journal of Medicine
Annals of Internal Medicine
Annals of Surgery
Arteriosclerosis Thrombosis and Vascular Biology
British Medical Journal
Cancer Research
Cardiovascular and Interventional Radiological
Cell
Circulation
Clinical Cancer Research
Clinical Endocrinology
Clinical Nuclear Medicine
Diabetes
Diabetes Care
Endocrinology
European Heart Journal
European Journal of Endocrinology
European Urology
Fertility and Sterility
Human Reproduction
Hypertension
International Journal of Cardiology
International Journal of Obesity
Journal of Bone Mineral Research
Journal of Clinical Endocrinology & Metabolism
Journal of Clinical Investigation
Journal of Clinical Oncology
Journal of Clinical Psychopharmacology
Journal of Hypertension
Journal of Immunology
Journal of Neurosurgery
Journal of Pediatric Surgery
Journal of the American College of Cardiology
Journal of the American College of Surgeons
Journal of the American Medical Association
Journal of the National Cancer Institute
Journal of Urology
Journal of Vascular and Interventional Radiology
Lancet
Metabolism
Modern Pathology
Nature
Neuroendocrinology

New England Journal of Medicine
Osteoporosis International
Pediatrics
Proceedings of the National Academy of Sciences of the United States of America
Surgery
Thyroid
Urology
World Journal of Surgery

STANDARD ABBREVIATIONS

The following terms are abbreviated in this edition: adrenocorticotropin hormone (ACTH); acquired immunodeficiency syndrome (AIDS); cardiopulmonary resuscitation (CPR); central nervous system (CNS); cerebrospinal fluid (CSF); computed tomography (CT); corticotropin-releasing hormone (CRH); deoxyribonucleic acid (DNA); electrocardiography (ECG); follicle-stimulating hormone (FSH); gonadotropin-releasing hormone (GnRH); growth hormone (GH); health maintenance organization (HMO); high-density lipoprotein (HDL); human immunodeficiency virus (HIV); insulin-dependent diabetes mellitus (IDDM); insulin-like growth factor I (IGF-I); intensive care unit (ICU); intermediate-density lipoprotein (IDL); intramuscular (IM); intravenous (IV); low-density lipoprotein (LDL); luteinizing hormone (LH); magnetic resonance (MR) imaging (MRI); multiple endocrine neoplasia (MEN); non-insulin-dependent diabetes mellitus (NIDDM); parathyroid hormone (PTH); prolactin (PRL); releasing hormone (RH); ribonucleic acid (RNA); thyrotropin-releasing hormone (TRH); thyroid-stimulating hormone or thyrotropin (TSH); thyroxine (T_4); triiodothyronine (T_3); ultrasound (US); and very-low-density lipoprotein (VLDL).

NOTE

The YEAR BOOK OF ENDOCRINOLOGY is a literature survey service providing abstracts of articles published in the professional literature. Every effort is made to assure the accuracy of the information presented in these pages. Neither the editor nor the publisher of the YEAR BOOK OF ENDOCRINOLOGY can be responsible for errors in the original materials. The editors' comments are their own opinions. Mention of specific products within this publication does not constitute endorsement.

To facilitate the use of the YEAR BOOK OF ENDOCRINOLOGY as a reference tool, all illustrations and tables included in this publication are now identified as they appear in the original article. This change is meant to help the reader recognize that any illustration or table appearing in the YEAR BOOK OF ENDOCRINOLOGY may be only one of many in the original article. For this reason, figure and table numbers appear to be out of sequence within the YEAR BOOK OF ENDOCRINOLOGY.

Introduction

It is my fourth year as Editor-in-Chief of the YEAR BOOK OF ENDOCRINOLOGY. For me and for the co-editors, it was as difficult as the years before to choose the best articles (in our eyes) for the YEAR BOOK. Just to give you an example: by using the quite limited key words "thyroid cancer" in PubMed, almost 2000 articles show up. Therefore, there is a high probability that the co-editors and I have not included key research articles that will prove to be of high importance in the future. On the other hand, this has been minimalized since an on-line system has been established by Elsevier in which articles undergo a process of preselection. This helps the editors to evaluate each research article and pick up the most important articles in the field. Out of the selected articles, this year's Editor's Choice is an article by Neumann et al.[1] The study describes a new small-molecule antagonist that inhibits Graves' disease (GD) antibody activation of the TSH receptor. GD is caused by persistent, unregulated stimulation of thyroid cells by thyroid-stimulating antibodies (TSAbs) that activate the TSH receptor (TSHR). In the present study, the authors optimized small molecule TSHR ligands. This study has a major clinical implication. None of the therapies applied thus far in GD patients is pathogenesis-based. All therapies do not inhibit the production of TSAbs or TSAb activation of TSHR signaling. This type of therapy with a small molecule might be more easily titrated to achieve a euthyroid state and might be used to treat recurrences associated with anti-thyroid drugs and radioactive iodine.

We hope that the selected articles and their accompanying editorial comments provide our readers fresh insight into endocrine problems encountered in everyday practice.

Matthias Schott, MD, PhD

Reference

1. Neumann S, Eliseeva E, McCoy JG, et al. A new small-molecule antagonist inhibits Graves' disease antibody activation of the TSH receptor. *J Clin Endocrinol Metab*. 2011;96:548-554.

1 Diabetes

Introduction

What were major topics in diabetes research in 2010?

There were very interesting basic-science findings on the pathogenesis of type 2 diabetes. One highlight is definitely the work by Ng and colleagues, who used a mouse model to investigate why diabetes runs in families. Beyond classic genetics, there are obviously epigenetic alterations that predispose individuals to development of diabetes. In their study, over-feeding of the fathers made the offspring prone to diabetes, even though the offspring were not obese themselves.

This finding in a mouse model opens the broad area of epigenetic programming: environmental factors like overnutrition can apparently alter the expression of genes, and this can even be inherited. There are also interesting epidemiologic data from humans pointing in the same direction.

After the landmark studies ACCORD, ADVANCE, and the 10-year follow-up of the UKPDS study have been published in 2008, the diabetes community is still sorting out sub-analysis on this data. In 2010, an extension of the ACCORD study and post hoc analyses have been published that attempt to explain the factors contributing to cardiovascular mortality (see the article by the ACCORD study group in this chapter).

Another major topic was the association of obesity and diabetes with cancer risk. There are now plenty of data from epidemiological studies (eg, Berrington de Gonzalez et al) demonstrating the association of several cancer entities with obesity and diabetes.

At the next stage, mechanistic studies are needed to test whether this is a causal relationship.

Sven Schinner, MD, PhD

Complications

Diabetes Mellitus, Fasting Glucose, and Risk of Cause-Specific Death

The Emerging Risk Factors Collaboration (Univ of Cambridge, UK; et al)
N Engl J Med 364:829-841, 2011

Background.—The extent to which diabetes mellitus or hyperglycemia is related to risk of death from cancer or other nonvascular conditions is uncertain.

Methods.—We calculated hazard ratios for cause-specific death, according to baseline diabetes status or fasting glucose level, from individual-participant data on 123,205 deaths among 820,900 people in 97 prospective studies.

Results.—After adjustment for age, sex, smoking status, and body-mass index, hazard ratios among persons with diabetes as compared with persons without diabetes were as follows: 1.80 (95% confidence interval [CI], 1.71 to 1.90) for death from any cause, 1.25 (95% CI, 1.19 to 1.31) for death from cancer, 2.32 (95% CI, 2.11 to 2.56) for death from vascular causes, and 1.73 (95% CI, 1.62 to 1.85) for death from other causes. Diabetes (vs. no diabetes) was moderately associated with death from cancers of the liver, pancreas, ovary, colorectum, lung, bladder, and breast. Aside from cancer and vascular disease, diabetes (vs. no diabetes) was also associated with death from renal disease, liver disease, pneumonia and other infectious diseases, mental disorders, nonhepatic digestive diseases, external causes, intentional self-harm, nervous-system disorders, and chronic obstructive pulmonary disease. Hazard ratios were appreciably reduced after further adjustment for glycemia measures, but not after adjustment for systolic blood pressure, lipid levels, inflammation or renal markers. Fasting glucose levels exceeding 100 mg per deciliter (5.6 mmol per liter), but not levels of 70 to 100 mg per deciliter (3.9 to 5.6 mmol per liter), were associated with death. A 50-year-old with diabetes died, on average, 6 years earlier than a counterpart without diabetes, with about 40% of the difference in survival attributable to excess nonvascular deaths.

Conclusions.—In addition to vascular disease, diabetes is associated with substantial premature death from several cancers, infectious diseases, external causes, intentional self-harm, and degenerative disorders, independent of several major risk factors. (Funded by the British Heart Foundation and others.)

▶ The glucose thresholds to define the diagnosis of diabetes mellitus (DM) are based on the risk for retinopathy. However, it has been shown in numerous studies that DM is associated with increased macrovascular complication and cardiovascular death.[1,2] This study investigates not only the effects of DM on nonvascular death but also the relationship of fasting plasma glucose levels with the risk of death. Even after adjustment for body mass index and other risk factors, DM was associated with a strong increase in the risk for not only cardiovascular death but also death by cancer. The latter is of particular interest, as the relationship between glycemic control and the antihyperglycemic medication and cancer risk has been intensively discussed. In fact, DM appears as an independent risk factor for a number of cancer entities. These include cancers of the liver, pancreas, ovary, colorectum, lung, bladder, and breast. In principle, the nature of this study is correlative. However, it is highly plausible that DM plays a causative role for the excessive risk of death even from cancer. Possible underlying mechanisms can of course not be explained by this study. Reasonable explanations are based on the fact that glucose and insulin can both promote tumor growth. It can, however, not be ruled out that the underlying causes for diabetes (nutrition, lack of physical activity) are themselves causal cofactors for the excess death.

Another interesting aspect of this study is the definition of the cutoff for the fasting plasma glucose level, namely 100 mg/dL, for the risk of death. Of note, this is well below the current diabetes definition and underlines furthermore the fact that the current diabetes definitions derive from retinopathy risk assessments (and not from macrovascular risk or risk of death).

S. Schinner, MD, PhD

References

1. Sarwar N, Gao P, Seshasai SR; The Emerging Risk Factors Collaboration. Diabetes mellitus, fasting blood glucose concentration, and risk of vascular disease: a collaborative meta-analysis of 102 prospective studies. *Lancet.* 2010;375:2215-2222.
2. Coutinho M, Gerstein HC, Wang Y, Yusuf S. The relationship between glucose and incident cardiovascular events. A metaregression analysis of published data from 20 studies of 95,783 individuals followed for 12.4 years. *Diabetes Care.* 1999;22:233-240.

Glycemic Control

Insulin degludec, an ultra-long-acting basal insulin, once a day or three times a week versus insulin glargine once a day in patients with type 2 diabetes: A 16-week, randomised, open-label, phase 2 trial

Zinman B, Fulcher G, Rao PV, et al (Univ of Toronto, Ontario, Canada; Royal North Shore Hosp and Univ of Sydney, New South Wales, Australia; Nizam's Inst of Med Sciences Univ, Hyderabad, India; et al)

Lancet 377:924-931, 2011

Background.—Insulin degludec is a new basal insulin that forms soluble multihexamer assemblies after subcutaneous injection, resulting in an ultra-long action profile. This study aimed to assess efficacy and safety of insulin degludec injected once a day or three times a week compared with insulin glargine once a day in insulin-naive people with type 2 diabetes, who were inadequately controlled with oral antidiabetic drugs.

Methods.—In this 16-week, randomised, open-label, parallel-group phase 2 trial, participants aged 18—75 years with type 2 diabetes and glycosylated haemoglobin (HbA_{1C}) of 7·0—11·0% were enrolled and treated at 28 clinical sites in Canada, India, South Africa, and the USA. Participants were randomly allocated in a 1:1:1:1 ratio by computer-generated block randomisation to receive insulin degludec either once a day or three times a week or insulin glargine once a day, all in combination with metformin. Investigators were masked to data until database release. The primary outcome was HbA_{1C} after 16 weeks of treatment. Analyses were done by intention to treat. This trial is registered with ClinicalTrials. gov, number NCT00611884.

Findings.—Of 367 patients screened, 245 were eligible for inclusion. 62 participants were randomly allocated to receive insulin degludec three times a week (starting dose 20 U per injection [1 U=9 nmol]), 60 to receive insulin degludec once a day (starting dose 10 U [1 U=6 nmol]; group A), 61 to receive insulin degludec once a day (starting dose 10 U [1 U=9 nmol]; group B), and 62 to receive insulin glargine (starting dose 10 U [1 U= 6 nmol]) once a day. At study end, mean HbA_{1C} levels were much the same across treatment groups, at $7 \cdot 3\%$ (SD $1 \cdot 1$), $7 \cdot 4\%$ ($1 \cdot 0$), $7 \cdot 5\%$ ($1 \cdot 1$), and $7 \cdot 2\%$ ($0 \cdot 9$), respectively. Estimated mean HbA_{1C} treatment differences from insulin degludec by comparison with insulin glargine were $0 \cdot 08\%$ (95% CI $-0 \cdot 23$ to $0 \cdot 40$) for the three dose per week schedule, $0 \cdot 17\%$ ($-0 \cdot 15$ to $0 \cdot 48$) for group A, and $0 \cdot 28\%$ ($-0 \cdot 04$ to $0 \cdot 59$) for group B. Few participants had hypoglycaemia and the number of adverse events was much the same across groups, with no apparent treatment-specific pattern.

Interpretation.—Insulin degludec provides comparable glycaemic control to insulin glargine without additional adverse events and might reduce dosing frequency due to its ultra-long action profile.

▶ The formulation of novel insulins with different pharmacokinetics has changed diabetes therapy over the past decades.[1-3] Here, a novel ultralong-acting insulin (degludec) has been investigated in a small and short-term study. Insulin degludec can be administered once daily or 3 times a week and was compared with insulin glargine once daily in this study.

The patients included had poorly controlled type 2 diabetes mellitus (glycosylated hemoglobin [HbA_{1c}], 8.8% at study entry). All patients were initially already treated with metformin, and this was continued in all study arms. The nature of the study was short term (16 weeks).

The authors report a comparable HbA_{1c} reduction (to approximately 7.5%) in all groups investigated. There were statistically comparably low rates of hypoglycemia in all groups, but there was a trend toward more hypoglycemia when insulin degludec was administered 3 times a week. This must be taken with caution, as the number of patients was small and the difference was not statistically significant. However, one might have expected an opposite trend. In conclusion, insulin degludec proves to be as efficient as insulin glargine in reducing HbA_{1c}. This is an interesting and important finding.

Nevertheless, it will be very important to see the true safety and side effect profile on a longer run in future studies. In addition, further studies will of course be needed to assess diabetes-related end points under insulin degludec treatment.

S. Schinner, MD, PhD

References

1. Horvath K, Jeitler K, Berghold A, et al. Long-acting insulin analogues versus NPH insulin (human isophane insulin) for type 2 diabetes mellitus. *Cochrane Database Syst Rev.* 2007;(2). CD005613.
2. Heise T, Pieber TR. Towards peakless, reproducible and long-acting insulins. An assessment of the basal analogues based on isoglycaemic clamp studies. *Diabetes Obes Metab.* 2007;9:648-659.
3. Jonassen I, Havelund S, Ribel U, et al. Insulin degludec is a new generation ultralong acting basal insulin with a unique mechanism of protraction based on multihexamer formation. *Diabetes.* 2010;59:A11.

Effects of Aerobic and Resistance Training on Hemoglobin A₁c Levels in Patients With Type 2 Diabetes: A Randomized Controlled Trial

Church TS, Blair SN, Cocreham S, et al (Louisiana State Univ System, Baton Rouge; Univ of South Carolina, Columbia; et al)
JAMA 304:2253-2262, 2010

Context.—Exercise guidelines for individuals with diabetes include both aerobic and resistance training although few studies have directly examined this exercise combination.

Objective.—To examine the benefits of aerobic training alone, resistance training alone, and a combination of both on hemoglobin A_{1c} (HbA_{1c}) in individuals with type 2 diabetes.

Design, Setting, and Participants.—A randomized controlled trial in which 262 sedentary men and women in Louisiana with type 2 diabetes and HbA_{1c} levels of 6.5% or higher were enrolled in the 9-month exercise program between April 2007 and August 2009.

Intervention.—Forty-one participants were assigned to the nonexercise control group, 73 to resistance training 3 days a week, 72 to aerobic exercise in which they expended 12 kcal/kg per week; and 76 to combined aerobic and resistance training in which they expended 10 kcal/kg per week and engaged in resistance training twice a week.

Main Outcome.—Change in HbA_{1c} level. Secondary outcomes included measures of anthropometry and fitness.

Results.—The study included 63.0% women and 47.3% nonwhite participants who were a mean (SD) age of 55.8 years (8.7 years) with a baseline HbA_{1c} level of 7.7% (1.0%). Compared with the control group, the absolute mean change in HbA_{1c} in the combination training exercise group was −0.34% (95% confidence interval [CI], −0.64% to −0.03%; $P=.03$). The mean changes in HbA_{1c} were not statistically significant in either the resistance training (−0.16%; 95% CI, −0.46% to 0.15%; $P=.32$) or the aerobic (−0.24%; 95% CI, −0.55% to 0.07%; $P=.14$) groups compared with the control group. Only the combination exercise group improved maximum oxygen consumption (mean, 1.0 mL/ kg per min; 95% CI, 0.5-1.5, $P<.05$) compared with the control group. All exercise groups reduced waist circumference from −1.9 to −2.8 cm compared with the control group. The resistance training group lost a mean of −1.4 kg fat mass (95% CI, −2.0 to −0.7 kg; $P<.05$) and combination training group lost a mean of −1.7 (−2.3 to −1.1 kg; $P<.05$) compared with the control group.

Conclusions.—Among patients with type 2 diabetes mellitus, a combination of aerobic and resistance training compared with the nonexercise control group improved HbA_{1c} levels. This was not achieved by aerobic or resistance training alone.

Trial Registration.—clinicaltrials.gov Identifier: NCT00458133.

▶ Sedentary lifestyle is one of the major problems in Western societies. Physical activity can prevent and cure metabolic disease. However, it is not clear how to motivate people to exercise and which type of exercise is most efficient. This study addressed the latter question. Patients with typical features of type 2 diabetes mellitus were included: The mean age was 55 years, hemoglobin A_{1c} (HbA_{1c}) level was 7.7%, and the body mass index (BMI) was 34.9 kg/m^2. These patients did not exercise regularly at study entry. Patients were enrolled to different exercise regimes: either aerobic or resistance training or a combination of both. The primary end point after 9 months was the change in HbA_{1c}. With every type of exercise, HbA_{1c} and related parameters (BMI, waist circumference, etc) were improved. However, only the combination of aerobic and resistance training reached statistical significance.

How were the exercise programs defined? Aerobic training aimed for consumption of 12 kcal/kg body weight per week. This was achieved after approximately 150 minutes of moderate training. Notably, the combined training group differed only slightly with respect to energy consumption (10 vs 12 kcal/kg body weight per week). Therefore, aerobic training was the major contribution for both treatment regimes. However, studies like this are important to translate findings from physiology and theoretical recommendations into clinical practice. Knowing an exact exercise plan might help to motivate patients to eventually take part in it. This study is very useful for clinicians, as it is one of the few publications in this field leading to clinical recommendations.

S. Schinner, MD, PhD

Long-Term Effects of Intensive Glucose Lowering on Cardiovascular Outcomes
The ACCORD Study Group (McMaster Univ and Hamilton Health Sciences, Ontario, Canada; Wake Forest Univ School of Medicine, Winston-Salem, NC; Case Western Reserve Univ, Cleveland, OH; et al)
N Engl J Med 364:818-828, 2011

Background.—Intensive glucose lowering has previously been shown to increase mortality among persons with advanced type 2 diabetes and a high risk of cardiovascular disease. This report describes the 5-year outcomes of a mean of 3.7 years of intensive glucose lowering on mortality and key cardiovascular events.

Methods.—We randomly assigned participants with type 2 diabetes and cardiovascular disease or additional cardiovascular risk factors to receive intensive therapy (targeting a glycated hemoglobin level below 6.0%) or standard therapy (targeting a level of 7 to 7.9%). After termination of the intensive therapy, due to higher mortality in the intensive-therapy group, the target glycated hemoglobin level was 7 to 7.9% for all participants, who were followed until the planned end of the trial.

Results.—Before the intensive therapy was terminated, the intensive-therapy group did not differ significantly from the standard-therapy group in the rate of the primary outcome (a composite of nonfatal myocardial infarction, nonfatal stroke, or death from cardiovascular causes)

(P=0.13) but had more deaths from any cause (primarily cardiovascular) (hazard ratio, 1.21; 95% confidence interval [CI], 1.02 to 1.44) and fewer nonfatal myocardial infarctions (hazard ratio, 0.79; 95% CI, 0.66 to 0.95). These trends persisted during the entire follow-up period (hazard ratio for death, 1.19; 95% CI, 1.03 to 1.38; and hazard ratio for nonfatal myocardial infarction, 0.82; 95% CI, 0.70 to 0.96). After the intensive intervention was terminated, the median glycated hemoglobin level in the intensive-therapy group rose from 6.4% to 7.2%, and the use of glucose-lowering medications and rates of severe hypoglycemia and other adverse events were similar in the two groups.

Conclusions.—As compared with standard therapy, the use of intensive therapy for 3.7 years to target a glycated hemoglobin level below 6% reduced 5-year nonfatal myocardial infarctions but increased 5-year mortality. Such a strategy cannot be recommended for high-risk patients with advanced type 2 diabetes. (Funded by the National Heart, Lung and Blood Institute; ClinicalTrials.gov number, NCT00000620.)

▶ This study reports on the extension of the observation period of the initial Action to Control Cardiovascular Risk in Diabetes (ACCORD) study. As reported in 2008, the intensified treatment group of the initial ACCORD study was stopped after 3.7 years because of increased mortality in this group. The study compared cardiovascular outcomes in patients with long-standing type 2 diabetes mellitus and a high burden of preexisting cardiovascular disease under conventional (glycated hemoglobin A_{1c} [HbA_{1c}] goal 7.0%-7.9%) versus intensified (HbA_{1c} goal < 6.0%) therapy.[1-3]

This study reports a follow-up of the patients who were initially ascribed to the intensified group and subsequently switched to a conventional treatment regime aiming for an HbA_{1c} target of 7.0% to 7.9%. Consequently, the mean HbA_{1c} level in these patients rose from 6.4% to 7.2%.

The outcomes were now assessed after a total of 5 years, of which 3.7 years were under an intensified glucose-lowering regime. As in the initial observation, the risk of death by any cause was slightly higher in the former intensified group, whereas the risk for nonfatal myocardial infarction was lower. The incidence of severe hypoglycemia was equal in both groups after the intensified group was switched to conventional treatment.

What is new in this study?

As expected, HbA_{1c} and hypoglycemia risk were now equal in both groups. Still, the initial trend with a decreased risk for myocardial infarction but increased risk of death was maintained.

How come?

Apparently, 3.7 years of intensive treatment prolonged by a 1.3-year postinterventional follow-up does not significantly improve cardiovascular outcomes. This is not surprising and in line with the follow-up study of the United Kingdom Prospective Diabetes Study. In the latter study, cardiovascular risk after stricter glucose control was reduced 10 years after the intervention was stopped. One major point that we learned from this study was that benefits for cardiovascular end points need time to develop.[4] Therefore, it is not surprising that 1.3 additional years of postinterventional follow-up does not change the overall trend of the initial study with respect to cardiovascular end points.

Why is the mortality still increased, although hypoglycemia risk is comparable between the 2 groups?

This finding does indeed argue against hypoglycemia as the major cause for increased mortality in the intensified group. Although it is still not clear, why patients initially under strict glucose control have still a higher mortality even after switching to standard therapy drug interactions might be one possible explanation.

Taken together, these data further argue against an HbA_{1c} target $< 6\%$ in patients with high cardiovascular risk and long-standing diabetes mellitus.

S. Schinner, MD, PhD

References

1. Gerstein HC, Miller ME, Byington RP, et al. Action to Control Cardiovascular Risk in Diabetes Study Group. Effects of intensive glucose lowering in type 2 diabetes. *N Engl J Med.* 2008;358:2545-2559.
2. Calles-Escandón J, Lovato LC, Simons-Morton DG, et al. Effect of intensive compared with standard glycemia treatment strategies on mortality by baseline subgroup characteristics: the Action to Control Cardiovascular Risk in Diabetes (ACCORD) trial. *Diabetes Care.* 2010;33:721-727.
3. Riddle MC, Ambrosius WT, Brillon DJ, et al. Epidemiologic relationships between A1C and all-cause mortality during a median 3.4-year follow-up of glycemic treatment in the ACCORD trial. *Diabetes Care.* 2010;33:983-990.
4. Holman RR, Paul SK, Bethel MA, Matthews DR, Neil HA. 10-Year follow-up of intensive glucose control in type 2 diabetes. *N Engl J Med.* 2008;359:1577-1589.

Pathogenesis

Separate and combined associations of body-mass index and abdominal adiposity with cardiovascular disease: collaborative analysis of 58 prospective studies

The Emerging Risk Factors Collaboration (Univ of Cambridge, UK; et al)
Lancet 377:1085-1095, 2011

Background.—Guidelines differ about the value of assessment of adiposity measures for cardiovascular disease risk prediction when information is available for other risk factors. We studied the separate and combined associations of body-mass index (BMI), waist circumference, and waist-to-hip ratio with risk of first-onset cardiovascular disease.

Methods.—We used individual records from 58 cohorts to calculate hazard ratios (HRs) per 1 SD higher baseline values ($4 \cdot 56$ kg/m^2 higher BMI, $12 \cdot 6$ cm higher waist circumference, and $0 \cdot 083$ higher waist-to-hip ratio) and measures of risk discrimination and reclassification. Serial adiposity assessments were used to calculate regression dilution ratios.

Results.—Individual records were available for 221 934 people in 17 countries (14 297 incident cardiovascular disease outcomes; $1 \cdot 87$ million person-years at risk). Serial adiposity assessments were made in up to 63 821 people (mean interval $5 \cdot 7$ years [SD $3 \cdot 9$]). In people with BMI of 20 kg/m^2 or higher, HRs for cardiovascular disease were $1 \cdot 23$ (95% CI $1 \cdot 17-1 \cdot 29$) with BMI, $1 \cdot 27$ ($1 \cdot 20-1 \cdot 33$) with waist circumference, and $1 \cdot 25$ ($1 \cdot 19-1 \cdot 31$) with waist-to-hip ratio, after adjustment for age, sex, and smoking status. After further adjustment for baseline systolic blood pressure, history of diabetes, and total and HDL cholesterol, corresponding HRs were $1 \cdot 07$ ($1 \cdot 03-1 \cdot 11$) with BMI, $1 \cdot 10$ ($1 \cdot 05-1 \cdot 14$) with waist circumference, and $1 \cdot 12$ ($1 \cdot 08-1 \cdot 15$) with waist-to-hip ratio. Addition of information on BMI, waist circumference, or waist-to-hip ratio to a cardiovascular disease risk prediction model containing conventional risk factors did not importantly improve risk discrimination (C-index changes of $-0 \cdot 0001$, $-0 \cdot 0001$, and $0 \cdot 0008$, respectively), nor classification of participants to categories of predicted 10-year risk (net reclassification improvement $-0 \cdot 19\%$, $-0 \cdot 05\%$, and $-0 \cdot 05\%$, respectively). Findings were similar when adiposity measures were considered in combination. Reproducibility was greater for BMI (regression dilution ratio $0 \cdot 95$, 95% CI $0 \cdot 93-0 \cdot 97$) than for waist circumference ($0 \cdot 86$, $0 \cdot 83-0 \cdot 89$) or waist-to-hip ratio ($0 \cdot 63$, $0 \cdot 57-0 \cdot 70$).

Interpretation.—BMI, waist circumference, and waist-to-hip ratio, whether assessed singly or in combination, do not importantly improve cardiovascular disease risk prediction in people in developed countries when additional information is available for systolic blood pressure, history of diabetes, and lipids.

▶ This meta-analysis used pooled data from more than 200 000 patients who were included in 58 prospective studies. At study entry, the mean age was 58 years and women were slightly in the majority (56%). A minimum time period for a follow-up was 1 year, but 60 000 patients were followed for approximately 6 years. Importantly, one inclusion criterion was the absence of cardiovascular or other macrovascular disease. The major aim was to evaluate the risk prediction for vascular events based on anthropometric assessment. Results were adjusted for age, sex, and smoking and additionally for hypertension, history of diabetes, and lipid profile when indicated.

Basically, risk for coronary heart disease showed a J-shaped profile when referred to the body mass index (BMI). A very interesting aspect of this study is the subgroup analysis of the effects of visceral obesity with different degrees of obesity. Thus, visceral obesity, even in the normal weight (BMI < 24.5 kg/m^2) and the overweight (BMI, 24.5-28 kg/m^2) subgroup, predicts cardiovascular events. This has major clinical implications, as it identifies a novel risk group of atherosclerotic complications, namely the relatively lean but viscerally obese. What are the underlying mechanisms? It has been known for several years that visceral adipocytes differ from subcutaneous adipocytes with respect to adipokine release.[1] Adipokines are fat cell—derived hormones. Their secretion pattern is altered in obesity, leading to wording of the dysfunctional adipocyte. In addition, visceral adipocytes show impaired response to insulin and impaired fatty acid storage under obese conditions. This leads to a spillover of fatty acids into organs where they are ectopically stored.

S. Schinner, MD, PhD

Reference

1. Deng Y, Scherer PE. Adipokines as novel biomarkers and regulators of the metabolic syndrome. *Ann N Y Acad Sci.* 2010;1212:E1-E19.

Chronic high-fat diet in fathers programs β-cell dysfunction in female rat offspring

Ng S-F, Lin RCY, Laybutt DR, et al (Univ of New South Wales, Sydney, Australia; Garvan Inst of Med Res, Sydney, Australia; et al)
Nature 467:963-966, 2010

The global prevalence of obesity is increasing across most ages in both sexes. This is contributing to the early emergence of type 2 diabetes and its related epidemic. Having either parent obese is an independent risk factor for childhood obesity. Although the detrimental impacts of diet-induced maternal obesity on adiposity and metabolism in offspring are well established, the extent of any contribution of obese fathers is unclear, particularly the role of non-genetic factors in the causal pathway. Here we show that paternal high-fat-diet (HFD) exposure programs β-cell 'dysfunction' in rat F_1 female offspring. Chronic HFD consumption in Sprague–Dawley fathers induced increased body weight, adiposity, impaired glucose tolerance and insulin sensitivity. Relative to controls, their female offspring had an early onset of impaired insulin secretion and glucose tolerance that worsened with time, and normal adiposity. Paternal HFD altered the expression of 642 pancreatic islet genes in adult female offspring ($P < 0.01$); genes belonged to 13 functional clusters, including cation and ATP binding, cytoskeleton and intracellular transport. Broader pathway analysis of 2,492 genes differentially expressed ($P < 0.05$) demonstrated involvement of calcium-, MAPK- and Wnt-signalling pathways, apoptosis and the cell cycle. Hypomethylation of the *Il13ra2* gene, which showed the highest fold difference in expression (1.76-fold increase), was demonstrated. This is the first report in mammals of non-genetic, intergenerational transmission of metabolic sequelae of a HFD from father to offspring.

▶ It is not surprising that obesity and type 2 diabetes run within families. The most probable explanation is the same lifestyle/nutrition of the family members. This is part of the family culture and certainly has a substantial degree of inheritance.

Another aspect of the inheritance of obesity and type2 diabetes is of course genetics, and there have been substantial advances of our understanding of the genetic contributions to these diseases in recent years.

Animal model offers possibilities to dissect these different contributions (lifestyle vs genes) to diabetes risk. This study by Ng and colleagues has identified another novel mechanism of diabetes inheritance. Basically, they found that paternal obesity increases the diabetes risk for daughters through mechanisms that are neither lifestyle related nor classical genetics related.

What was the design of the study?

The authors induced obesity in male wild-type rats by feeding them a high-fat diet. Normal fed animals served as controls. The lean and obese males were crossed with lean wild-type female rats. The offspring was then analyzed with respect to metabolic changes. Interestingly, the offspring of both groups of fathers did not differ in body weight. However, analysis of glucose metabolism revealed impaired glucose tolerance in offspring of obese males. Further molecular investigations showed that these animals, albeit lean themselves, had defects in β-cell function. Microarray results showed altered expression of genes involved in various signal transduction pathways in β-cells of these animals.

How can paternal obesity result in differential gene expression in the offspring?

A proof of principle experiment showed differences in the methylation status of 1 gene in β-cells between the 2 groups. Thus, epigenetic changes, induced by metabolic derangements in spermatids of obese male, are thought to be transmitted to the next generation.

This is an exciting article. It suggests a novel mechanism of transmission of disease from one generation to the other. The study raises further questions: Are the epigenetic changes in the offspring reversible? By diet and lifestyle? By pharmacologic interventions? Can these findings be translated into clinical medicine? If the same was true for humans, enormous increases of obesity and diabetes were possible consequences over the next generations.

For further reading, reference the articles by Skinner,[1] Skinner et al,[2] and Ozanne and Hales.[3]

S. Schinner, MD, PhD

References

1. Skinner MK. Metabolic disorders: Fathers' nutritional legacy. *Nature*. 2010;467: 922-923.
2. Skinner MK, Manikkam M, Guerrero-Bosagna C. Epigenetic transgenerational actions of environmental factors in disease etiology. *Trends Endocrinol Metab*. 2010;21:214-222.
3. Ozanne SE, Hales CN. Early programming of glucose-insulin metabolism. *Trends Endocrinol Metab*. 2002;13:368-373.

Developmental Programming: Differential Effects of Prenatal Testosterone Excess on Insulin Target Tissues
Nada SE, Thompson RC, Padmanabhan V (Univ of Michigan, Ann Arbor)
Endocrinology 151:5165-5173, 2010

Polycystic ovarian syndrome (PCOS) is the leading cause of infertility in reproductive-aged women with the majority manifesting insulin resistance. To delineate the causes of insulin resistance in women with PCOS, we determined changes in the mRNA expression of insulin receptor (IR) isoforms and members of its signaling pathway in tissues of adult control (n = 7) and prenatal testosterone (T)-treated (n = 6) sheep (100 mg/kg twice a week from d 30—90 of gestation), the reproductive/metabolic characteristics of which are similar to women with PCOS. Findings revealed that prenatal T excess reduced ($P < 0.05$) expression of IR-B isoform (only isoform detected), insulin receptor substrate-2 (*IRS-2*), protein kinase B (*AKt*), peroxisome proliferator-activated receptor-γ (*PPARγ*), hormone-sensitive lipase (*HSL*), and mammalian target of rapamycin (*mTOR*) but increased expression of rapamycin-insensitive companion of mTOR (rictor), and eukaryotic initiation factor 4E (*eIF4E*) in the liver. Prenatal T excess increased ($P < 0.05$) the IR-A to IR-B isoform ratio and expression of *IRS-1*, glycogen synthase kinase-3α and -β (*GSK-3α* and -β), and rictor while reducing ERK1 in muscle. In the adipose tissue, prenatal T excess increased the expression of *IRS-2*, phosphatidylinositol 3-kinase (*PI3K*), *PPARγ*, and *mTOR mRNAs*. These findings provide evidence that prenatal T excess modulates in a tissue-specific manner the expression levels of several genes involved in mediating insulin action. These changes are consistent with the hypothesis that prenatal T excess disrupts the insulin sensitivity of peripheral tissues, with liver and muscle being insulin resistant and adipose tissue insulin sensitive.

▶ There is a complex interplay between hyperandrogenemia and glucose metabolism in women. It is well established that insulin resistance, mostly because of obesity, is a common cause for the polycystic ovarian syndrome.[1] This syndrome is characterized by excessive androgen production from the ovaries. An often-used treatment modality targets, in fact, insulin resistance by using metformin.

This study asks the question the other way around: What is the effect of hyperandrogenemia on insulin sensitivity? More specifically, the authors tested the effect of prenatal exposure to androgens in female animals (sheep) on insulin signaling in liver, skeletal muscle, and adipose tissue.

As a result of prenatal testosterone treatment, insulin sensitivity in these animals decreased. The authors tried to attribute this effect to the respective insulin sensitive organ by quantifying the expression of genes involved in insulin signal transduction. Unfortunately, the authors did not look at the phosphorylation state of these molecules, although this is a crucial regulatory step. However, their data indicate that liver and muscle but not adipose tissue develop insulin resistance in response to prenatal androgen exposure.

This is an interesting finding, as it demonstrates tissue-specific effects of prenatal programming. The underlying mechanisms and pathophysiological implications are not understood.

Another important question of clinical importance arises from these data: Is insulin resistance inheritable by epigenetic changes?

This study suggests that women with hyperandrogenemia (often caused by obesity and insulin resistance) might transmit this metabolic derangement to the next generation.

S. Schinner, MD, PhD

Reference

1. Ng SF, Lin RC, Laybutt DR, Barres R, Owens JA, Morris MJ. Chronic high-fat diet in fathers programs β-cell dysfunction in female rat offspring. *Nature*. 2010;467:963-966.

Basal α-Cell Up-Regulation in Obese Insulin-Resistant Adolescents

Weiss R, D'Adamo E, Santoro N, et al (Hebrew Univ School of Medicine, Jerusalem, Israel; Yale Univ School of Medicine, New Haven, CT)
J Clin Endocrinol Metab 96:91-97, 2011

Context.—The aim of this analysis was to evaluate glucagon and c-peptide concentrations in two scenarios: euglycemic hyperinsulinemia and hyperglycemic hyperinsulinemia. We postulated that worsening obesity and insulin resistance will be reflected as an up-regulated (less suppressible) islet secretion profile.

Methods.—Eighty-two [34 obese with normal glucose tolerance (NGT), 30 obese with impaired glucose tolerance (IGT), and 18 nonobese with NGT] subjects underwent a euglycemic-hyperinsulinemic clamp (EHC) and a hyperglycemic clamp. C-peptide and glucagon were evaluated at basal and steady-state (SS) conditions.

Results.—Basal glucagon was significantly elevated in obese insulin-resistant and obese IGT subjects as was basal c-peptide. SS glucagon and c-peptide levels during the EHC were lower in the lean and obese insulin-sensitive subjects compared with the obese insulin-resistant subjects with NGT or IGT. Fasting glucagon was the only significant determinant ($\beta = 0.66, P < 0.001$) of SS glucagon during the EHC ($R^2 = 0.57$). In a longitudinal follow-up of a subsample, those who converted from normal to IGT significantly increased their fasting glucagon concentration in comparison with those who remained with NGT.

Conclusions.—Islet up-regulation manifesting as basal elevated glucagon and c-peptide secretion that determines the suppressive effects of hyperinsulinemia appears early in the course of deteriorating glucose tolerance.

▶ The role of glucagon in the development of type 2 diabetes is still incompletely understood. It has been known for decades that hyperglucagonemia is a typical feature of diabetes. Insulin is a strong suppressor of glucagon gene transcription and glucagon release from α-cells. α-cells express insulin receptors, and the intracellular insulin signal transduction cascade has been characterized in α-cells. The clinical impact of hyperglucagonemia to hyperglycemia is clearly established. Glucagon-like peptide (GLP)-1 based therapies as novel treatment modalities for type 2 diabetes target glucagon release, and there are data showing that this is a major part of the glucose lowering effect.[1]

However, there are few clinical studies on the regulation of glucagon release in response to obesity and insulin resistance.

This study demonstrates that basal glucagon was elevated in obese insulin-resistant subjects despite stimulated c-peptide.

This finding provokes the hypothesis of insulin resistance of pancreatic α-cells. There are indeed data from in vitro studies supporting this hypothesis. It has been shown that chronic insulin treatment induces insulin resistance of pancreatic α-cells. It must be considered that α-cells reside in direct proximity to β-cells in pancreatic islets, thus being exposed to high insulin concentrations. Furthermore, studies on the insulin signaling cascade in α-cells revealed reduced expression and activity of the insulin receptor and the insulin receptor substrate.

Further studies will be needed to investigate whether the same mechanisms are responsible for the induction of insulin resistance in α-cells like those in liver and muscle.

This study is interesting for our pathophysiological understanding of diabetes mellitus. The clinical impact of glucagon as a therapeutic target has been highlighted since the development of GLP-1 based therapies.

S. Schinner, MD, PhD

Reference

1. González M, Böer U, Dickel C, et al. Loss of insulin-induced inhibition of glucagon gene transcription in hamster pancreatic islet alpha cells by long-term insulin exposure. *Diabetologia.* 2008;51:2012-2021.

2 Lipoproteins and Atherosclerosis

Introduction

The complexities and controversies in the area of lipids, lipoproteins, and atherosclerosis are compounding rapidly. There is little controversy as to whether lipids and lipoproteins play diverse roles in atherogenesis. Low-density lipoproteins are established as causal in atherogenesis. In contrast, the relationship of high-density lipoproteins (HDLs) to risk for atherogenesis is more complex. In this edition of the YEAR BOOK OF ENDOCRINOLOGY, a number of reports investigating the relationship between HDL/apoA-I are evaluated and reveal a complex, decidedly mixed picture. The Framingham investigators show that a low HDL-C is associated with increased risk for coronary heart disease (CHD) only in the presence of insulin resistance. Investigators from the Copenhagen Heart Study were unable to demonstrate any impact on risk for CHD in subjects with a variety of single-nucleotide polymorphisms that are associated with increases in serum levels of HDL-C or apoA-I. Some patients develop antibodies to their own apoA-I. Serum levels of anti-apoA-I IgG antibodies correlate with severity of coronary atherosclerotic disease and appear to potentiate the intensity of intravascular inflammatory tone. It is well established that tight glycemic control helps to reduce risk for the development and progression of diabetic retinopathy. In a study by Sasongko and coworkers, it is shown that there is an inverse relationship between risk for retinopathy and serum levels of apoA-I. In one of the most important investigations in the field of lipidology over the past year, Khera and coworkers demonstrate that the capacity of HDL to promote reverse cholesterol transport impacts risk for both carotid and coronary atherosclerosis and is a significant predictor of risk for CHD-related morbidity and mortality. Relatively speaking, it will be some time before we have a truly comprehensive and accurate understanding of how and under what circumstances HDLs either prevent or promote atherosclerotic disease.

The recent announcement by the National Institutes of Health that the Atherothrombosis Intervention in Metabolic syndrome with low HDL/high triglycerides: Impact on Global Health outcomes (AIMH-High) study was terminated because of futility has brought the question of the therapeutic value of HDL-C management into sharp focus. Cannon and coworkers demonstrate that the cholesteryl ester transfer protein inhibitor anacetrapib does not induce hypertension, increase aldosterone levels, or cause electrolyte disturbances, and its use is associated with a trend toward fewer cardiovascular events compared with placebo. They also show that this medication can raise HDL-C 138%. Clinical trials exploring the efficacy of anacetrapib and dalcetrapib will help to further delineate the value of raising HDL-C in high-risk patients. Apart from the various off target toxicities precipitated by torcetrapib, another CETP inhibitor, Xing et al suggest that elevated HDL_2 may precipitate toxicity by stimulating the production of aldosterone synthase and aldosterone by adrenocortical cells.

Obesity is a burgeoning issue throughout the world. Metabolic differences among adipose tissue depots are a focus of considerable study. Investigators from the Jackson Heart Study demonstrate that both visceral and subcutaneous adipose tissue contribute significantly to risk for CHD in African American men and women. In contrast, Swedish investigators show that visceral adipose tissue portends increased risk for CHD, while increased gynoid (femorogluteal) fat deposition is protective against CHD in both men and women. Adipose tissue also appears to play a significant role in HDL biogenesis. Adipocytes can express SR-BI and ABCA1, two important cell surface receptors that can lipidate nascent discoidal HDL particles. In the setting of insulin resistance, these cell surface receptors are down-regulated, resulting in less HDL lipidation and maturation.

The JUPITER trial results have certainly impacted cardiovascular care significantly. The JUPITER investigators show that reducing LDL-C <50 mg/dL is associated with a significantly lower risk for CHD-related events than lowering it to >50 mg/dL. The initial finding that rosuvastatin therapy was associated with a 25% increase in risk for new onset type 2 diabetes mellitus was unexpected. However, subsequent meta-analyses confirmed that this is a class effect for the statin drugs. In an important analysis of serum samples from the STELLAR trial, it is shown that high-dose atorvastatin and rosuvastatin therapy is associated with increases in serum glucose and insulin and a reduction in adiponectin. As shown by Kojima et al, low serum adiponectin is associated with increased necrotic core volumes in human coronary atherosclerotic plaques. Rein et al show that the severity of albuminuria portends a graded, more severe degree of obstructive coronary disease.

Fatty acids also continue to garner much-needed attention. Two studies with the omega-3 fish oils were negative. In a small study, Skulas Ray et al fail to demonstrate any capacity of high-dose fish oil to improve vasoreactivity or lower serum markers of inflammation. Norwegian investigators were unable to detect a dose-response relationship between amount of fish consumed and risk for CAD. In a fascinating study, investigators were able to demonstrate that an omega-3 fatty acid receptor mediates insulin sensitization and reduces serum levels of insulin. The Framingham investigators also established that serum levels of specific fatty acids constitute a signature of sorts and can be used to predict risk for insulin resistance and diabetes mellitus. These investigators also showed that 5 fatty acids (highly unsaturated with long carbon chain length) are protective against insulin resistance and diabetes.

Clearly, this has been a very exciting year for lipids and atherosclerosis research. Questions abound. The development of novel drugs continues and new lipid pathways regulating normal physiology and disease continue to be identified. It will be exciting to see how these new insights impact clinical care in the years ahead.

Peter P. Toth, MD, PhD

Epidemiology and Diagnosis

Impact of Abdominal Visceral and Subcutaneous Adipose Tissue on Cardiometabolic Risk Factors: The Jackson Heart Study

Liu J, Fox CS, Hickson DA, et al (Jackson State Univ, MS; Harvard Med School, Boston, MA; et al)
J Clin Endocrinol Metab 95:5419-5426, 2010

Objective.—Obesity is a major driver of cardiometabolic risk. Abdominal visceral adipose tissue (VAT) and sc adipose tissue (SAT) may confer differential metabolic risk profiles. We investigated the relations of VAT and SAT with cardiometabolic risk factors in the Jackson Heart Study cohort.

Methods.—Participants from the Jackson Heart Study (n = 2477; 64% women; mean age, 58 yr) underwent multidetector computed tomography, and the volumetric amounts of VAT and SAT were assessed between 2007 and 2009. Cardiometabolic risk factors were examined by sex in relation to VAT and SAT.

Results.—Men had a higher mean volume of VAT (873 vs. 793 cm^3) and a lower mean volume of SAT (1730 *vs.* 2659 cm^3) than women ($P = 0.0001$). Per 1-SD increment in either VAT or SAT, we observed elevated levels of fasting plasma glucose and triglyceride, lower levels of high-density lipoprotein-cholesterol, and increased odds ratios for hypertension, diabetes, and metabolic syndrome. The effect size of VAT in women was larger than that of SAT [fasting plasma glucose, 5.51 ± 1.0 *vs.* 3.36 ± 0.9; triglyceride, 0.17 ± 0.01 *vs.* 0.05 ± 0.01; high-density lipoprotein-cholesterol, -5.36 ± 0.4 vs. -2.85 ± 0.4; and odds ratio for hypertension, 1.62 (1.4–1.9) *vs.* 1.40 (1.2–1.6); diabetes, 1.82 (1.6–2.1) *vs.* 1.58 (1.4–1.8); and metabolic syndrome, 3.34 (2.8–4.0) *vs.* 2.06 (1.8–2.4), respectively; $P < 0.0001$ for difference between VAT and SAT]. Similar patterns were also observed in men. Further more, VAT remained associated with most risk factors even after accounting for body mass index (P ranging from 0.006–0.0001). The relationship of VAT to most risk factors was significantly different between women and men.

Conclusions.—Abdominal VAT and SAT are both associated with adverse cardiometabolic risk factors, but VAT remains more strongly associated with these risk factors. The results from this study suggest that relations with cardiometabolic risk factors are consistent with a pathogenic role of abdominal adiposity in participants of African ancestry (Tables 1, 3 and 4).

▶ Visceral adipose tissue (VAT) is receiving considerable attention because of its correlation with increased risk for diabetes mellitus, metabolic syndrome, and coronary artery disease. VAT is metabolically highly active and represents a source of free fatty acids, interleukins, cytokines, and angiotensinogen, among a large number of other adipokines. When present in high mass/volume and there is significant infiltration of the VAT with macrophages, VAT can become dysregulated and resistant to the effects of insulin. In the setting of insulin resistance, hormone-sensitive lipase provides a constitutive source of free fatty acids. Excess fatty acid availability can promote systemic insulin resistance and the steatosis of multiple organs, including the pancreas, heart, liver, and skeletal muscle. Excess fatty acid availability coupled with insulin resistance drives the development of atherogenic dyslipidemia with high serum very-low-density lipoprotein, triglyceride and low-density lipoprotein cholesterol levels, and low levels of high-density lipoprotein (HDL). As insulin resistance progresses, the patient makes the transition from impairments in fasting glucose to frank diabetes secondary to the loss of pancreatic insulin secretory capacity. In the setting of excess VAT and insulin resistance, blood pressure can rise secondary to diffuse endothelial dysfunction, increased angiotensin II production, expanded intravascular volume, and increased central sympathetic outflow. Excess VAT is thus highly detrimental to human health.

The Jackson Heart Study is a prospective observational study of African Americans enrolled from Jackson, Mississippi. In this analysis, 2477 subjects underwent abdominal CT to quantify subcutaneous adipose tissue (SAT) and VAT. Not surprisingly, men had more VAT and less SAT compared with women (Table 1). Both VAT and SAT contributed to cardiometabolic risk

TABLE 1.—Clinical Characteristics of Study Participants who Underwent CT Assessment of VAT and SAT

	Women (n = 1596)	Men (n = 881)
Age (yr)	59 ± 11	58 ± 11
Abdominal VAT (cm^3)	793.7 ± 364.8	873.0 ± 412.2
Abdominal SAT (cm^3)	2659.3 ± 966.8	1729.5 ± 815.3
BMI (kg/m^2)	32.7 ± 6.9	29.9 ± 5.2
WC (cm)	103.1 ± 14.2	102.4 ± 13.5
Triglyceride (mmol/liter)[a]	0.97 (0.70, 1.33)	1.05 (0.73, 1.57)
HDL-C (mmol/liter)	1.50 ± 0.4	1.25 ± 0.3
Total cholesterol (mmol/liter)	5.17 ± 1.0	4.94 ± 1.0
Fasting glucose (mmol/liter)	5.83 ± 2.0	5.90 ± 1.7
Systolic BP (mm Hg)	127 ± 18	125 ± 17
Diastolic BP (mm Hg)	76 ± 10	79 ± 10
Current smoking (%)	4.9	9.7
Obesity (BMI ≥30) (%)	60.7	44.4
Diabetes mellitus (%)	23.7	22.1
Metabolic syndrome (%)	57.9	50.2
Hypertension (%)	74.6	66.4

All values are number (percentage) or mean ± SM.
[a]Median (25th, 75th percentile).

TABLE 3.—Multivariable[a] Adjusted Regression Coefficients of Abdominal Adiposity (Per 1-SD Increase) With Metabolic Risk Factors

	Women					Men					P for Sex Interaction
	MV	P[b]	P[c]	MV+BMI	P	MV	P[b]	P[c]	MV+BMI	P	
SBP											
VAT	0.70±0.5	0.15		0.47±0.6	0.42	1.30±0.6	0.02	0.04	1.06±0.7	0.12	0.0005
SAT	0.44±0.5	0.35				1.36±0.8	0.07				0.0001
DBP											
VAT	0.42±0.3	0.13		0.63±0.3	0.06	0.79±0.3	0.02	0.22	0.75±0.4	0.07	0.0001
SAT	0.22±0.3	0.41				0.44±0.4	0.32				0.0001
FPG											
VAT	5.51±1.0	0.0001	0.0001	5.88±1.0	0.0001	3.58±1.0	0.005	0.01	3.52±1.3	0.006	0.0001
SAT	3.36±0.9	0.0005				2.39±1.3	0.08				0.10
Log TG											
VAT	0.17±0.01	0.0001	0.0001	0.19±0.02	0.0001	0.19±0.02	0.0001	0.0001	0.20±0.02	0.0001	0.0293
SAT	0.05±0.01	0.0005				0.12±0.03	0.0001				0.0001
HDL-C											
VAT	−5.36±0.4	0.0001	0.0003	−4.21±0.5	0.0001	−3.72±0.4	0.0001	0.53	−2.71±0.5	0.0001	0.0001
SAT	−2.85±0.4	0.0001				−3.63±0.6	0.0001				0.0001

For BP, FPG, TG, HDL, and low-density lipoprotein (LDL), an additional covariate of antihypertensive medication, antidiabetic medication, or lipid-lowering medication was included in the model. MV, Multivariable adjusted; FPG, fasting plasma glucose; SBP, systolic BP; DBP, diastolic BP; TG, triglycerides.

[a] Adjusted for age, smoking, and alcohol use.
[b] P for VAT or SAT in the model.
[c] P for difference in effect size between VAT and SAT.

TABLE 4.—Multivariable[a] Adjusted Odds Ratio for Hypertension, Diabetes, and Metabolic Syndrome with Per 1-SD Increase in Abdominal VAT or SAT

	Women					Men					P for sex interaction
	MV	P[b]	P[c]	MV+BMI	P	MV	P[b]	P[c]	MV+BMI	P	
HTN											
VAT	1.62 (1.4–1.9)	0.0001	0.0001	1.29 (1.1–1.5)	0.006	1.55 (1.3–1.8)	0.0001	0.0001	1.34 (1.1–1.6)	0.003	0.051
SAT	1.40 (1.2–1.6)	0.0001				1.45 (1.2–1.8)	0.0002				0.005
DM											
VAT	1.82 (1.6–2.1)	0.0001	0.0001	1.40 (1.2–1.7)	0.0001	1.69 (1.4–2.0)	0.0002	0.0001	1.41 (1.2–1.7)	0.0004	0.087
SAT	1.58 (1.4–1.8)	0.0001				1.78 (1.5–2.2)	0.0001				0.59
MetS											
VAT	3.34 (2.8–4.0)	0.0001	0.0001	2.41 (2.0–2.9)	0.0001	3.46 (2.8–4.3)	0.0001	0.0001	2.53 (2.0–3.2)	0.0001	0.0001
SAT	2.06 (1.8–2.4)	0.0001				3.57 (2.8–4.6)	0.0001				0.0004

For BP, fasting plasma glucose (FPG), triglycerides (TG), HDL, and LDL, an additional covariate of antihypertensive medication, antidiabetic medication, or lipid-lowering medication was included in the model. MV, Multivariable adjusted; HTN, hypertension; DM, diabetes; MetS, metabolic syndrome.

[a]Adjusted for age, smoking, and alcohol use.
[b]P for VAT or SAT in the model.
[c]P for difference in effect size between VAT and SAT.

and independently increased risk for hyperglycemia, metabolic syndrome, diabetes mellitus, hypertension, hypertriglyceridemia, and low HDL cholesterol, though VAT contributed more strongly to adverse metabolic changes than SAT (Table 3). Of particular interest are the observations that increased SAT elevated risk for hypertension (odds ratio [OR], 1.4 vs 1.45), metabolic syndrome (OR, 1.58 vs 1.75), and diabetes mellitus (OR, 2.06 vs 3.57) in women and men, respectively. VAT correlated with adverse metabolic features independent of body mass index (Table 4).

These are important results. There has been enormous emphasis in recent years on visceral adiposity (omental, perimesenteric, perinephric, and other fat depots within the abdominal cavity) and its relationship to cardiometabolic risk. This study highlights the important contribution that SAT makes to all features of cardiometabolic risk. At least in African Americans, it appears that general adiposity and not just assessments of VAT should guide approaches to intervention. That SAT contributes so strongly to cardiometabolic risk is particularly interesting, given the fact that these smaller adipocytes with less expression of adrenergic receptors are in general sources of adiponectin and are less involved in continuous free fatty acid release. The relationship between SAT and cardiometabolic risk in people of European American ancestry has been substantially more mixed. Studies such as the Jackson Heart Study will continue to lend important new insights into how best to define racial differences in identifying and managing cardiometabolic risk.

P. P. Toth, MD, PhD

Genetically Elevated Apolipoprotein A-I, High-Density Lipoprotein Cholesterol Levels, and Risk of Ischemic Heart Disease
Haase CL, Tybjærg-Hansen A, Grande P, et al (Univ of Copenhagen, Denmark)
J Clin Endocrinol Metab 95:E500-E510, 2010

Context.—Epidemiologically, levels of high-density lipoprotein (HDL) cholesterol and its major protein constituent, apolipoprotein A-I (apoA-I), are inversely related to risk of ischemic heart disease (IHD).

Objective.—We tested whether common genetic variation in the *apolipoprotein A1* gene (*APOA1*) contributes to apoA-I and HDL cholesterol levels and risk of IHD in the general population.

Design.—We resequenced the regulatory and coding regions of *APOA1* in 190 individuals from the Copenhagen City Heart Study with the lowest 1% (n = 95) and highest 1% (n = 95) apoA-I levels. Two single-nucleotide polymorphisms (SNPs) were subsequently genotyped in the Copenhagen City Heart Study (n = 10,273) and in 2361 cases with IHD (the Copenhagen Ischemic Heart Disease Study).

Results.—In total, 13 genetic variants were identified. Three SNPs, g.−560A→C, g.−151C→T, and *181A→G, determined a haplotype that differed between high and low apoA-I groups (6 *vs.* 1%, P = 0.002). Genotype combinations of two SNPs, the g.−560A→C (tagging the g.−560A→C/g.−151C→T/*181A→G haplotype) and g.−310G→A (situated near a potential functional promoter site), were associated with increases in apoA-I and HDL cholesterol levels of up to 6.6 and 8.5%, respectively, resulting in theoretically predicted reductions in risk of 9 and 8% for IHD and 14 and 12% for myocardial infarction (MI). Despite this, these same genotype combinations were not associated with decreased risk of IHD or MI.

Conclusion.—Common genetic variation in *APOA1* associated with increased apoA-I and HDL cholesterol levels did not associate with decreased risk of IHD or MI.

▶ Epidemiologically the relationship between serum high-density lipoprotein cholesterol (HDL-C) levels and risk for coronary artery disease (CAD) is an inverse one: As HDL-C levels rise, risk for CAD decreases. Based on a large amount of epidemiologic investigation as well as in vitro evidence supporting the conclusion that HDL exerts multiple beneficial functions within blood vessel walls (eg, reverse cholesterol transport, anti-inflammatory, antioxidative, antithrombotic, and antiapoptotic effects among others), considerable interest is now focused on the development of novel therapeutic agents to raise HDL-C in a more robust and predictable manner. In addition, a number of large-scale, prospective, randomized studies are either underway or being designed to test the HDL hypothesis in a more rigorous manner. Although a considerable amount of data are consistent with HDL playing a vasculoprotec-tive role, a growing number of exceptions are being identified. In patients with CAD or heightened systemic inflammatory tone, HDL particles can be pro-oxidative and proinflammatory.[1,2] Among patients expressing apo A-I-Milano or apo A-I-Paris, HDL-C levels are frequently quite low, yet these patients are not predisposed to premature onset of CAD.[3] The low risk of these subjects is believed to be because of the augmented functionality of these apo A-I vari-ants. A very high HDL-C may also not necessarily be atheroprotective.[4] It is becoming increasingly apparent that much of the relationship between HDL-C and risk for coronary heart disease (CHD) depends on the specific genetic and metabolic background of a subject.

Haase and coworkers tested 2 hypotheses in subjects enrolled in the Copenhagen City Heart Study and the Copenhagen Ischemic Heart Disease Study: (1) Do single nucleotide polymorphisms (SNPs) in the gene for apopro-tein A1 impact lipids and lipoproteins, and (2) do these SNPs for apo A-I adjust risk for ischemic heart disease (IHD) and myocardial infarction (MI)? The coding and regulatory sequences for apo A-I were sequenced for subjects in the highest and lowest 1% for apo A-I. Thirteen SNPs were identified that corre-lated with high and low apo A-I. Genetic variants and combinations of variants associated with increased apo A-I and HDL-C had no impact on risk for IHD (Fig 2 in the original article) or MI (Fig 3 in the original article).

This study is quite interesting. There are variants of apo A-I that are associ-ated with reduced risk for CAD, IHD, and MI. One concern with this study is that the predicted effect size of the variants evaluated by these investigators ranges from only approximately 8%-14%. It is possible that this study did not include an adequate number of patients or monitor them long enough to detect such a relatively small change in risk. These authors suggest that it is not the circulating level of apo A-I or HDL-C that portends risk but rather serum levels of triglycerides and circulating levels of remnant lipoproteins. This, too, is controversial because triglycerides are only inconsistently associated with increased risk for CHD. Sorting out the role of HDL in atherogenesis is an enormously complex undertaking and involves hundreds and perhaps thousands of genetic polymorphisms. This is an issue that will not likely yield simple answers.

P. P. Toth, MD, PhD

References

1. Ansell BJ, Fonarow GC, Fogelman AM. High-density lipoprotein: is it always atheroprotective? *Curr Atheroscler Rep.* 2006;8:405-411.
2. Heinecke JW. The HDL proteome: a marker—and perhaps mediator—of coronary artery disease. *J Lipid Res.* 2009;50:S167-S171.
3. Toth PP, Davidson MH. Therapeutic interventions targeted at the augmentation of reverse cholesterol transport. *Curr Opin Cardiol.* 2004;19:374-379.
4. Barter P, Kastelein J, Nunn A, Hobbs R, Future Forum Editorial Board. High density lipoproteins (HDLs) and atherosclerosis; the unanswered questions. *Atherosclerosis.* 2003;168:195-211.

Insulin Resistance and the Relationship of a Dyslipidemia to Coronary Heart Disease: The Framingham Heart Study

Robins SJ, Lyass A, Zachariah JP, et al (Boston Univ School of Medicine, MA)
Arterioscler Thromb Vasc Biol 31:1208-1214, 2011

Objective.—The goal of this study was to examine the effect of insulin resistance (IR) in subjects without diabetes on the relationship of a dyslipidemia with high triglycerides and low high-density lipoprotein cholesterol (HDL-C) to the development of coronary heart disease (CHD).

Methods and Results.—Lower and higher fasting plasma HDL-C and triglyceride concentrations (defined at the study population median) and presence or absence of IR (defined by upper quartile Homeostatic Model Assessment values) were related to the development of myocardial infarction or CHD death in Framingham Heart Study participants without diabetes or a history of CHD (n=2910) attending the 1991 to 1995 examination. During follow-up (mean, 14 years), 128 participants experienced an incident CHD event. With Kaplan-Meier plots, the incidence of CHD was significantly greater with than without IR at either the lowest HDL-C or the highest triglycerides ($P<0.001$). In multivariable Cox models adjusted for major CHD risk factors, including waist circumference, only subgroups with IR had a significantly higher incidence of CHD. Compared with a reference group without IR and with higher-than-median HDL-C or lower-than-median triglycerides, the hazard ratio (HR) for incident events was significant with only IR and a lower HDL-C (HR 2.83, $P<0.001$) or higher triglycerides (HR 2.50, $P<0.001$). These findings were similar in men and women.

Conclusion.—In this community-based sample exclusive of diabetes, incident CHD risk associated with plasma HDL-C or triglycerides was significantly increased only in the presence of IR.

▶ Insulin resistance (IR) induces multiple changes in lipid and lipoprotein metabolism. In the setting of IR, there is increased hepatic secretion of triglyceride enriched very low-density lipoproteins (VLDLs). Under normal conditions, the triglycerides in these VLDLs are lipolyzed by lipoprotein lipase, resulting in the release of glycerol and fatty acids. With progressive lipolysis, the VLDLs are converted into intermediate-density lipoproteins and then low-density lipoproteins. IR is associated with reduced lipoprotein lipase activity, resulting in hypertriglyceridemia and hyperVLDLemia. To off-load this excess triglyceride mass, cholesterol ester transfer protein engages in a stoichiometric 1:1 exchange reaction of cholesterol ester for triglyceride, resulting in the enrichment of high-density lipoprotein (HDL) particles with triglycerides. This reaction converts the HDL particles into better substrates for lipolysis by hepatic lipase, which catabolizes HDL and results in low serum levels of this lipoprotein. Although elevated triglyceride level and low HDL cholesterol (HDL-C) are most commonly attributable to IR,[1] there are many genetic polymorphisms that can give rise to hypertriglyceridemia and hypoalphalipoproteinemia independent of IR.

Robins and coworkers evaluated an important extant issue in the Framingham Heart Study cohort: Do hypertriglyceridemia and hypoalphalipoproteinemia increase risk for cardiovascular events in both the presence and absence of IR? As anticipated, IR was most prevalent in subjects with low HDL-C and high triglyceride levels (Fig 1 in the original article). With a mean follow-up of 14 years in 2910 subjects, these investigators showed that the incidence of a cardiovascular event (nonfatal myocardial infarction or cardiovascular death) was highest for patients with IR and the lowest HDL-C and highest triglyceride levels (Fig 2 in the original article). In the absence of IR, low HDL-C and high triglyceride levels were associated with significantly less risk for cardiovascular events. Interestingly, subjects with mean HDL-C of 55 mg/dL and IR had higher risk than subjects with mean HDL-C of 42 mg/dL and no IR. Similarly, among patients without IR, a high triglyceride level had virtually the same risk as low triglyceride level (Fig 2 in the original article). High (mean 174 mg/dL) or low (mean 90 mg/dL) triglyceride levels in the presence of IR were both associated with increased cardiovascular risk compared with the same groups with no IR. These findings applied to both men and women even after adjustment for major risk factors and waist circumference.

These findings from the Framingham Heart Study highlight the significant impact of IR on cardiovascular risk. The Framingham investigators also call into question if hypertriglyceridemia and low HDL-C are risk factors for cardiovascular disease in the absence of IR. The latter finding is most certainly a complex issue, given that some forms of hypoalphalipoproteinemia portend increased risk for cardiovascular disease, while others do not.[2,3] Similarly, increased serum levels of triglycerides are only inconsistently associated with heightened risk for cardiovascular events.[4] At the least, these findings accentuate the importance of relieving IR in patients with high triglyceride levels and low HDL-C in any approach to reducing cardiovascular risk. Much further work is necessary to more fully elucidate the genetic and metabolic backgrounds that most strongly correlate low HDL-C and high triglyceride levels with increased cardiovascular risk.

P. P. Toth, MD, PhD

References

1. Rashid S, Watanabe T, Sakaue T, Lewis GF. Mechanisms of HDL lowering in insulin resistant, hypertriglyceridemic states: the combined effect of HDL triglyceride enrichment and elevated hepatic lipase activity. *Clin Biochem.* 2003;36: 421-429.
2. Willer CJ, Sanna S, Jackson AU, et al. Newly identified loci that influence lipid concentrations and risk of coronary artery disease. *Nat Genet.* 2008;40:161-169.
3. Frikke-Schmidt R, Nordestgaard BG, Stene MC, et al. Association of loss-of-function mutations in the ABCA1 gene with high-density lipoprotein cholesterol levels and risk of ischemic heart disease. *JAMA.* 2008;299:2524-2532.
4. Sarwar N, Danesh J, Eiriksdottir G, et al. Triglycerides and the risk of coronary heart disease: 10,158 incident cases among 262,525 participants in 29 Western prospective studies. *Circulation.* 2007;115:450-458.

Relation of Albuminuria to Angiographically Determined Coronary Arterial Narrowing in Patients With and Without Type 2 Diabetes Mellitus and Stable or Suspected Coronary Artery Disease
Rein P, Vonbank A, Saely CH, et al (Vorarlberg Inst for Vascular Investigation and Treatment, Feldkirch, Austria; et al)
Am J Cardiol 107:1144-1148, 2011

Albuminuria is associated with atherothrombotic events and all-cause mortality in patients with and without diabetes. However, it is not known whether albuminuria is associated with atherosclerosis per se in the same manner. The present study included 914 consecutive white patients who had been referred for coronary angiography for the evaluation of established or suspected stable coronary artery disease (CAD). Albuminuria was defined as a urinary albumin/creatinine ratio ≥ 30 µg/mg. Microalbuminuria was defined as 30 to 300 µg albumin/mg creatinine, and macroalbuminuria as a urinary albumin/creatinine ratio of ≥ 300 µg/mg. The prevalence of stenoses of $\geq 50\%$ was significantly greater in patients with albuminuria than in those with normoalbuminuria (66% vs 51%; $p < 0.001$). Logistic regression analysis, adjusted for age, gender, diabetes, smoking, hypertension, low-density lipoprotein cholesterol, high-density lipoprotein cholesterol, C-reactive protein, body mass index, estimated glomerular filtration rate, and the use of angiotensin-converting enzyme inhibitors/angiotensin II antagonists, aspirin, and statins, confirmed that albuminuria was significantly associated with stenoses $\geq 50\%$ (standardized adjusted odds ratio [OR] 1.68, 95% confidence interval [CI] 1.15 to 2.44; $p = 0.007$). The adjusted OR was 1.54 (95% CI 1.03 to 2.30;

p = 0.034) for microalbuminuria and 2.55 (95% CI 1.14 to 5.72; p = 0.023) for macroalbuminuria. This association was significant in the subgroup of patients with type 2 diabetes (OR 1.66, 95% CI 1.01 to 2.74; p = 0.045) and in those without diabetes (OR 1.42, 95% CI 1.05 to 1.92; p = 0.023). An interaction term urinary albumin/creatinine ratio*diabetes was not significant (p = 0.579). In conclusion, micro- and macroalbuminuria were strongly associated with angiographically determined coronary atherosclerosis in both patients with and those without type 2 diabetes mellitus, independent of conventional cardiovascular risk factors and the estimated glomerular filtration rate (Fig 1).

▶ Microalbuminuria is a widely acknowledged adverse prognostic indicator of increased risk for cardiovascular events in patients with and without diabetes mellitus.[1,2] Albuminuria is a manifestation of glomerular injury and systemic endothelial dysfunction. Endothelial dysfunction potentiates a large number of pathophysiologic changes within arterial walls, ultimately resulting in heightened intravascular inflammation and atherogenesis. In this study by Rein et al, the magnitude of albuminuria is correlated with risk of angiographically determined obstructive coronary artery disease (CAD) in 914 consecutive patients referred for coronary angiography. These investigators found a dose-response relationship between severity of albuminuria and prevalence of coronary plaques that were ≥50% obstructive (normoalbuminuria, 51%; microalbuminuria, 65%; and macroalbuminuria, 71%) (Fig 1). Moreover, microalbuminuria was an

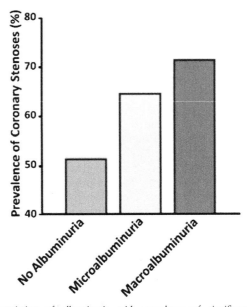

FIGURE 1.—Association of albuminuria with prevalence of significant coronary stenoses (p_{trend} = 0.001). (Reprinted from Rein P, Vonbank A, Saely CH, et al. Relation of albuminuria to angiographically determined coronary arterial narrowing in patients with and without type 2 diabetes mellitus and stable or suspected coronary artery disease. *Am J Cardiol.* 2011;107:1144-1148, Copyright 2011, with permission from Elsevier.)

independent risk factor for obstructive disease after adjusting for age, gender, diabetes status, smoking, hypertension, low-density lipoprotein cholesterol, high-density lipoprotein cholesterol, C-reactive protein, and body mass index. The relationship of microalbuminuria to risk of obstructive CAD remained significant after further adjusting for estimated glomerular filtration rate and use of angiotensin converting enzyme inhibitors, angiotensin receptor blockers, statins, and aspirin. Compared with patients with normoalbuminuria, the presence of microalbuminuria and macroalbuminuria correlated with odds ratios for obstructive CAD of 1.54 ($P = .034$) and 2.55 ($P = .023$) compared with normoalbuminuria. These relationships held in patients who either had or did not have diabetes mellitus.

Microalbuminuria and its progression to macroalbuminuria/proteinuria are associated with increased risk for cardiovascular events as well as chronic kidney disease, end-stage renal disease, and need for dialysis/transplantation in diabetics and nondiabetics. This study shows that micro/macroalbuminuria also correlate with risk for obstructive CAD even after adjusting for all other established CAD risk factors and background medications. An important next step will be to determine in a prospective randomized manner as to whether or not albuminuria/proteinuria reduction either slows or halts the progression of angiographically identifiable CAD.

P. P. Toth, MD, PhD

References

1. Arnlöv J, Evans JC, Meigs JB, et al. Low-grade albuminuria and incidence of cardiovascular disease events in nonhypertensive and nondiabetic individuals: the Framingham Heart Study. *Circulation.* 2005;112:969-975.
2. Gerstein HC, Mann JF, Yi Q, et al. Albuminuria and risk of cardiovascular events, death, and heart failure in diabetic and nondiabetic individuals. *JAMA.* 2001;286: 421-426.

Low-Density Lipoprotein Cholesterol and the Risk of Cancer: A Mendelian Randomization Study
Benn M, Tybjærg-Hansen A, Stender S, et al (Copenhagen Univ Hosp, Denmark)
J Natl Cancer Inst 103:508-519, 2011

Background.—Low plasma levels of low-density lipoprotein (LDL) cholesterol are associated with an increased risk of cancer, but whether this association is causal is unclear.

Methods.—We studied 10613 participants in the Copenhagen City Heart Study (CCHS) and 59 566 participants in the Copenhagen General Population Study, 6816 of whom had developed cancer by May 2009. Individuals were genotyped for *PCSK9* R46L (rs11591147), *ABCG8* D19H (rs11887534), and *APOE* R112C (rs429358) and R158C (rs7412) polymorphisms, all of which are associated with lifelong reduced plasma LDL cholesterol levels. Plasma LDL cholesterol was calculated using the Friedewald equation in samples in which the triglyceride level was less than 354 mg/dL and measured directly by colorimetry for samples with higher triglyceride levels. Risk of cancer was estimated prospectively using Cox proportional hazards regression analyses and cross-sectionally by logistic regression analyses. Causality was studied using instrumental variable analysis. All statistical tests were two-sided.

Results.—In the CCHS, compared with plasma LDL cholesterol levels greater than the 66th percentile (>158 mg/dL), those lower than the 10th percentile (<87 mg/dL) were associated with a 43% increase (95% confidence interval [CI] = 15% to 79% increase) in the risk of cancer. The polymorphisms were associated with up to a 38% reduction (95% CI = 36% to 41% reduction) in LDL cholesterol levels but not with increased risk of cancer. The causal odds ratio for cancer for a 50% reduction in plasma LDL cholesterol level due to all the genotypes in both studies combined was 0.96 (95% CI = 0.87 to 1.05), whereas the hazard ratio of cancer for a 50% reduction in plasma LDL cholesterol level in the CCHS was 1.10 (95% CI = 1.01 to 1.21) (P for causal odds ratio vs observed hazard ratio = .03).

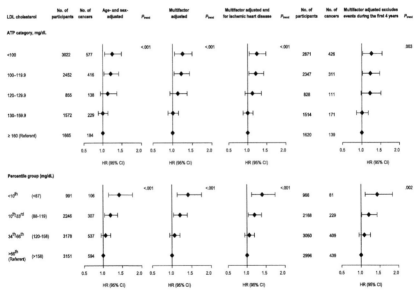

FIGURE 1.—Risk of any cancer as a function of plasma low-density lipoprotein (LDL) cholesterol level in the Copenhagen City Heart Study. Plasma LDL cholesterol levels were measured in 11 110 individuals who partic-ipated in the 1991—1994 or the 2001—2003 examinations of the Copenhagen City Heart Study and were subsequently followed up for a median of 15 years with respect to incident cancer. Individuals with cancer before study entry were excluded, explaining why the number of participants is lower than the overall number of participants with a LDL measurement. Multifactor adjustment was for age, sex, body mass index, hypertension, diabetes mellitus, current smoking, and statin use. **Black diamonds** represent the hazard ratios, and **error bars** indicate the 95% confidence intervals (CIs). P values for trend are two-sided and were estimated by Cuzick extension of a Wilcoxon rank-sum test. ATP = adult treatment panel III. (Reprinted from Benn M, Tybjærg-Hansen A, Stender S, et al. Low-Density Lipoprotein Cholesterol and the Risk of Cancer: A Mendelian Randomization Study. *J Natl Cancer Inst.* 2011;103:508-519, with permission from The Author 2011. Published by Oxford University Press.)

Conclusion.—Low plasma LDL cholesterol levels were robustly associated with an increased risk of cancer, but genetically decreased LDL cholesterol was not. This finding suggests that low LDL cholesterol levels per se do not cause cancer (Fig 1, Table 2).

▶ There is concern on the part of many physicians that lowering low-density lipoprotein cholesterol (LDL-C) below some as yet inadequately defined threshold may be harmful. A number of prospective observational studies have suggested a possible link between low serum cholesterol and increased risk for cancer.[1,2] Concern about this possible association once again came to the fore with publication of the Simvastatin and Ezetimibe in Aortic Stenosis trial, which suggested an increased risk for cancer among patients randomized to lipid-lowering therapy.[3] A subsequent meta-analysis refuted this finding and suggested it was attributable to chance.[4] In general, as shown by the Cholesterol Treatment Trialists' Collaborators, among 90 000 patients enrolled in randomized prospective statin trials, and there is no relationship discernible between either attained LDL-C or duration of statin therapy and risk of cancer.

Benn and coworkers evaluated the relationship between serum LDL-C and risk for cancer in the Copenhagen City Heart Study (CCHS) and Copenhagen General Population Study. Risk for cancer was assessed in a mendelian randomization study that quantified the impact of lifelong reduction in serum LDL-C from single nucleotide polymorphisms (SNPs) in the genes for *PCSK9*, *ABCG8*, and apolipoprotein E. Risk estimates were adjusted for age, gender, body mass index, hypertension, diabetes mellitus, smoking status, and statin use. Low serum LDL-C was associated with an increased risk for cancer in both cohorts (Fig 1 for the CCHS). In the CCHS, a 50% reduction in LDL-C was associated with a 10% ($P = .003$) increase in risk for cancer even after adjustment. None of the SNPs were associated with an increased risk for cancer (Table 2). Although low LDL-C appeared to correlate with increased risk for cancer, genetically determined lifelong lower LDL-C did

TABLE 2.—Studies Summary of the Causal Effect of Reduced Low-Density Lipoprotein (LDL) Cholesterol on Increased Risk of Cancer*

Model	F	R^2, %	Relative Risk[†] (95% CI) of Cancer for a 50% Reduction in LDL Cholesterol Level	P[‡]	P[§]
Observational estimate	—	—	1.10 (1.01 to 1.21)	.003	—
Instrumental variable estimate					
All genotypes combined	474	6.5	0.96 (0.87 to 1.05)	.31	.03
PCSK9 R46L	131	0.4	1.33 (0.59 to 2.97)	.30	.42
ABCG8 D19H	23	0.1	2.28 (0.43 to 12.11)	.73	.23
APOE genotype	844	5.9	0.92 (0.75 to 1.10)	.39	.02

*F statistics (evaluation of strength of instrument) and R^2 (contribution of genotype to variation in LDL cholesterol levels in percent) are from the first-stage regression analysis. — = not applicable; CI = confidence interval.
†The observational estimate of risk is a hazard ratio; the instrumental variable estimates of risk are odds ratios.
‡For the statistical significance of the hazard ratio or odds ratio from Cox proportional hazards or logistic regression analysis (two-sided).
§For the observational estimate from conventional epidemiology vs the causal estimate from instrumental variable analysis by the method Altman and Bland (36) (two-sided).

not. In this study, a 50% reduction in LDL-C caused by SNPs was not associated with an increase in risk for cancer overall or for any specific type of cancer (ie, gastrointestinal, hematologic, etc). The investigators conclude that low LDL-C per se is not oncogenic.

The cardiovascular benefit of LDL-C lowering is one of the most highly investigated issues in modern medicine. The magnitude of LDL-C reduction correlates with the magnitude of risk reduction. It is reassuring that an additional well-done analysis incorporating mendelian randomization in 2 large cohorts confirms that genetically determined, clinically meaningful, lifelong reduction in LDL-C is not associated with increased risk for any type of cancer.

P. P. Toth, MD, PhD

References

1. Sherwin RW, Wentworth DN, Cutler JA, Hulley SB, Kuller LH, Stamler J. Serum cholesterol levels and cancer mortality in 361,662 men screened for the Multiple Risk Factor Intervention Trial. *JAMA.* 1987;257:943-948.
2. Strasak AM, Pfeiffer RM, Brant LJ, et al. Time-dependent association of total serum cholesterol and cancer incidence in a cohort of 172,210 men and women: a prospective 19-year follow-up study. *Ann Oncol.* 2009;20:1113-1120.
3. Rossebo AB, Pedersen TR, Boman K, et al. Intensive lipid lowering with simvastatin and ezetimibe in aortic stenosis. *N Engl J Med.* 2008;359:1343-1356.
4. Peto R, Emberson J, Landray M, et al. Analyses of cancer data from three ezetimibe trials. *N Engl J Med.* 2008;359:1357-1366.

Metabolic Syndrome

Abdominal and gynoid adipose distribution and incident myocardial infarction in women and men

Wiklund P, Toss F, Jansson J-H, et al (Umeå Univ, Sweden; Skellefteå County Hosp, Sweden)
Int J Obes 34:1752-1758, 2010

Objective.—The relationships between objectively measured abdominal and gynoid adipose mass with the prospective risk of myocardial infarction (MI) has been scarcely investigated. We aimed to investigate the associations between fat distribution and the risk of MI.

Subjects.—Total and regional fat mass was measured using dual-energy X-ray absorptiometry (DEXA) in 2336 women and 922 men, of whom 104 subsequently experienced an MI during a mean follow-up time of 7.8 years.

Results.—In women, the strongest independent predictor of MI was the ratio of abdominal to gynoid adipose mass (hazard ratio (HR) = 2.44, 95% confidence interval (CI) 1.79—3.32 per s.d. increase in adipose mass), after adjustment for age and smoking. This ratio also showed a strong association with hypertension, impaired glucose tolerance and hypertriglyceridemia ($P<0.01$ for all). In contrast, the ratio of gynoid to total adipose mass was associated with a reduced risk of MI (HR = 0.57, 95% CI 0.43—0.77), and reduced risk of hypertension, impaired glucose tolerance and hypertriglyceridemia ($P<0.001$ for all). In men, gynoid fat mass was associated with a decreased risk of MI (HR = 0.69, 95% CI 0.48–0.98), and abdominal fat mass was associated with hypertriglyceridemia (*P* for trend 0.02).

Conclusion.—In summary, fat distribution was a strong predictor of the risk of MI in women, but not in men. These different results may be explained by the associations found between fat distribution and hypertension, impaired glucose tolerance and hypertriglyceridemia (Tables 1-3).

▶ Wiklund and coworkers also provide important new insights into the impact of anatomical variation in adiposity and risk for myocardial infarction (MI) as well as for hypertension, impaired glucose tolerance, and hypertriglyceridemia. The study included 2280 women and 874 men from northern Sweden. Gynoid adipose tissue is defined as femorogluteal fat. Abdominal and gynoid fat estimates were performed using dual-energy x-ray absorptiometry. Over 7.8 years of follow-up, 104 subjects sustained an MI. Among women, short stature, abdominal adipose tissue mass, abdominal/gynoid adipose mass, gynoid/

TABLE 1.—Physical Characteristics, Adipose Distribution and Background Data at Baseline in Relation to Whether the Female and Male Subjects Suffered an MI or Not During Follow-Up

Females	No MI During Follow-Up (N = 2280)	MI During Follow-Up (N = 56)
Age (years)	56.2 ± 13.2	57.9 ± 7.9
Weight (kg)	67.7 ± 12.9	68.3 ± 13.0
Height (m)	1.63 ± 0.07	1.61 ± 0.06**
BMI (kgm^{-2})	25.5 ± 4.5	26.4 ± 4.7
Total adipose mass (kg)	26.2 ± 9.7	27.5 ± 9.0
Abdominal adipose mass (g)	1510 ± 536	1726 ± 508**
Gynoid adipose mass (g)	2679 ± 841	2651 ± 770
Abdominal/gynoid adipose mass	0.56 ± 0.12	0.66 ± 0.14***
Gynoid/total adipose mass	0.11 ± 0.01	0.010 ± 0.01***
Diabetes (%)	4.6	30.4***
Hypertension (%)	27.4	65.5***
Hyperlipidemia (%)	9.0	24.0*
Current smoking (%)	20.4	22.2
Males	No MI during follow-up (N = 874)	MI during follow-up (N = 48)
Age (years)	51.8 ± 13.1	54.3 ± 8.6
Weight (kg)	81.6 ± 12.6	78.5 ± 12.5
Height (m)	1.77 ± 0.07	1.75 ± 0.05
BMI (kgm^{-2})	26.0 ± 3.6	25.5 ± 3.9
Total adipose mass (kg)	21.0 ± 7.7	20.3 ± 10.1
Abdominal adipose mass (g)	1484 ± 458	1473 ± 607
Gynoid adipose mass (g)	1856 ± 588	1754 ± 774
Abdominal/gynoid adipose mass	0.81 ± 0.15	0.85 ± 0.14*
Gynoid/total adipose mass	0.09 ± 0.01	0.09 ± 0.01
Diabetes (%)	9.8	35.4**
Hypertension (%)	30.4	48.9*
Hypertriglyceridemia (%)	15.6	30.8
Current smoking (%)	17.8	26.8

Abbreviations: BMI, body mass index; MI, myocardial infarction. Means and s.d. are presented.
*P<0.05.
**P<0.01.
***P<0.001.

TABLE 2.—Associations Between Quartiles of the Different Adipose Mass Estimates and Hypertension or Treatment for Hypertension, Diabetes or Impaired Glucose Tolerance and Treatment for Hypertriglyceridemia or Hypertriglyceridemia After Adjustment for the Influence of Age and Smoking

Women	Hypertension			Impaired Glucose Tolerance			Hypertriglyceridemia		
	OR	95% CI	P-Value	OR	95% CI	P-Value	OR	95% CI	P-Value
BMI	2.26	1.50–3.43	0.001	2.46	1.37–4.42	0.01	3.67	1.91–7.03	<0.001
Total adipose mass	2.62	1.70–4.03	<0.001	2.05	1.14–3.67	0.03	3.45	1.83–6.50	<0.001
Abdominal adipose mass	2.89	1.85–4.51	<0.001	2.93	1.59–5.38	0.001	8.39	3.48–20.20	<0.001
Gynoid adipose mass	1.89	1.26–2.86	0.02	1.55	0.89–2.71	0.37	1.69	0.95–3.01	0.07
Abdominal/gynoid adipose mass	2.54	1.63–3.97	<0.001	2.88	1.62–5.12	<0.001	8.48	3.50–20.57	<0.001
Gynoid/total adipose mass	0.40	0.26–0.61	<0.001	0.31	0.18–0.54	<0.001	0.10	0.04–0.24	<0.001

Men	Hypertension			Impaired Glucose Tolerance			Hypertriglyceridemia		
	OR	95% CI	P for Trend	OR	95% CI	P for Trend	OR	95% CI	P for Trend
BMI	1.29	0.69–2.39	0.85	0.92	0.43–1.98	0.40	2.46	1.15–5.26	0.04
Total adipose mass	1.42	0.76–2.67	0.25	1.18	0.50–2.79	0.81	2.78	1.20–6.44	0.08
Abdominal adipose mass	1.59	0.84–3.01	0.49	0.98	0.42–2.30	0.61	3.01	1.29–7.05	0.02
Gynoid adipose mass	1.27	0.68–2.36	0.73	1.06	0.48–2.38	0.85	1.98	0.89–4.41	0.31
Abdominal/gynoid adipose mass	0.82	0.42–1.59	0.56	0.97	0.40–2.44	0.97	1.46	0.60–3.52	0.40
Gynoid/total adipose mass	0.53	0.27–1.06	0.22	0.95	0.38–2.35	0.83	0.37	0.16–0.86	0.12

Abbreviations: BMI, body mass index; CI, confidence interval; MI, myocardial infarction; OR, odds ratio. ORs and 95% CIs are presented for the fourth vs the first quartiles of the different fat estimates in 1040 women and 388 men. *P*-values are presented.

TABLE 3.—HRs for the Risk of MI per s.d. Increase in the Adipose Variables, Adjusted for Age and Smoking in 1439 Subjects Including 41 Males and 49 Females who Later Sustained an MI

	Women			Men		
	HR	95% CI	*P*-Value	HR	95% CI	*P*-Value
BMI	1.18	0.85–1.62	0.32	0.84	0.60–1.18	0.31
Total adipose mass	1.07	0.78–1.47	0.67	0.71	0.50–1.02	0.07
Abdominal adipose mass	1.53	1.10–2.12	0.01	0.80	0.55–1.17	0.25
Gynoid adipose mass	0.88	0.65–1.20	0.43	0.69	0.48–0.98	0.04
Abdominal/gynoid adipose mass	2.44	1.79–3.32	<0.01	1.29	0.89–1.85	0.18
Gynoid/total adipose mass	0.57	0.43–0.77	<0.01	1.05	0.75–1.48	0.78

Abbreviations: BMI, body mass index; CI, confidence interval; HR, hazard ratio; MI, myocardial infarction. The 95% CIs and *P*-values are presented.

total adipose tissue mass, diabetes mellitus, hyperlipidemia, and hypertension all correlated with risk for MI (Table 1). Among men, abdominal/gynoid adipose mass, diabetes, and hypertension correlated with risk for MI (Table 1). In women, body mass index (BMI), total adipose mass, abdominal adipose mass, and abdominal/gynoid adipose mass all correlated positively with risk for hypertension, hypertriglyceridemia, and impaired glucose tolerance (Table 2). Gynoid adipose tissue mass was protective against each of these metabolic derangements. In men, BMI and adipose tissue mass correlated with hypertriglyceridemia, but none of the other adipose tissue measures achieved statistical significance for metabolic derangement. Adipose tissue distribution affected risk for MI. Among women, increased abdominal/gynoid adipose mass was associated with a 2.4-fold higher risk, while increased gynoid/total adipose tissue mass was protective against MI (hazard ratio [HR], 0.57; Table 3). Among men, gynoid adipose tissue mass reduced risk for MI, with an HR of 0.69 ($P = .04$).

The relationship between adiposity and cardiovascular risk was stronger for women than men in this study. Moreover, none of the adiposity indices usually associated with increased risk for cardiovascular disease achieved statistical significance in men. Visceral adiposity did increase risk for MI in women. Gynoid adipose tissue was protective in both men and women. The lack of correlation between events and visceral adipose tissue in men may be attributable to the small sample size, although a correlation between these variables has not been consistently found. It is possible that the apparent protectiveness of gynoid adipose tissue is attributable to higher capacity for adiponectin production, better insulin sensitivity, and less responsiveness to circulating catecholamines, resulting in less release of free fatty acid mass and injurious adipocytokines. This study certainly suggests that region-specific fat depots affect risk for metabolic derangements and cardiovascular events in different and quantifiable ways. Much work remains to be done in this area before the relationships between the volume/mass of specific adipose tissue depots, insulin resistance, and risk for cardiovascular events can be quantified in a reliable and generalizable manner.

P. P. Toth, MD, PhD

Hypercholesterolemia and hypoadiponectinemia are associated with necrotic core-rich coronary plaque

Kojima S, Kojima S, Maruyoshi H, et al (Kumamoto Univ, Japan; et al)
Int J Cardiol 147:371-376, 2011

Background.—Hypercholesterolemia is a risk factor for coronary artery disease and closely linked to unstable plaque. Hypoadiponectinemia is frequently observed in patients with metabolic syndrome complicated with macroangiopathy and predicts poor clinical outcome. Spectral analysis of intravascular ultrasonography radiofrequency (IVUS-Virtual Histology [VH]) allows quantitative analysis of plaque composition. The purpose of this study was to verify the effects of low-density lipoprotein (LDL) cholesterol level on plaque morphology, and test the hypothesis that adiponectin influences coronary plaque volume and composition.

Methods.—Preintervention IVUS-VH using a continuous pullback was performed in 92 coronary vessels in 92 patients with coronary artery disease. The morphological distribution of plaque was evaluated prospectively in a 60-mm segment of coronary vessels containing the culprit lesion.

Results.—Serum LDL cholesterol levels correlated positively with necrotic core volume ($r = 0.217, P = 0.037$) and percent necrotic core tissue ($r = 0.308, P = 0.003$), while plasma adiponectin levels correlated negatively with plaque volume ($r = -0.297, P = 0.004$) and necrotic core volume ($r = -0.306, P = 0.003$). Multiple regression analyses showed close association between necrotic core volume and statin-use ($\beta = -21.68, P = 0.004$) and adiponectin levels ($\beta = -31.25, P = 0.038$), and that percent necrotic core tissue was influenced by statin-use ($\beta = -4.595, P = 0.026$) and LDL cholesterol levels ($\beta = 0.092, P = 0.031$).

Conclusions.—Adiponectin is closely linked to coronary plaque volume. Hypercholesterolemia and hypoadiponectinemia correlate with necrotic core lesions and may contribute to increased risk of coronary plaque vulnerability. Statins can affectively prevent necrotic core plaque formation associated with hypercholesterolemia and hypoadiponectinemia (Figs 2 and 3).

▶ Adiponectin is a beneficial adipocyte-derived cytokine that promotes systemic insulin sensitization. Adiponectin levels decrease in the setting of metabolic syndrome and type 2 diabetes mellitus. Reductions in circulating levels of adiponectin portend increased risk for cardiovascular events and increased severity of coronary artery disease.[1,2] Atherogenesis in its earliest phase is driven by the scavenging of oxidatively modified lipoprotein particles by monocyte-derived macrophages in the subendothelial space. The resulting foam cells can undergo apoptosis. Apoptotic foam cells can fragment, and the histologic debris produced can be cleared in an orderly manner by other phagocytic cells. However, if the rate of debris clearance cannot keep up with the rate of debris formation, then a necrotic core develops within the atherosclerotic plaque that comprises lipid and cellular fragments.[3] As the

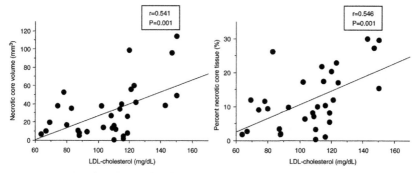

FIGURE 2.—Correlation between low-density lipoprotein (LDL) cholesterol levels and necrotic core plaque in patients with acute coronary syndrome (ACS). (Reprinted from Kojima S, Kojima S, Maruyoshi H, et al. Hypercholesterolemia and hypoadiponectinemia are associated with necrotic core-rich coronary plaque. *Int J Cardiol.* 2011;147:371-376, Copyright 2011, with permission from Elsevier.)

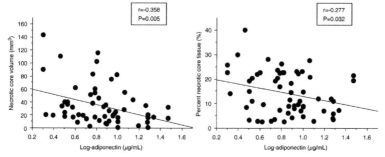

FIGURE 3.—Correlation between plasma adiponectin levels and necrotic core plaque in patients with stable angina pectoris (SAP). (Reprinted from Kojima S, Kojima S, Maruyoshi H, et al. Hypercholesterolemia and hypoadiponectinemia are associated with necrotic core-rich coronary plaque. *Int J Cardiol.* 2011;147:371-376, Copyright 2011, with permission from Elsevier.)

necrotic core expands, it can destabilize the plaque and promote plaque rupture and acute coronary luminal obstruction.

In this investigation by Kojima and coworkers, the role of adiponectin in human coronary atherosclerotic plaque constitution is evaluated using intravascular ultrasonographic virtual histology. Not surprisingly, serum low-density lipoprotein cholesterol correlated with both necrotic core volume and percent necrotic core tissue and statin therapy reduced both of these parameters (Fig 2). Of interest is the observation that adiponectin levels correlated inversely with both necrotic core volume and percent necrotic core tissue (Fig 3).

Metabolic syndrome and insulin resistance are associated with a large number of risk factors that increase risk for acute cardiovascular events, including impairments in glucose metabolism, hypertension, and dyslipidemia. This work suggests that the hypoadiponectinemia associated with insulin resistance is also an important risk factor because it can influence atherosclerotic plaque volume, histologic organization, and, presumptively, stability. Whether adiponectin directly or indirectly impacts macrophage viability and scavenging capacity in active plaque is yet to be determined. This work supports the conclusion that hypoadiponectinemia is associated with increased risk for large necrotic core volumes and plaque instability among patients with established coronary artery disease.

P. P. Toth, MD, PhD

References

1. Toth PP. Adiponectin and high-density lipoprotein: a metabolic association through thick and thin. *Eur Heart J.* 2005;26:1579-1581.
2. Dekker JM, Funahashi T, Nijpels G, et al. Prognostic value of adiponectin for cardiovascular disease and mortality. *J Clin Endocrinol Metab.* 2008;93: 1489-1496.
3. Tabas I. Consequences and therapeutic implications of macrophage apoptosis in atherosclerosis: the importance of lesion stage and phagocytic efficiency. *Arterioscler Thromb Vasc Biol.* 2005;25:2255-2264.

Adipocyte Modulation of High-Density Lipoprotein Cholesterol

Zhang Y, McGillicuddy FC, Hinkle CC, et al (Univ of Pennsylvania School of Medicine, Philadelphia; et al)
Circulation 121:1347-1355, 2010

Background.—Adipose harbors a large depot of free cholesterol. However, a role for adipose in cholesterol lipidation of high-density lipoprotein (HDL) in vivo is not established. We present the first evidence that adipocytes support transfer of cholesterol to HDL in vivo as well as in vitro and implicate ATP-binding cassette subfamily A member 1 (ABCA1) and scavenger receptor class B type I (SR-BI), but not ATP-binding cassette subfamily G member 1 (ABCG1), cholesterol transporters in this process.

Methods and Results.—Cholesterol efflux from wild-type, ABCA1$^{-/-}$, SR-BI$^{-/-}$, and ABCG1$^{-/-}$ adipocytes to apolipoprotein A-I (apoA-I) and HDL3 were measured in vitro. 3T3L1 adipocytes, labeled with ^{3}H-cholesterol, were injected intraperitoneally into wild-type, apoA-I transgenic, and apoA-I$^{-/-}$ mice, and tracer movement onto plasma HDL was monitored. Identical studies were performed with labeled wild-type, ABCA1$^{-/-}$, or SR-BI$^{-/-}$ mouse embryonic fibroblast adipocytes. The effect of tumor necrosis factor-α on transporter expression and cholesterol efflux was monitored during adipocyte differentiation. Cholesterol efflux to apoA-I and HDL3 was impaired in ABCA1$^{-/-}$ and SR-BI$^{-/-}$ adipocytes, respectively, with no effect observed in ABCG1$^{-/-}$ adipocytes. Intraperitoneal injection of labeled 3T3L1 adipocytes resulted in increased HDL-associated ^{3}H-cholesterol in apoA-I transgenic mice but reduced levels in apoA-I$^{-/-}$ animals. Intraperitoneal injection of labeled ABCA1$^{-/-}$ or SR-BI$^{-/-}$ adipocytes reduced plasma counts relative to their respective controls. Tumor necrosis factor-_ reduced both ABCA1 and SR-BI expression and impaired cholesterol efflux from partially differentiated adipocytes.

Conclusions.—These data suggest a novel metabolic function of adipocytes in promoting cholesterol transfer to HDL in vivo and implicate adipocyte SR-BI and ABCA1, but not ABCG1, in this process. Furthermore, adipocyte modulation of HDL may be impaired in adipose inflammatory disease states such as type 2 diabetes mellitus.

▶ High-density lipoproteins (HDLs) are known to originate from a number of cell types. Chylomicrons secreted by jejunal enterocytes are enriched with apoprotein AI (apo AI), the primary apoprotein building block of HDLs. In serum, as chylomicrons are lipolyzed, surface coat constituents composed of apo AI and phospholipid can be released. The surface coat constituents can be further lipidated to form nascent discoidal HDL and HDL3 via the activity of lecithin—cholesterol acyltransferase. The adenosine triphosphate—binding membrane cassette transport protein A1 (ABCA1) is a sterol transport protein that can bind poorly lipidated apo AI on the surface of hepatocytes, jejunocytes, and macrophages and promote the formation of HDLs.[1] ABCA1 binds apo AI, nascent discoidal HDL, and small spherical HDLs (HDL3). ABCG1 is another cholesterol translocator on the surface of macrophages that binds and lipidates larger, more-mature, spherical HDL particles labeled HDL2.[2] Lipidated HDL particles become progressively more enriched with cholesterol ester and participate in reverse cholesterol transport (RCT) and the delivery of cholesterol esters for steroidogenesis to scavenger receptor class B type I (SR-BI) on the surface of hepatocytes and steroidogenic tissues, respectively. SR-BI selectively delipidates HDL particles and releases them back into the circulation.[3] In macrophages, SR-BI can also function as a bidirectional cholesterol translocator and can participate in net HDL lipidation. Adipose tissue comprises a large storage depot for lipids and cholesterol. To date, the role of adipose tissue in the genesis of HDL had not been studied.

In this fascinating paper by Zhang and coworkers, HDL dynamics within adipose tissues were evaluated. Using a variety of homozygous knockout mice, these investigators demonstrated that adipose tissue lipidates apo AI and HDL3 via ABCA1 and SR-BI, respectively. This was confirmed in cultured murine and human adipocytes. They found no evidence of a role in HDL lipidation and biogenesis by ABCG1. Consistent with the capacity of adipocytes to lipidate HDLs, adipose tissue—derived cholesterol was found to move into plasma on HDL particles and then into the liver and feces, consistent with adipocytes participating in RCT. Insulin resistance is at least partially induced by tumor necrosis factor α (TNF-α). In this model, TNF-α impaired ABCA1 and SR-BI expression and reduced cholesterol efflux and HDL biogenesis by adipocytes (Fig 1 in the original article).

These findings raise a number of issues. In recent years, much work has focused on adipose tissue as a reservoir of fatty acids, which can potentiate insulin resistance and promote ectopic fat deposition in a diverse number of tissues, including the pancreas, liver, heart, and skeletal muscle, among others. Little focus had been placed on adipose tissue as a sterol source. This work suggests that adipose tissue is an important regulator of serum HDL concentrations. Serum HDL levels appear to be regulated by the gut, liver, adipose tissue, serum triglyceride levels, lipoprotein lipolysis in serum, and, to a small degree, macrophages in the subendothelial space. Of particular interest is the fact that TNF-α impaired adipocyte cholesterol mobilization and translocation on to HDL particles and also reduced adipocyte expression of peroxisomal proliferator receptor γ, adiponectin, and lipoprotein lipase. All these are adverse metabolic changes. This investigation also suggests that serum HDL reductions are a result of reduced HDL production by insulin-resistant dysregulated adipose tissue and not just increased HDL catabolism driven by hepatic lipase.

P. P. Toth, MD, PhD

References

1. Brewer HB Jr, Remaley AT, Neufeld EB, Basso F, Joyce C. Regulation of plasma high-density lipoprotein levels by the ABCA1 transporter and the emerging role of high-density lipoprotein in the treatment of cardiovascular disease. *Arterioscler Thromb Vasc Biol.* 2004;24:1755-1760.
2. Vaughan AM, Oram JF. ABCG1 redistributes cell cholesterol to domains removable by high density lipoprotein but not by lipid-depleted apolipoproteins. *J Biol Chem.* 2005;280:30150-30157.
3. Rigotti A, Miettinen HE, Krieger M. The role of the high-density lipoprotein receptor SR-BI in the lipid metabolism of endocrine and other tissues. *Endocr Rev.* 2003;24:357-387.

Lipid profiling identifies a triacylglycerol signature of insulin resistance and improves diabetes prediction in humans
Rhee EP, Cheng S, Larson MG, et al (Massachusetts General Hosp (MGH), Boston; Boston Univ (BU) School of Medicine, Framingham; et al)
J Clin Invest 121:1402-1411, 2011

Dyslipidemia is an independent risk factor for type 2 diabetes, although exactly which of the many plasma lipids contribute to this remains unclear. We therefore investigated whether lipid profiling can inform diabetes prediction by performing liquid chromatography/mass spectrometry–based lipid profiling in 189 individuals who developed type 2 diabetes and 189 matched disease-free individuals, with over 12 years of follow up in the Framingham Heart Study. We found that lipids of lower carbon number and double bond content were associated with an increased risk of diabetes, whereas lipids of higher carbon number and double bond content were associated with decreased risk. This pattern was strongest for triacylglycerols (TAGs) and persisted after multivariable adjustment for age, sex, BMI, fasting glucose, fasting insulin, total triglycerides, and HDL cholesterol. A combination of 2 TAGs further improved diabetes prediction. To explore potential mechanisms that modulate the distribution of plasma lipids, we performed lipid profiling during oral glucose tolerance testing, pharmacologic interventions, and acute exercise testing. Levels of TAGs associated with increased risk for diabetes decreased in response to insulin action and were elevated in the setting of insulin resistance. Conversely, levels of TAGs associated with decreased diabetes risk rose in response to insulin and were poorly correlated with insulin resistance. These studies identify a relationship between lipid acyl chain content and diabetes risk and demonstrate how lipid profiling could aid in clinical risk assessment (Table 2).

▶ The human lipidome and the functional range of many of its constituent lipids are extraordinarily complex. The lipidome comprises many types of cholesterol esters, phospholipids, sphingolipids, cerebrosides, gangliosides, monoacylglycerols, diacylglycerols, and triacylglycerols. Standard lipid profiles measure total cholesterol, high-density lipoprotein cholesterol (HDL-C), low-density lipoprotein cholesterol, and triglycerides (triacylglycerols). The latter are quite varied, as their specific chemical identity depends on the specific chain length (ie, carbon number) and degree of saturation/unsaturation. Many combinations of acyl chains along positions sn-1, sn-2, and sn-3 are known to exist. The biochemical distribution of acyl chains depends on specific types of fat and lipid consumed in the diet and absorbed within the gastrointestinal tract as well as on patterns of hepatic lipoprotein uptake and biochemical disposal and metabolism.

Rhee and coworkers develop a model of lipid profiling using liquid chromatography and mass spectrometry to improve prediction of risk for insulin resistance and diabetes mellitus. This analysis is a nested case-control study of the Framingham Offspring Cohort comparing patients who did and did not develop diabetes over 12 years of follow-up. After multivariable adjustment for gender, age, body mass index, fasting insulin and glucose, triglycerides, and HDL-C, 15 lipid moieties achieved statistical significance (Table 2). Ten lipids were associated with increased risk for diabetes, and each standard deviation (SD) increase in log marker correlated with a 1.35- to 1.94-fold increase in risk for diabetes. Among persons in the highest quartile of these analytes, risk for diabetes increased 1.35- to 4.19-fold. Five lipid species were associated with reduced risk for diabetes, with each SD increment in log marker correlating with a 0.67- to 0.78-fold reduced risk for new-onset diabetes. Persons in the highest quartile for these protective lipids had a 0.30- to 0.56-fold risk of developing diabetes over the follow-up period. Lipids correlating with increased risk for diabetes comprised primarily of saturated and monounsaturated fatty acids of low carbon number and double bond content. In contrast, protective lipids were composed primarily of polyunsaturated fats of high carbon number and double bond content. Interestingly, based on dietary questionnaires, no relationship was found between the percentages of total fat intake from saturated or polyunsaturated fats.

These data show that complex specific lipidomic signatures are associated with insulin resistance and increased risk for diabetes mellitus. This work most certainly extends the risk for metabolic syndrome, diabetes, and cardiovascular disease associated with triglycerides to a novel range. The metabolic alterations and causal chains giving rise to these specific graded levels of risk have yet to be elucidated, especially because changes in levels of particular lipids did not depend on the distribution of dietary saturated and unsaturated fat. Insulin resistance gives rise to a very complex biochemical milieu. It will be important to elucidate whether these complex changes in acyl chain distributions contribute to the development of insulin resistance/diabetes mellitus or are simply a manifestation

TABLE 2.—Relationship of Individual Baseline Lipid Levels to Risk of Future Diabetes

Lipid	OR per SD	P Value	OR 1st Quartile	OR 2nd Quartile	OR 3rd Quartile	OR 4th Quartile	P Value for Trend
TAG 52:1	1.94 (1.18–3.20)	0.009	1.0	2.21 (1.01–4.83)	1.74 (0.72–4.21)	4.19 (1.39–12.62)	0.032
TAG 50:0	1.74 (1.19–2.57)	0.005	1.0	2.02 (0.95–4.29)	1.95 (0.87–4.37)	3.86 (1.43–10.41)	0.016
PC 34:2	1.47 (1.06–2.04)	0.021	1.0	2.12 (1.00–4.49)	2.45 (1.07–5.58)	2.89 (1.16–7.20)	0.035
TAG 48:1	1.47 (1.05–2.05)	0.026	1.0	1.34 (0.63–2.84)	1.32 (0.65–2.67)	2.91 (1.23–6.91)	0.023
TAG 46:1	1.44 (1.01–2.06)	0.043	1.0	1.10 (0.53–2.30)	1.32 (0.63–2.76)	2.23 (0.95–5.22)	0.054
TAG 48:0	1.41 (1.01–1.95)	0.042	1.0	0.79 (0.39–1.59)	1.04 (0.52–2.10)	2.15 (0.96–4.78)	0.051
TAG 44:1	1.41 (1.02–1.94)	0.036	1.0	0.94 (0.47–1.85)	1.35 (0.66–2.77)	1.61 (0.74–3.48)	0.17
LPE 18:2	1.39 (1.07–1.81)	0.016	1.0	1.73 (0.86–3.51)	1.86 (0.90–3.88)	2.67 (1.30–5.46)	0.001
SM 22:0	1.38 (1.05–1.81)	0.022	1.0	1.09 (0.54–2.20)	1.62 (0.85–3.10)	2.56 (1.18–5.56)	0.015
PC 36:2	1.35 (1.02–1.80)	0.039	1.0	1.18 (0.61–2.30)	1.72 (0.83–3.53)	1.35 (0.61–2.99)	0.35
TAG 58:10	0.67 (0.50–0.89)	0.006	1.0	0.56 (0.30–1.07)	0.49 (0.26–0.95)	0.30 (0.14–0.67)	0.003
LPC 22:6	0.69 (0.53–0.90)	0.006	1.0	0.76 (0.42–1.36)	0.57 (0.30–1.09)	0.38 (0.18–0.79)	0.008
TAG 56:9	0.70 (0.52–0.94)	0.017	1.0	0.89 (0.46–1.69)	0.57 (0.29–1.10)	0.46 (0.21–1.01)	0.019
TAG 60:12	0.74 (0.58–0.96)	0.022	1.0	0.51 (0.27–0.97)	0.74 (0.41–1.35)	0.56 (0.28–1.11)	0.17
PC 38:6	0.78 (0.61–1.00)	0.049	1.0	0.78 (0.43–1.40)	0.63 (0.34–1.20)	0.51 (0.26–1.00)	0.041
TAG 50:0+TAG 58:10	2.72 (1.55–4.76)	0.001	1.0	2.50 (1.04–6.01)	4.64 (1.96–11.01)	4.30 (1.75–10.58)	0.001

Values are ORs (95% confidence intervals) for diabetes, from conditional logistic regressions. All models adjusted for age, sex, BMI, fasting glucose, fasting insulin, triglycerides, and HDL cholesterol. Analytes are ordered by OR per SD values. The trend test used integers for quartile values. Each individual was assigned to a quartile based on the cut-off point values calculated in the control sample. For the combination of TAGs 50:0 and 58:10, values represent results for a weighted score comprised of coefficients for each TAG that were estimated from individually fitted models.

of these metabolic derangements. The fact that 5 lipids were protective against the development of impairments in glucose metabolism is noteworthy. Further intensive investigation into the biogenesis of these lipids and whether they can be therapeutically manipulated is warranted.

P. P. Toth, MD, PhD

Nutrition and Nutritional Supplements

Dietary intake of n—3 long-chain polyunsaturated fatty acids and coronary events in Norwegian patients with coronary artery disease

Manger MS, Strand E, Ebbing M, et al (Univ of Bergen, Norway; Haukeland Univ Hosp, Bergen, Norway; et al)
Am J Clin Nutr 92:244-251, 2010

Background.—Consumption of fish and n—3 (omega-3) long-chain polyunsaturated fatty acids (LCPUFAs) has been associated with reduced risk of coronary artery disease (CAD) mortality.

Objective.—The aim was to examine the relation between dietary intake of n—3 LCPUFAs or fish and risk of future coronary events or mortality in patients with well-characterized CAD.

Design.—This was a substudy of 2412 participants in the Western Norway B Vitamin Intervention Trial with a median follow-up time of 57 mo. Patients aged >18 y diagnosed with CAD (81% men) completed a food-frequency questionnaire at baseline, from which daily intakes of eicosapentaenoic, docosapentaenoic, and docosahexaenoic acids as well as fish were estimated on the basis of diet and intakes of supplements including fish and cod liver oils. The main endpoint was a composite of coronary events, including coronary death, nonfatal acute myocardial infarction, and unstable angina pectoris.

Results.—The mean (± SD) intakes of n—3 LCPUFAs in quartiles 1—4 were 0.58 ± 0.29, 0.83 ± 0.30, 1.36 ± 0.44, and 2.64 ± 1.18 g/d, respectively. We found no dose-response relation between quartiles of n—3 LCPUFAs (based on intake as percentage of total energy) or fish and coronary events or separate endpoints. A post hoc additive proportional hazards model showed a slightly increased risk of coronary events at an intake of n—3 LCPUFAs < ≈0.30 g/d.

Conclusion.—Among Norwegian patients with CAD consuming relatively high amounts of n—3 LCPUFAs and fish, there were no significant trends toward a reduced risk of coronary events or mortality with increasing intakes. This trial was registered at clinicaltrials.gov as NCT00354081 (Tables 1 and 4).

▶ The ω-3 fish oils (eicosapentaenoic acid and docosahexaenoic acid) are used to reduce serum levels of triglycerides in patients with hypertriglyceridemia[1] and are also used to treat patients who have sustained a myocardial infarction (MI) because of demonstrable reductions in risk for reinfarction and mortality.[2] Current guidelines by the American Heart Association also recommend that

TABLE 1.—Baseline Characteristics of Participants by Quartiles of N−3 Long-chain Polyunsaturated Fatty Acid (LCPUFA) Intake (N = 2412)[1]

	Quartiles of N-3 LCPUFA Intake (%TE)[2]				P for trend[3]
	1	2	3	4	
n−3 LCPUFAs (%TE)	0.15 ± 0.06[4]	0.34 ± 0.06	0.57 ± 0.08	1.15 ± 0.40	<0.001
Age (y)	60.1 ± 10.5	61.6 ± 9.7	62.3 ± 9.3	62.6 ± 9.1	<0.001
Male sex [n (%)]	482 (79.9)	486 (80.6)	484 (80.3)	489 (81.1)	0.66
BMI (kg/m²)	26.7 ± 3.9	26.6 ± 3.5	27.2 ± 3.6	26.8 ± 3.7	0.17
LVEF 50% [n (%)]	65 (10.8)	57 (9.5)	65 (10.8)	67 (11.1)	0.68
Hemoglobin (g/dL)	14.4 ± 1.3	14.4 ± 1.1	14.4 ± 1.2	14.4 ± 1.1	0.99
Creatinine (μmol/L)	92.0 ± 17.4	91.0 ± 15.7	91.6 ± 17.0	91.4 ± 14.4	0.68
Total cholesterol (mmol/L)	5.2 ± 1.4	5.0 ± 1.1	5.1 ± 1.2	4.9 ± 1.1	0.02
HDL cholesterol (mmol/L)	1.2 ± 0.3	1.2 ± 0.3	1.2 ± 0.3	1.3 ± 0.4	0.005
LDL cholesterol (mmol/L)	3.1 ± 1.1	3.0 ± 1.0	3.2 ± 1.1	3.0 ± 1.0	0.15
Triglycerides (mmol/L)	1.9 ± 1.0	1.8 ± 1.1	1.8 ± 1.0	1.6 ± 1.0	<0.001
CRP (mg/L)[5]	2.1 (1.0, 5.0)	1.8 (0.9, 4.1)	2.0 (0.9, 3.8)	1.4 (0.8, 3.3)	0.09
Cardiovascular history and risk factors [n (%)]					
Myocardial infarction	244 (40.5)	237 (39.3)	242 (40.1)	271 (44.9)	0.11
Percutaneous coronary intervention	136 (22.6)	121 (20.1)	124 (20.6)	140 (23.2)	0.74
Coronary artery bypass graft surgery	59 (9.8)	88 (14.6)	84 (13.9)	104 (17.2)	0.001
Diabetes mellitus	55 (9.1)	63 (10.4)	60 (10.0)	80 (13.3)	0.03
Hypertension[6]	267 (44.3)	265 (43.9)	289 (47.9)	297 (49.3)	0.04
Current smoker[7]	195 (32.3)	188 (31.2)	131 (21.7)	104 (17.2)	<0.001
Clinical diagnosis before baseline coronary angiography [n (%)]					
Stable angina pectoris	485 (80.4)	507 (84.1)	526 (87.2)	524 (86.9)	0.001
Acute coronary syndrome[8]	110 (18.2)	86 (14.3)	68 (11.3)	75 (12.4)	0.001
Aortic valve stenosis	8 (1.3)	10 (1.7)	9 (1.5)	4 (0.7)	0.30
Extent of CAD at baseline coronary angiography [n (%)]					
No or nonsignificant CAD	66 (10.9)	82 (13.6)	58 (9.6)	62 (10.3)	0.30
One-vessel disease	196 (32.5)	181 (30.0)	176 (29.2)	170 (28.2)	0.10
Two-vessel disease	168 (27.9)	153 (25.4)	155 (25.7)	175 (29.0)	0.64
Three-vessel disease	173 (28.7)	187 (31.0)	214 (35.5)	196 (32.5)	0.06
Medication after baseline coronary angiography [n (%)]					
Acetylsalicylic acid	546 (90.5)	548 (90.9)	535 (88.7)	543 (90.0)	0.50
Statins	533 (88.4)	541 (89.7)	535 (88.7)	537 (89.1)	0.86
β-Blockers	473 (78.4)	479 (79.4)	448 (74.3)	479 (79.4)	0.78

ACE inhibitors/ARBs	169 (28.0)	178 (29.5)	210 (34.8)	204 (33.8)	0.007
Calcium channel blockers	137 (22.7)	134 (22.2)	144 (23.9)	133 (22.1)	0.97
Loop diuretics	59 (9.8)	48 (8.0)	69 (11.4)	47 (7.8)	0.64

[1]%TE, percentage of total energy; LVEF, left ventricular ejection fraction; CRP, C-reactive protein; CAD, coronary artery disease; ACE, angiotensinconverting enzyme; ARBs, angiotensin receptor blockers.
[2]$n = 603$ in each quartile.
[3]Calculated by using linear regression for continuous variables and logistic regression for binary variables.
[4]Mean ± SD (all such values).
[5]$n = 599, 603, 603,$ and 597 for quartiles 1–4, respectively; values are medians (25th, 75th percentiles).
[6]Receiving medical treatment of hypertension.
[7]Current smoker or <1 mo since quitting.
[8]Includes acute myocardial infarction and unstable angina pectoris.

TABLE 4.—Hazard Ratios for Endpoints by Quartiles of Total Fish Intake[1]

| | Quartiles of Total Fish Intake (G)[2] | | | | P for trend | Quartiles 2–4 vs quartile 1 |
	1	2	3	4		
Total fish intake (g)	41.1 ± 16.3[3]	81.4 ± 9.3	118.0 ± 12.4	198.0 ± 63.8		
Person-months	34,341	33,832	34,358	34,256		
Coronary events[4]						
No. of events	71	75	76	70		
Age-and sex-adjusted	1.00	1.04 (0.75, 1.45)[5]	1.04 (0.75, 1.44)	0.98 (0.70, 1.36)	0.88	1.02 (0.78, 1.34)
Multivariate[6]	1.00	1.08 (0.78, 1.50)	1.07 (0.77, 1.48)	1.04 (0.74, 1.45)	0.86	1.06 (0.81, 1.40)
All-cause death						
No. of events	35	32	38	32		
Age-and sex-adjusted	1.00	0.82 (0.51, 1.33)	0.94 (0.59, 1.49)	0.87 (0.53, 1.42)	0.72	0.88 (0.59, 1.30)
Multivariate[6]	1.00	0.85 (0.52, 1.37)	0.97 (0.61, 1.55)	0.95 (0.58, 1.55)	0.98	0.92 (0.62, 1.36)
Coronary death						
No. of events	21	17	19	19		
Age-and sex-adjusted	1.00	0.72 (0.38, 1.38)	0.77 (0.41, 1.44)	0.85 (0.45, 1.60)	0.67	0.78 (0.47, 1.30)
Multivariate[6]	1.00	0.79 (0.42, 1.51)	0.83 (0.44, 1.56)	1.03 (0.54, 1.94)	0.94	0.87 (0.52, 1.46)
AMI (fatal and nonfatal)						
No. of events	53	55	55	47		
Age-and sex-adjusted	1.00	0.99 (0.68, 1.45)	0.96 (0.65, 1.41)	0.84 (0.56, 1.25)	0.39	0.93 (0.68, 1.28)
Multivariate[6]	1.00	1.05 (0.72, 1.53)	1.01 (0.69, 1.49)	0.93 (0.63, 1.40)	0.72	1.00 (0.73, 1.38)
Stable angina with angiographic progression of CAD						
No. of events	66	79	63	90		
Age-and sex-adjusted	1.00	1.24 (0.89, 1.72)	0.95 (0.67, 1.35)	1.37 (0.99, 1.89)	0.17	1.18 (0.90, 1.56)
Multivariate[6]	1.00	1.24 (0.89, 1.72)	0.93 (0.66, 1.32)	1.34 (0.97, 1.85)	0.23	1.17 (0.88, 1.54)

[1]AMI, acute myocardial infarction; CAD, coronary artery disease. Hazard ratios and 95% CIs were calculated by using Cox proportional hazards.

[2]n = 604, 602, 603, and 603 in quartiles 1–4, respectively.

[3]Mean ± SD (all such values).

[4]Composite of coronary death, nonfatal AMI, and unstable angina pectoris (excluding procedure-related AMI).

[5]Hazard ratio; 95% CI in parentheses (all such values).

[6]Multivariate model adjusted for age (continuous), sex, left ventricular ejection fraction (continuous), diabetes mellitus (yes or no), hypertension (yes or no), current smoker (still smoking at baseline or <1 mo since quitting), acute coronary syndrome (yes or no), and current use of statins.

patients increase their intake of oily fish or use purified fish oil supplements to reduce risk for cardiovascular events in both the primary and secondary prevention settings.[3]

Manger and coworkers evaluated the capacity of fish consumption to reduce risk for cardiovascular events in 2412 Norwegian patients with established coronary artery disease (CAD) enrolled in Western Norway B Vitamin Intervention Trial. Follow-up was for approximately 5 years. Analysis was by quartile of fish and fish oil supplement consumption. Groups were evenly matched for severity of CAD (1-, 2-, or 3-vessel disease) and other baseline factors (Table 1). Patients were on intensive background therapy with aspirin, statins, and β-blockade. Approximately one-third of patients were also being treated with an angiotensin-converting enzyme (ACE) inhibitor. These investigators found no dose-response relationship between fish/fish oil consumption and risk for coronary or all-cause mortality, fatal or nonfatal MI, or stable angina with angiographic evidence for CAD progression (Table 4). There was a significant increase in risk for events below a threshold value of 0.30 g fish/d (Fig 1 in the original article). Above this threshold, increased fish/fish oil consumption conferred no benefit on cardiovascular outcomes nor on rates of CAD progression. There were no associations between the consumption of fatty, lean, or processed fish, nor between users and nonusers of fish oil or cod liver oil. Of note is the observation that even among the consumers of the largest amount of fish, no harm was observed.

Many of these patients were enrolled from coastal regions of Western Norway where lifelong fish oil consumption is high. There is, consequently, no significant change in exposure to fish during the course of the study. Fish consumption is estimated at time of intake with a nutritional questionnaire. This is a very different scenario from studies that randomized patients to a fish oil supplement versus placebo and then followed cohorts prospectively.[4,5] The capacity to detect a difference between groups may have also been dampened by the intensity of background therapy with drugs known to beneficially impact risk for cardiovascular events, including aspirin, statins, β-blockers, and ACE inhibitors. Given these results and other recent negative studies with fish oils, it would be of interest to conduct a randomized study to determine whether or not these agents reduce risk for cardiovascular events in the setting of current standards of care for patients with CAD with and without hypertriglyceridemia.

P. P. Toth, MD, PhD

References

1. Toth PP, Dayspring TD, Pokrywka GS. Drug therapy for hypertriglyceridemia: fibrates and omega-3 fatty acids. *Curr Atheroscler Rep.* 2009;11:71-79.
2. Marchioli R, Barzi F, Bomba E, et al. Early protection against sudden death by n-3 polyunsaturated fatty acids after myocardial infarction: time-course analysis of the results of the Gruppo Italiano per lo Studio Della Sopravvivenza nell'Infarto Miocardico (GISSI)-Prevenzione. *Circulation.* 2002;105:1897-1903.
3. Kris-Etherton P, Daniels SR, Eckel RH, et al. AHA scientific statement: summary of the Scientific Conference on Dietary Fatty Acids and Cardiovascular Health. Conference summary from the Nutrition Committee of the American Heart Association. *J Nutr.* 2001;131:1322-1326.

4. Yokoyama M, Origasa H, Matsuzaki M, et al. Effects of eicosapentaenoic acid on major coronary events in hypercholesterolaemic patients (JELIS): a randomised open-label, blinded endpoint analysis. *Lancet.* 2007;369:1090-1098.
5. Dietary supplementation with n-3 polyunsaturated fatty acids and vitamin E after myocardial infarction: results of the GISSI-Prevenzione trial. Gruppo Italiano per lo Studio della Sopravvivenza nell'Infarto miocardico. *Lancet.* 1999;354:447-455.

Pharmacologic Therapy

Aldosterone Production in Human Adrenocortical Cells Is Stimulated by High-Density Lipoprotein 2 (HDL2) through Increased Expression of Aldosterone Synthase (CYP11B2)

Xing Y, Cohen A, Rothblat G, et al (Med College of Georgia, Augusta; Children's Hosp of Philadelphia, PA; et al)
Endocrinology 152:751-763, 2011

Adrenal aldosterone production is regulated by physiological agonists at the level of early and late rate-limiting steps. Numerous studies have focused on the role of lipoproteins including high-density lipoprotein (HDL) as cholesterol providers in this process; however, recent research suggests that HDL can also act as a signaling molecule. Herein, we used the human H295R adrenocortical cell model to study the effects of HDL on adrenal aldosterone production and *CYP11B2* expression. HDL, especially HDL2, stimulated aldosterone synthesis by increasing expression of *CYP11B2*. HDL treatment increased *CYP11B2* mRNA in both a concentration-and time-dependent manner, with a maximal19-fold increase (24 h, 250 μg/ml of HDL). Effects of HDL on *CYP11B2* were not additive with natural agonists including angiotensin II or K^+. HDL effects were likely mediated by a calcium signaling cascade, because a calcium channel blocker and a calmodulin kinase inhibitor abolished the *CYP11B2*-stimulating effects. Of the two subfractions of HDL, HDL2 was more potent than HDL3 in stimulating aldosterone and *CYP11B2*. Further studies are needed to identify the active components of HDL, which regulate aldosterone production.

▶ The therapeutic inhibition of cholesteryl ester transfer protein (CETP) is an area of ferocious investigation. CETP inhibition can give rise to very large elevations in high-density lipoprotein cholesterol (HDL-C), a shift in lipoprotein metabolism that is hoped to dramatically reduce the residual risk associated with statin monotherapy. Work with 2 CETP inhibitors (dalcetrapib and anacetrapib) is ongoing, and both are being studied mechanistically as well as in large scale, randomized, prospective clinical trials. CETP inhibition reduces the 1:1 stoichiometric exchange of cholesterol esters out of HDL particles for triglycerides from apoprotein B_{100} containing lipoproteins such as very-low-density lipoprotein receptor and intermediate-density lipoprotein. This reduces the flux of cholesterol through the indirect route for reverse cholesterol transport, a reaction that depends on hepatic cholesterol uptake via the low-density lipoprotein receptor (LDL) receptor and the LDL receptor—related protein. Torcetrapib was a CETP inhibitor in late-stage trials when it was withdrawn from development when it was apparent that it increased mortality despite striking elevations in HDL-C and reductions in LDL-C.[1,2] Torcetrapib therapy was associated with significant elevations in blood pressure as well as a number of electrolyte disturbances. Subsequent investigation showed that torcetrapib therapy induced large increases in aldosterone production, likely yielding the aforementioned off-target toxicities.[3] It has been assumed that torcetrapib stimulated this surge of aldosterone directly.

HDL particles deliver cholesterol to steroidogenic tissues such as the adrenals, testes, ovaries, and placenta via scavenger receptor, class B type I (SR-BI). SR-BI modulates the selective delipidation of the HDL particle and then releases it back into the circulation to participate in lipid scavenging and exchange.[4] Aldosterone is formed from deoxycorticosterone by the mitochondrial enzyme aldosterone synthase (CYP11B2). Aldosterone is synthesized within the zona glomerulosa and its production is regulated by angiotensin II. By virtue of their mechanism of action, the CETP inhibitors have a propensity to increase serum levels of large, cholesteryl ester–rich HDL subfraction 2 (HDL_2) particles. Xing and coworkers show that HDL_2 particles activate a calcium signaling cascade in a human adrenocortical cell model, which increases nuclear expression and transcription of aldosterone synthase and aldosterone (Fig in the original article).

This elegant study suggests that HDL_2 may have been the offending agent responsible for increasing adrenal aldosterone production. This is yet to be confirmed in an in vivo model. If this is the case in vivo, then it is possible that high levels of HDL_2 could be involved in blood pressure regulation and electrolyte balance. This would certainly complicate current views of HDL. According to this scenario, HDL_2 could conceivably induce hypertension or electrolyte imbalances. To date, HDL_2 has been shown to be associated with net benefit for reducing cardiovascular events.[5] Neither dalcetrapib nor anacetrapib are associated with increases in aldosterone production or hypertension.[6] It would be of interest to compare the capacity of HDL species obtained from patients treated with each of these CETP inhibitors and determine whether or not they induce different levels of aldosterone synthase activity.

P. P. Toth, MD, PhD

References

1. Tall AR, Yvan-Charvet L, Wang N. The failure of torcetrapib: was it the molecule or the mechanism? *Arterioscler Thromb Vasc Biol.* 2007;27:257-260.
2. Toth PP. Torcetrapib and atherosclerosis: what happened and where do we go from here? *Future Lipidol.* 2007;2:277-284.
3. Barter PJ, Caulfield M, Eriksson M, et al. Effects of torcetrapib in patients at high risk for coronary events. *N Engl J Med.* 2007;357:2109-2122.
4. Rigotti A, Miettinen HE, Krieger M. The role of the high-density lipoprotein receptor SR-BI in the lipid metabolism of endocrine and other tissues. *Endocr Rev.* 2003;24:357-387.
5. Brunzell JD, Hokanson JE. Low-density and high-density lipoprotein subspecies and risk for premature coronary artery disease. *Am J Med.* 1999;107:16S-18S.
6. Toth PP. Pharmacomodulation of high-density lipoprotein metabolism as a therapeutic intervention for atherosclerotic disease. *Curr Cardiol Rep.* 2010;12: 481-487.

Lipid-lowering intensification and low-density lipoprotein cholesterol achievement from hospital admission to 1-year follow-up after an acute coronary syndrome event: Results from the Medications Applied aNd SusTAINed Over Time (MAINTAIN) registry

Melloni C, Shah BR, Ou F-S, et al (Duke Univ Med Ctr, Durham, NC; et al)
Am Heart J 160:1121-1129.e1, 2010

Background.—Current American College of Cardiology/American Heart Association guidelines recommend initiation or intensification of statin therapy to achieve low-density lipoprotein cholesterol (LDL-C) goals after an acute coronary syndrome (ACS), yet little is known about the actual practice of intensifying lipid-lowering (LL) therapy and LDL-C achievement from hospital admission to 1-year follow-up.

Methods.—The MAINTAIN registry enrolled ACS patients from January 2006 through September 2007, collecting data on statin formulation, dose, and lipid profiles at both baseline and 12 months. Statin intensity (estimated LDL-C lowering) was categorized by formulation and dose as either moderate (b40%) or intensive (≥40%). In-hospital LL intensification is described and LDL goal attainment is reported for patients with complete baseline and 12-month lipid panels.

Results.—Of the 788 patients without contraindications to LL, 40% were on LL therapy before admission, and 89% at discharge. Among patients on LL therapy with LDL-C N100 mg/dL at admission, only 37% (n = 38) had their LL therapy intensified. Among 382 patients with 12 months of data, 89% (n = 341) were discharged on a statin. Of these, 89% were still on a statin at 12-month follow-up. A LDL-C goal of ≤100 mg/dL was achieved in 71% of patients, but the optional LDL-C goal ≤70 mg/dL was achieved in only 31%.

Conclusions.—Most high-risk ACS patients are prescribed statin therapy at hospital discharge and remain on therapy at 12-month follow-up. Despite this, the LDL-C goal of ≤70 mg/dL is achieved in a small minority. There is substantial opportunity to intensify LL therapy after ACS to achieve guideline LDL-C goals and prevent future morbidity and mortality (Table 4).

▶ In 2004, the National Cholesterol Education Panel (NCEP) issued a white paper supplement that defined the new category of very high cardiovascular risk. These patients include those with acute coronary syndromes (ACS; unstable angina, non-ST segment elevation myocardial infarction [NSTEMI], and ST segment elevation myocardial infarction). For these patients, NCEP recommended a low-density lipoprotein cholesterol (LDL-C) target of < 100 mg/dL with a therapeutic option of lowering it to < 70 mg/dL.[1] The lower therapeutic option was justified largely based on the results of the Pravastatin or Atorvastatin Evaluation and Infection Therapy Thrombolysis in Myocardial Infarction 22 trial.[2,3] A subsequent meta-analysis confirmed that more intensive LDL-C lowering with high-dose statin therapy is associated with greater relative risk reductions for cardiovascular events.[4] Concerns about toxicity with high-dose statin therapy

TABLE 4.—Patient Characteristics and Secondary Prevention by 12-Month LDL-C Goal Attainment*

	Overall (n = 382)	12-m LDL-C ≤70 mg/dL (n = 117)	12-m LDL-C >70 mg/dL (n = 265)	P
Age (y)[†]	60 (54, 69)	60 (53, 69)	61 (54, 69)	.728
Female sex	28.3	21.4	32.3	.073
Race				.630
White	82.7	82.9	82.6	
African American	11.5	10.3	12.1	
Other	5.8	6.8	5.3	
Insurance status				.087
HMO/private	55.8	64.1	52.1	
Medicare	28.8	24.8	30.6	
Self/none	6.8	4.3	7.9	
Other	7.3	6.8	7.5	
Medical history				
Hypertension	61.0	54.7	63.8	.094
Diabetes mellitus	25.9	28.2	24.9	.481
Peripheral artery disease	7.6	4.3	9.1	.104
Prior myocardial infarction	20.9	12.8	24.5	.009
Any prior revascularization	27.8	18.8	31.7	.009
Prior stroke	5.2	4.3	5.7	.576
Prior congestive heart failure	6.3	2.6	7.9	.046
Discharge medication counseling				
Medication list and instructions	90.7	96.3	88.1	.483
Medication explanation	89.5	96.3	86.4	.318
Postdischarge prevention				
Postdischarge cardiac rehabilitation program	26.7	31.6	24.5	.167
Diet/exercise program	41.1	46.2	38.9	.212
Patient—provider communication				
Appointment with primary care physician after discharge	84.8	88.9	83.0	.184
Appointment with cardiologist	80.1	84.6	78.1	.180
Health care provider talks in a language I understand	92.3	94.1	91.5	.706
Medication adherence[‡]				
Aspirin	69.3	75.5	66.5	.140
Clopidogrel	66.3	76.5	61.2	.046
β-Blocker	69.0	77.7	65.0	.015
ACEI/ARB	65.5	69.7	63.5	.441
Any statin	66.7	76.0	62.2	.042
Non-statin medication	43.4	51.5	39.7	.085
Any LL medication	67.3	75.9	63.1	.056

*All data reported as percentages unless otherwise specified.
[†]Presented as median (25th, 75th percentiles).
[‡]Defined as never or rarely missing a dose of the drug.

persist among physicians and patients, despite a large number of trials that clearly delineate a large benefit to risk ratio, particularly in secondary prevention. Despite recent efforts to emphasize risk-stratified targets of LDL-C and non—high-density lipoprotein cholesterol, to increase statin titration rates, and to encourage the use of adjuvant therapy to increase goal attainment, success has been mixed.[5] Melloni and coworkers evaluated goal attainment rates among patients with a history of ACS enrolled in the Medications Applied and Sustained Over Time (MAINTAIN) registry. Patients with ACS are among the highest risk patients because they have manifested coronary disease with unstable features. Only 89% of these patients were prescribed a statin at time of discharge. Patients already on lipid-lowering therapy with LDL-C >100 mg/dL had their therapy intensified only 37% of the time. The LDL-C goals of <100 mg/dL and <70 mg/dL were attained 71% and 31% of the time, respectively. When comparing the groups achieving LDL-C above or below 70 mg/dL, there were no differences in discharge medication counseling, explanation of medications, enrollment in cardiac rehabilitation, diet and exercise programs, or postdischarge appointments with the patients' primary care physician or cardiologist (Table 4). Of interest is the finding that among patients with LDL-C >70 mg/dL, adherence with clopidogrel, β-blockade, and statin therapy was lower compared with patients who achieved an LDL level <70 mg/dL.

Adopting a therapeutic option can certainly generate confusion because it frames a therapeutic target as somewhat equivocal and wobbly. In the next iteration of NCEP, it would be helpful if the <70-mg/dL LDL-C target for very-high-risk patients is converted to a hard target, not an optional one. This will lend clarity and specificity. The MAINTAIN registry data also show that for a sizeable percentage of patients who are discharged subsequent to ACS, lipid-lowering therapy is not intensified in patients whose LDL-C level exceeds 100 mg/dL despite clear data showing that when it comes to LDL-C, lower is better. There is also significant nonadherence in the group whose LDL-C >70 mg/dL as demonstrated by reduced compliance with other life-saving drugs, including thienopyridines and β-blockers. The precise causes for nonadherence (medication cost, side effects, not understanding importance of medication, among others) need to be more precisely defined. Very-high-risk patients, especially those sustaining an ACS, warrant much more careful attention to appropriately intensify LDL-C—lowering therapy and improve long-term adherence with all components of the pharmacologic regimen.

P. P. Toth, MD, PhD

References

1. Grundy SM, Cleeman JI, Merz CN, et al. Implications of recent clinical trials for the National Cholesterol Education Program Adult Treatment Panel III guidelines. *Circulation.* 2004;110:227-239.
2. Cannon CP, Braunwald E, McCabe CH, et al. Intensive versus moderate lipid lowering with statins after acute coronary syndromes. *N Engl J Med.* 2004;350: 1495-1504.
3. Cannon CP, McCabe CH, Belder R, Breen J, Braunwald E. Design of the pravastatin or atorvastatin evaluation and infection therapy (PROVE IT)-TIMI 22 trial. *Am J Cardiol.* 2002;89:860-861.
4. Cannon CP, Steinberg BA, Murphy SA, Mega JL, Braunwald E. Meta-analysis of cardiovascular outcomes trials comparing intensive versus moderate statin therapy. *J Am Coll Cardiol.* 2006;48:438-445.
5. Davidson MH, Maki KC, Pearson TA, et al. Results of the national cholesterol education (NCEP) program evaluation project utilizing novel E-technology (NEPTUNE) II survey and implications for treatment under the recent NCEP writing group recommendations. *Am J Cardiol.* 2005;96:556-563.

Dose-response effects of omega-3 fatty acids on triglycerides, inflammation, and endothelial function in healthy persons with moderate hypertriglyceridemia
Skulas-Ray AC, Kris-Etherton PM, Harris WS, et al (Pennsylvania State Univ, Univ Park; Univ of South Dakota, Vermillion; et al)
Am J Clin Nutr 93:243-252, 2011

Background.—Eicosapentaenoic acid (EPA) and docosahexaenoic acid (DHA) have been shown to reduce cardiovascular mortality at a dose of ≈ 1 g/d. Studies using higher doses have shown evidence of reduced inflammation and improved endothelial function. Few studies have compared these doses.

Objective.—The objective of this study was to compare the effects of a nutritional dose of EPA+DHA (0.85 g/d) with those of a pharmaceutical dose (3.4 g/d) on serum triglycerides, inflammatory markers, and endothelial function in healthy subjects with moderately elevated triglycerides.

Design.—This was a placebo-controlled, double-blind, randomized, 3-period crossover trial (8 wk of treatment, 6 wk of washout) that compared the effects of 0.85 and 3.4 g EPA+DHA/d in 23 men and 3 postmenopausal women with moderate hypertriglyceridemia (150–500 mg/dL).

Results.—The higher dose of EPA+DHA lowered triglycerides by 27% compared with placebo (mean ± SEM: 173 ± 17.5 compared with 237 ± 17.5 mg/dL; $P = 0.002$), whereas no effect of the lower dose was observed on lipids. No effects on cholesterol (total, LDL, and HDL), endothelial function [as assessed by flow-mediated dilation, peripheral arterial tonometry/EndoPAT (Itamar Medical Ltd, Caesarea, Israel), or Doppler measures of hyperemia], inflammatory markers (interleukin-1β, interleukin-6, tumor necrosis factor-α, and high-sensitivity C-reactive protein), or the expression of inflammatory cytokine genes in isolated lymphocytes were observed.

Conclusion.—The higher dose (3.4 g/d) of EPA+DHA significantly lowered triglycerides, but neither dose improved endothelial function or inflammatory status over 8 wk in healthy adults with moderate hypertriglyceridemia. The trial was registered at clinicaltrials.gov as NCT00504309 (Tables 3 and 4).

▶ The fish oils eicosapentaenoic acid (EPA) and docosahexaenoic acid (DHA) have been shown to reduce risk for acute cardiovascular events in secondary prevention trials and to provide incremental cardiovascular benefit when given in addition to a statin.[1,2] In the Gruppo Italiano per lo Studio della Sopravvivenza nell'Infarto Miocardico 3 trial, fish oils had demonstrable capacity to significantly reduce risk for reinfarction and sudden cardiovascular death.[3] Fish oils have been ascribed roles in reducing inflammation, thrombosis, and arrhythmogenesis. The ω-3 fish oils are widely used to treat severe hypertriglyceridemia (triglycerides > 500 mg/dL) and are catabolized to form a variety of prostaglandins and leukotrienes. The ω-3 fish oils appear to reduce serum triglyceride levels by promoting intrahepatic mitochondrial β-oxidation, inhibiting triglyceride biosynthesis, and activating lipoprotein lipase.

TABLE 3.—Effects of Treatment on Plasma and Serum Measures $(n = 26)$[1]

	0 g/d	EPA+DHA 0.85 g/d	3.4 g/d	P value for Treatment Effect[2]
Lipids and lipoproteins				
TG (mg/dL)	237.3 ± 17.5^a	215.3 ± 17.5^a	173.7 ± 17.5^b	0.002
TC (mg/dL)	209.0 ± 7.9	212.1 ± 7.9	207.9 ± 7.9	0.60
LDL-C (mg/dL)	123.3 ± 7.6	127.6 ± 7.6	130.3 ± 7.6	0.21
HDL-C (mg/dL)	42.6 ± 1.9	42.7 ± 1.9	43.2 ± 1.9	0.76
non-HDL-C (mg/dL)	166.4 ± 7.1	169.4 ± 7.1	164.7 ± 7.1	0.54
non-HDL-C:HDL-C	4.03 ± 0.2	4.04 ± 0.2	3.95 ± 0.2	0.74
LDL-C:HDL-C	2.94 ± 0.2	3.00 ± 0.2	3.11 ± 0.2	0.15
TC:HDL-C	5.03 ± 0.2	5.04 ± 0.2	4.95 ± 0.2	0.74
Glucose metabolism				
Glucose (mg/dL)	96.1 ± 2.0	98.0 ± 1.9	99.2 ± 1.9	0.14
Insulin (μIU/mL)	14.6 ± 1.4	15.5 ± 1.4	15.0 ± 1.4	0.31
HOMA-IR	3.55 ± 0.4	3.75 ± 0.4	3.64 ± 0.4	0.46
QUICKI	0.14 ± 0.002	0.14 ± 0.002	0.14 ± 0.002	0.36
Markers of inflammation (plasma protein concentrations)				
hs-CRP (mg/L)	1.45 ± 0.2	1.32 ± 0.2	1.29 ± 0.2	0.72
IL-1β (pg/mL)	0.15 ± 0.02	0.15 ± 0.02	0.14 ± 0.02	0.89
IL-6 (pg/mL)	0.87 ± 0.15	0.85 ± 0.15	0.87 ± 0.15	0.89
TNF-α (pg/mL)	1.16 ± 0.07	1.07 ± 0.07	1.10 ± 0.07	0.20
Markers of inflammation (normalized gene expression in isolated PBMCs)				
IL-1β expression	1.10 ± 0.09	1.06 ± 0.09	1.08 ± 0.09	0.92
IL-6 expression	0.73 ± 0.16	0.73 ± 0.16	0.69 ± 0.16	0.70
TNF-α expression	1.00 ± 0.07	0.94 ± 0.07	0.97 ± 0.07	0.82
Liver enzymes (IU/L)				
AST	20.3 ± 1.1	21.1 ± 1.1	21.9 ± 1.1	0.18
ALT	27.4 ± 3.1	30.4 ± 3.1	32.4 ± 3.1	0.11
Erythrocyte omega-3 fatty acid content (% by weight)				
EPA	0.57 ± 0.09^a	1.15 ± 0.09^b	2.30 ± 0.09^c	< 0.0001
DPA	2.74 ± 0.08^a	3.04 ± 0.08^b	3.40 ± 0.08^c	< 0.0001
DHA	4.39 ± 0.15^a	5.34 ± 0.15^b	6.49 ± 0.15^c	< 0.0001
Omega-3 index	4.96 ± 0.21^a	6.49 ± 0.21^b	8.79 ± 0.21^c	< 0.0001

[1]All values are as means ± SEMs. LDL-C, LDL cholesterol; HDL-C, HDL cholesterol; TG, triglycerides; TC, total cholesterol; hs-CRP, high-sensitivity C-reactive protein; IL, interleukin; TNF, tumor necrosis factor; AST, aspartate aminotransferase; ALT, alanine aminotransferase; HOMA-IR, homeostatic model of insulin resistance; QUICKI, quantitative insulin-sensitivity check index; EPA, eicosapentaenoic acid; DPA, docosapentaenoic acid (n−3); DHA, docosahexaenoic acid; PBMCs, peripheral blood mononuclear cells. Values with different superscript letters are significantly different, $P < 0.05$ (Tukeyadjusted values from post hoc tests).
[2]P values are for the main effect of treatment based on the MIXED procedure (version 9.2; SAS Institute Inc, Cary, NC). Lipids and lipoproteins are the average of 2 samples taken on 2 separate days.

The investigation by Skulas-Ray and coworkers was designed to evaluate the impact of high (3.4 g/d) and low (0.85 g/d) dose ω-3 fatty acids on measures of serum lipids and lipoproteins, markers of inflammation, and arterial vasoreactivity compared with placebo. Sample size was relatively small at 26 patients who were mildly hypertriglyceridemic with baseline triglycerides of 223 mg/dL. High-dose fish oils reduced serum triglycerides by 27%, but other components of the lipid profile were unchanged (Table 3). The low dose of fish oil had no impact of any component of the lipid profile. Serum glucose and insulin levels were not affected relative to placebo at either dose. Levels of inflammatory mediators (C-reactive protein, interleukins 1 and 6, and tumor necrosis factor α) were unchanged in plasma, and no changes were noted in rates of monocyte gene expression at either dose of fish oil, despite the fact that high

TABLE 4.—Effects of Treatment on Measures of Endothelial Function $(N = 26)$[1]

	EPA+DHA			P value[2] For Treatment Effect	For Period Effect
	0 g/d	0.85 g/d	3.4 g/d		
Reactive hyperemia outcomes from FMD					
FMD (% change in artery diameter)	5.00 ± 0.48	4.03 ± 0.48	4.14 ± 0.48	0.11	0.73
ΔArtery diameter (mm, peak-base)	0.24 ± 0.02	0.19 ± 0.02	0.19 ± 0.02	0.07	0.80
Peak flow:resting flow[3]	6.28 ± 0.44	6.59 ± 0.45	6.84 ± 0.44	0.55	0.001
RHI from EndoPAT					
RHI	1.84 ± 0.10	1.82 ± 0.10	1.86 ± 0.10	0.86	0.02
Framingham RHI	0.28 ± 0.06	0.27 ± 0.07	0.33 ± 0.07	0.66	0.17
Pulse wave properties and HR from EndoPAT					
AI	−9.33 ± 1.6	−9.52 ± 1.6	−9.25 ± 1.6	0.97	0.56
AI standardized for HR of 75 bpm	−16.9 ± 1.6	−17.5 ± 1.5	−18.1 ± 1.5	0.53	0.91
Heart rate (beats/min)[4]	62.9 ± 1.6	62.7 ± 1.6	61.0 ± 1.6	0.09	0.03
Resting artery diameter and blood flow values (Doppler ultrasound)					
Artery diameter (mm)[5]	4.83 ± 0.13	4.92 ± 0.13	4.87 ± 0.13	0.09	0.005
Velocity time integral (m)[5]	0.17 ± 0.01	0.17 ± 0.01	0.18 ± 0.01	0.88	0.003
Maximum velocity (m/s)	0.98 ± 0.06	0.95 ± 0.06	1.00 ± 0.06	0.49	0.10
Average flow velocity (m/s)[5]	0.19 ± 0.02	0.19 ± 0.02	0.20 ± 0.02	0.84	0.01
Flow (mL/min)[5]	201 ± 17.5	207 ± 17.7	206 ± 17.5	0.94	0.0007
Postocclusion artery diameter and blood flow values (Doppler ultrasound)					
Artery diameter (mm)[5]	5.07 ± 0.13	5.10 ± 0.13	5.06 ± 0.13	0.55	0.01
Velocity time integral (m)	0.97 ± 0.05	0.99 ± 0.05	1.02 ± 0.05	0.45	0.43
Maximum velocity (m/s)	1.76 ± 0.07	1.76 ± 0.07	1.78 ± 0.07	0.83	0.22
Average flow velocity (m/s)	1.02 ± 0.04	1.01 ± 0.04	1.02 ± 0.04	0.83	0.57
Flow (mL/min)	1193 ± 77	1219 ± 77	1238 ± 77	0.68	0.47

[1] Values are expressed as means ± SEMs. EndoPAT, Itamar Medical Ltd, Caesarea, Israel. RHI, Reactive Hyperemia Index; AI, Augmentation Index; HR, heart rate; FMD, flow-mediated dilation; EPA, eicosapentaenoic acid; DHA, docosahexaenoic acid.

[2] P values are for the main effect of treatment and period based on the MIXED procedure with both fixed effects in the model when period effects were significant (version 9.2; SAS Institute Inc, Cary, NC). When the period was nonsignificant, it was removed from the model to determine treatment effects. None of the Tukey-adjusted P values for pairwise comparisons for treatment effects were significant $(P > .05)$.

[3] First-visit values were significantly greater than visit 2 and visit 3 values $(P < 0.005,$ Tukey-adjusted).

[4] First-visit values were significantly lower than visit 3 values $(P = 0.04,$ Tukey-adjusted).

[5] First-visit values were significantly lower than visit 2 and visit 3 values $(P < 0.05,$ Tukey-adjusted).

levels of ω-3 fish oils were taken up by red cell membranes. No improvement in endothelial function or in vasoreactivity were noted (Table 4).

The reduction in serum triglycerides is expected at the high dose of fish oils given the fact that these agents are indicated in the management of sever hypertriglyceridemia. The findings do not support previous conclusions that the fish oils reduce systemic inflammatory tone and improve arterial vasoreactivity. The sample size was small and the severity of hypertriglyceridemia was mild. It is possible that to detect the types of alterations in inflammation and endothelial function these investigators were trying to assess, a larger sample size of patients with much more substantial elevations in serum triglycerides might constitute a more appropriate study population. Moreover, 8 weeks of treatment may not be enough to adequately correct endothelial dysfunction and heightened systemic inflammatory tone. This study does not negate the considerable benefit the ω-3 fish oils confer on patients with dyslipidemia in both the primary and secondary prevention settings.

P. P. Toth, MD, PhD

References

1. Burr ML, Fehily AM, Gilbert JF, et al. Effects of changes in fat, fish, and fibre intakes on death and myocardial reinfarction: diet and reinfarction trial (DART). *Lancet.* 1989;2:757-761.
2. Yokoyama M, Origasa H, Matsuzaki M, et al. Effects of eicosapentaenoic acid on major coronary events in hypercholesterolaemic patients (JELIS): A randomised open-label, blinded endpoint analysis. *Lancet.* 2007;369:1090-1098.
3. Marchioli R, Barzi F, Bomba E, et al. Early protection against sudden death by n-3 polyunsaturated fatty acids after myocardial infarction: Time-course analysis of the results of the gruppo italiano per lo studio della sopravvivenza nell'infarto miocardico (gissi)-prevenzione. *Circulation.* 2002;105:1897-1903.

GPR120 Is an Omega-3 Fatty Acid Receptor Mediating Potent Anti-inflammatory and Insulin-Sensitizing Effects

Oh DY, Talukdar S, Bae EJ, et al (Univ of California, San Diego, La Jolla; et al)
Cell 142:687-698, 2010

Omega-3 fatty acids (ω-3 FAs), DHA and EPA, exert anti-inflammatory effects, but the mechanisms are poorly understood. Here, we show that the G protein-coupled receptor 120 (GPR120) functions as an ω-3 FA receptor/sensor. Stimulation of GPR120 with ω-3 FAs or a chemical agonist causes broad anti-inflammatory effects in monocytic RAW 264.7 cells and in primary intraperitoneal macrophages. All of these effects are abrogated by GPR120 knockdown. Since chronic macrophage-mediated tissue inflammation is a key mechanism for insulin resistance in obesity, we fed obese WT and GPR120 knockout mice a high-fat diet with or without ω-3 FA supplementation. The ω-3 FA treatment inhibited inflammation and enhanced systemic insulin sensitivity in WT mice, but was without effect in GPR120 knockout mice. In conclusion, GPR120 is a functional ω-3 FA receptor/sensor and mediates potent insulin sensitizing and antidiabetic effects in vivo by repressing macrophage-induced tissue inflammation (Figs 2 and 5).

▶ Fatty acid (FA) metabolism is complex. Saturated FAs can promote inflammation,[1] and some evidence suggests that the ω-3 FAs can suppress inflammation.[2] In this fascinating study by Oh and workers, the interaction of docosahexaenoic acid (DHA) and eicosapentaenoic acid (EPA) is characterized in both macrophages and adipocytes in a murine model. These cell types were chosen because the infiltration of visceral adipose tissue with macrophages induces inflammation, with a significant rise in the local expression of interleukins and cytokines. As this occurs, the adipose tissue becomes progressively more resistant to the effects of insulin. These investigators found that EPA and DHA bind to macrophages and adipocytes via a G protein—coupled receptor, GPR120, which functions as a cell surface FA sensor. When GPR120 binds to one of its FA agonists, downstream intracellular signaling is activated via β-arrestin2.

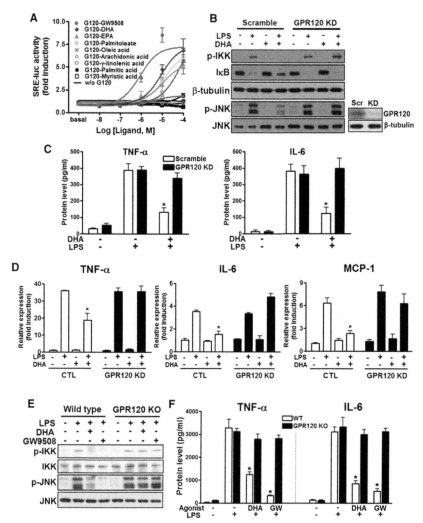

FIGURE 2.—Omega-3 FA Stimulates GPR120 and Mediates Anti-inflammatory Effects. (A–D) GPR120-mediated SRE-luc activity after treatment with various FAs. Results are fold activities over basal. Each data point represents mean ± SEM of three independent experiments performed in triplicate. Black lines indicate SREluc activities without GPR120 transfection or with non-stimulating FAs. DHA inhibits LPS-induced inflammatory signaling (B), cytokine secretion (C), and inflammatory gene mRNA expression level (D) in RAW 264.7 cells, but not in GPR120 knockdown cells. (E and F) GPR120 stimulation inhibits LPS-induced inflammatory response in WT primary macrophage. Data are expressed as the mean ± SEM of three independent experiments. *$p < 0.05$ versus LPS treatment in scrambled siRNA transfected cells or WT IPMacs. See also Figure S2. (Reprinted from Oh DY, Talukdar S, Bae EJ, et al. GPR120 is an omega-3 fatty acid receptor mediating potent anti-inflammatory and insulin-sensitizing effects. *Cell.* 2010;142:687-698, Copyright 2010, with permission from Cell Press.)

The ω-3 FAs suppress the production of tumor necrosis factor α, interleukins 1 and 6, and monocyte chemoattractant protein-1 by macrophages (Fig 2). The binding of ω-3 FAs to GPR120 activates glucose transport protein-4 expression

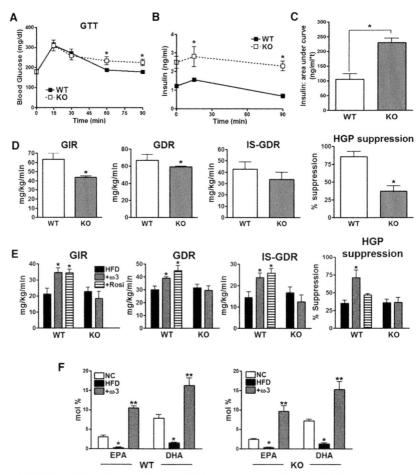

FIGURE 5.—In Vivo Metabolic Studies in GPR120 KO Mice. (A) GTT in NC-fed WT and GPR120 KO mice. n = 7 per group. (B and C) Insulin concentration was measured at the indicated time points and (C) area-under-curve analysis of the insulin data shows a significant difference between WT and GPR120 KO mice on NC. (D) Hyperinsulinemic/euglycemic clamp studies in chow-fed WT and GPR120 KO mice. (E) Clamp studies in HFD, ω-3 FA supplemented (+ω3), and Rosiglitazone treated HFD mice (+Rosi). n = 8 per group, $^*p < 0.05$ compared to HFD-fed WT group. (F) Mean ± SEM plasma concentration (mole (%)) of DHA and EPA for each diet in WT and GPR120 KO mice. n = 7 per each group. $^*p < 0.05$, compared to NC, and $^{**}p < 0.05$ compared to HFD. Data are represented as mean ± SEM. See also Figure S4, Figure S5, Figure S6, and Table S2. (Reprinted from Oh DY, Talukdar S, Bae EJ, et al. GPR120 is an omega-3 fatty acid receptor mediating potent anti-inflammatory and insulin-sensitizing effects. *Cell.* 2010;142:687-698, Copyright 2010, with permission from Cell Press.)

and cell surface translocation and is associated with increased glucose uptake by adipocytes. In a GPR120 knockout mouse model, mice became hyperinsulinemic and hyperglycemic and experienced increased hepatic glucose production. In obese, insulin-resistant wild-type mice given ω-3 FAs, the animals experienced improved insulin sensitivity, glucose disposal, and less hepatic glucose production and had less hepatic steatosis (Fig 5). These effects were not observed when obese, insulin-resistant GPR120 knockout mice were so treated. Treatment with either rosiglitazone or ω-3 FAs gave equal improvement in insulin and glycemic indices. The ω-3 FAs also reduced both adipose tissue macrophage density and inflammatory mediator release by adipose tissue in wild-type mice but not the GPR120 knockout mice.

It would be fascinating to determine whether the ω-3 fish oils help to regulate glucose internalization capacity by adipocytes and skeletal myocytes and improve systemic insulin sensitization in humans. The observation that treatment with a thiazolidinedione and the ω-3 FAs gave equal levels of improvement in hyperinsulinemia and serum glucose levels is surprising. It would also be valuable to ascertain if the ω-3 FAs reduce visceral adipose tissue macrophage infiltration and inflammation. Given the fact that the ω-3 FAs exert no known toxicity, it would be important to try to reproduce these results in a randomized prospective trial of humans with early insulin resistance.

P. P. Toth, MD, PhD

References

1. Calder PC. Polyunsaturated fatty acids and inflammation. *Biochem Soc Trans.* 2005;33:423-427.
2. Lee JY, Plakidas A, Lee WH, et al. Differential modulation of Toll-like receptors by fatty acids: preferential inhibition by n-3 polyunsaturated fatty acids. *J Lipid Res.* 2003;44:479-486.

Effects of Maximal Atorvastatin and Rosuvastatin Treatment on Markers of Glucose Homeostasis and Inflammation
Thongtang N, Ai M, Otokozawa S, et al (Jean Mayer United States Dept of Agriculture Human Nutrition Res Ctr on Aging at Tufts Univ, Boston, MA; et al)
Am J Cardiol 107:387-392, 2011

Studies have reported an increased risk of developing diabetes in subjects receiving statins versus placebo. Our purpose was to compare the effects of maximum doses of rosuvastatin and atorvastatin on the plasma levels of the insulin, glycated albumin, adiponectin, and C-reactive protein compared to baseline in hyperlipidemic patients. We studied 252 hyperlipidemic men and women who had been randomized to receive atorvastatin 80 mg/day or rosuvastatin 40 mg/day during a 6-week period. Atorvastatin and rosuvastatin were both highly effective in lowering the low-density lipoprotein cholesterol and triglyceride levels, with rosuvastatin more effective than atorvastatin in increasing high-density lipoprotein cholesterol. Atorvastatin and rosuvastatin at the maximum dosage both significantly ($p < 0.05$) increased the median insulin levels by 5.2% and 8.7%, respectively, from baseline. However, only atorvastatin increased the glycated albumin levels from baseline (+0.8% for atorvastatin vs −0.7% for rosuvastatin, $p = 0.002$). Both atorvastatin and rosuvastatin caused significant ($p < 0.001$) and similar median reductions

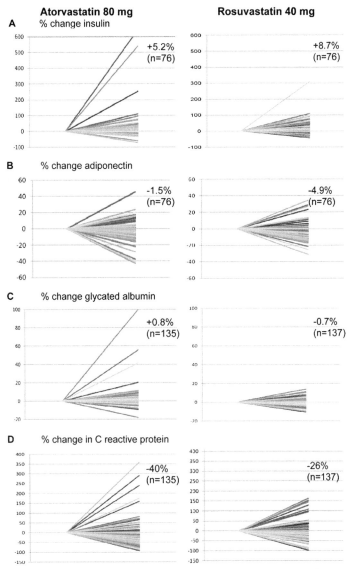

FIGURE 1.—Individual responses and median percentage of change from baseline after treatment of *(A)* insulin, *(B)* ADN, *(C)* GA, and *(D)* CRP. (Reprinted from Thongtang N, Ai M, Otokozawa S, et al. Effects of Maximal Atorvastatin and Rosuvastatin Treatment on Markers of Glucose Homeostasis and Inflammation. *Am J Cardiol.* 2011;107:387-392, Copyright 2011, with permission from Elsevier.)

in the C-reactive protein level of −40% and −26% compared to the baseline values. However, no statistically significant difference was found between the 2 groups in the adiponectin changes from baseline (−1.5% vs −4.9%, p = 0.15). In conclusion, our data have indicated that the maximum dosage

TABLE 1.—Glucose Homeostasis and Inflammatory Markers after Treatment of Subjects with Glycated Albumin <16.5%

Variable	Atorvastatin 80 mg/day		Rosuvastatin 40 mg/day	
	6-wk Level	P Value*	6-wk Level	P Value*
Insulin (μIU/ml)[†]	7.5 (2.6–35.8)	0.007	8.6 (2.5–25.5)	0.026
Adiponectin (μg/ml)[†]	11.0 (4.0–35.9)	0.262	9.8 (2.4–60.2)	0.005
Glycated albumin (%)[‡]	13.4 (10.6–18.7)	0.53	13.1 (10.1–16.4)	0.0017
C-reactive protein (mg/L)[‡]	1.1 (0.1–33.5)	<0.001	1.6 (0.1–25.7)	<0.001

Data are presented as median (interquartile range).
*p Values were based on an analysis comparing the changes from baseline.
[†]Number of subjects analyzed was 72 for both atorvastatin and rosuvastatin.
[‡]Number of subjects analyzed was 129 for atorvastatin and 130 for rosuvastatin groups.

of atorvastatin or rosuvastatin therapy significantly lower C-reactive protein levels but also moderately increase insulin levels (Fig 1, Table 1).

▶ The issue of how statins affect glycemic control has had a complex series of twists and turns. Initially, based on the West of Scotland Coronary Prevention Study,[1] there was some inclination to believe that statins perhaps reduced risk for new-onset type 2 diabetes mellitus (DM). Subsequently, a subgroup analysis from the Pravastatin or Atorvastatin Evaluation and Infection Therapy—Thrombolysis in Myocardial Infarction 22 trial suggested that high-dose atorvastatin is associated with a worsening of glycemic control. The issue was then subjected to greater scrutiny with publication of the Justification for the Use of Statins in Prevention: an Interventional Trial Evaluating Rosuvastatin trial, which demonstrated an increased risk of 25% relative to placebo for developing new-onset DM among subjects with high-sensitivity C-reactive protein (CRP) level $\geq$2 mg/L and low-density lipoprotein cholesterol level $\leq$130 mg/dL.[2] Subsequently, a meta-analysis confirmed that statins increase risk for DM and that it is a class effect.[3] Little is known about the relative risk for inducing DM as a function of statin dose. It has been suggested that statins may impair glycemic control to a small degree via their capacity to inhibit isoprenoid metabolism. The isoprenoids are by-products of 3-hydroxy-3-methylglutaryl coenzyme A and include farnesyl pyrophosphate, geranylgeranyl pyrophosphate, and coenzyme Q, a component of the mitochondrial electron transfer chain. The isoprenoids are involved in the production and translocation of glucose transport protein 4 (Glut4), a protein that regulates glucose uptake in multiple cell types. It is believed that reduced availability of the isoprenoids may decrease the cell surface expression of Glut4.

Thongtang and coworkers evaluated a variety of glycemic indices in patients randomized to the highest doses of atorvastatin (80 mg daily) and rosuvastatin (40 mg daily) in the Statin Therapies for Elevated Lipid Levels Compared Across Doses to Rosuvastatin trial. Both statins at these doses increased glycated albumin significantly over the 6-week observation period (Table 1). Both drugs also increased serum insulin level and decreased adiponectin and CRP levels, although there was considerable variability in the response to therapy with these analytes (Fig 1).

The changes noted occurred in just 6 weeks. The rise in insulin level, the reduction in adiponectin level, and the increase in glycated albumin level are all consistent with statin therapy somehow compromising glucose metabolism. However, the response by individual patients to these drugs varies widely. It will be important to conduct more studies directed at the precise molecular mechanisms regulating these derangements. In addition, it will be important to perform a prospective randomized study to more fully delineate what happens to glucose metabolism and the endocrine axis regulating glucose control as a function of time after statin therapy is initiated. In the meantime, statin therapy should not be withheld from patients out of concern that they may precipitate diabetes. It is clear that diabetics derive as much benefit from statins as do nondiabetic patients.[4,5]

P. P. Toth, MD, PhD

References

1. Shepherd J, Cobbe SM, Ford I, et al. Prevention of coronary heart disease with pravastatin in men with hypercholesterolemia. West of Scotland Coronary Prevention Study Group. *N Engl J Med*. 1995;333:1301-1307.
2. Ridker PM, Danielson E, Fonseca FA, et al. Rosuvastatin to prevent vascular events in men and women with elevated c-reactive protein. *N Engl J Med*. 2008;359:2195-2207.
3. Sattar N, Preiss D, Murray HM, et al. Statins and risk of incident diabetes: a collaborative meta-analysis of randomised statin trials. *Lancet*. 2010;375: 735-742.
4. Baigent C, Keech A, Kearney PM, et al. Efficacy and safety of cholesterol-lowering treatment: prospective meta-analysis of data from 90,056 participants in 14 randomised trials of statins. *Lancet*. 2005;366:1267-1278.
5. Kearney PM, Blackwell L, Collins R, et al. Efficacy of cholesterol-lowering therapy in 18,686 people with diabetes in 14 randomised trials of statins: a meta-analysis. *Lancet*. 2008;371:117-125.

Safety of Anacetrapib in Patients with or at High Risk for Coronary Heart Disease
Cannon CP, for the DEFINE Investigators (Brigham and Women's Hosp, Boston, MA; et al)
N Engl J Med 363:2406-2415, 2010

Background.—Anacetrapib is a cholesteryl ester transfer protein inhibitor that raises high-density lipoprotein (HDL) cholesterol and reduces low-density lipoprotein (LDL) cholesterol.

Methods.—We conducted a randomized, double-blind, placebo-controlled trial to assess the efficacy and safety profile of anacetrapib in patients with coronary heart disease or at high risk for coronary heart disease. Eligible patients who were taking a statin and who had an LDL cholesterol level that was consistent with that recommended in guidelines were assigned to receive 100 mg of anacetrapib or placebo daily for 18 months. The primary end points were the percent change from baseline in LDL cholesterol at 24 weeks (HDL cholesterol level was a secondary end point) and the safety and side-effect profile of anacetrapib through 76 weeks. Cardiovascular events and deaths were prospectively adjudicated.

Results.—A total of 1623 patients underwent randomization. By 24 weeks, the LDL cholesterol level had been reduced from 81 mg per deciliter (2.1 mmol per liter) to 45 mg per deciliter (1.2 mmol per liter) in the anacetrapib group, as compared with a reduction from 82 mg per deciliter (2.1 mmol per liter) to 77 mg per deciliter (2.0 mmol per liter) in the placebo group (P<0.001) — a 39.8% reduction with anacetrapib beyond that seen with placebo. In addition, the HDL cholesterol level increased from 41 mg per deciliter (1.0 mmol per liter) to 101 mg per deciliter (2.6 mmol per liter) in the anacetrapib group, as compared with an increase from 40 mg per deciliter (1.0 mmol per liter) to 46 mg per deciliter (1.2 mmol per liter) in the placebo group (P<0.001) — a 138.1% increase with anacetrapib beyond that seen with placebo. Through 76 weeks, no changes were noted in blood pressure or electrolyte or aldosterone levels with anacetrapib as compared with placebo. Prespecified adjudicated cardiovascular events occurred in 16 patients treated with anacetrapib (2.0%) and 21 patients receiving placebo (2.6%) (P=0.40). The prespecified Bayesian analysis indicated that this event distribution provided a predictive probability (confidence) of 94% that anacetrapib would not be associated with a 25% increase in cardiovascular events, as seen with torcetrapib.

Conclusions.—Treatment with anacetrapib had robust effects on LDL and HDL cholesterol, had an acceptable side-effect profile, and, within the limits of the power of this study, did not result in the adverse cardiovascular effects observed with torcetrapib. (Funded by Merck Research Laboratories; ClinicalTrials.gov number, NCT00685776.) (Tables 3 and 4).

▶ Therapeutic cholesterol ester transfer protein (CETP) inhibition is a controversial issue. Based on epidemiologic investigation, reduced CETP activity is associated with both increased[1] and decreased[2] risk for acute cardiovascular events. Conceptually, CETP inhibition is based on the assumption that the resulting rise in serum levels of high-density lipoprotein cholesterol (HDL-C) will be beneficial. However, CETP inhibition also decreases the throughput of cholesterol ester to the liver via indirect reverse cholesterol transport. The impact of the latter phenomenon on cardiovascular risk is as yet uncharacterized. Torcetrapib was widely considered to be a promising therapeutic option for high-risk patients because it substantially inhibited CETP, decreased low-density lipoprotein cholesterol (LDL-C), and significantly increased HDL-C. Despite these seemingly beneficial changes, torcetrapib therapy was associated with a significant increase in mortality.[3] Torcetrapib increased blood pressure, increased adrenal cortical production of aldosterone and cortisol, and induced adverse alterations in serum electrolytes. Torcetrapib also had no impact on rates of carotid atherosclerosis disease progression.[4,5] In light of these findings, there have been understandable misgivings surrounding the development of other candidate CETP inhibitors. Two of these, anacetrapib and dalcetrapib, remain in clinical development. Neither of these drugs increase serum aldosterone levels or appear to exert the off-target toxicities observed with torcetrapib.

TABLE 3.—Rates of Adverse Events and Safety Variables of Interest through Week 76*

Adverse Event or Safety Variable	Anacetrapib	Placebo	Absolute Difference Percentage Points (95% CI)	P Value
	No./Total No. (%)			
Adverse events				
Drug-related adverse event	92/808 (11.4)	86/804 (10.7)	0.7 (−2.4 to 3.8)	
Clinical adverse event leading to discontinuation of study drug	44/808 (5.4)	46/804 (5.7)	−0.2 (−2.5 to 2.2)	
Drug-related adverse event leading to discontinuation of study drug	22/808 (2.7)	18/804 (2.2)	0.5 (−1.1 to 2.1)	
Serious adverse event	123/808 (15.2)	119/804 (14.8)	0.2 (−3.3 to 3.7)	
Drug-related serious adverse event	2/808 (0.2)	4/804 (0.5)	−0.2 (−1.1 to 0.5)	
Safety variables of interest				
Elevation in systolic BP ≥10 mm Hg	502/802 (62.6)	514/797 (64.5)	−1.9 (−6.6 to 2.8)	0.43
Elevation in systolic BP ≥15 mm Hg	354/802 (44.1)	377/797 (47.3)	−3.2 (−8.0 to 1.7)	0.20
Elevation in diastolic BP ≥10 mm Hg	326/802 (40.6)	319/797 (40.0)	0.6 (−4.2 to 5.4)	0.80
Serum sodium >ULN	86/800 (10.8)	84/797 (10.5)	0.2 (−2.8 to 3.2)	0.89
Serum chloride >ULN	23/800 (2.9)	27/797 (3.4)	−0.5 (−2.3 to 1.2)	0.56
Serum bicarbonate >ULN	11/800 (1.4)	17/797 (2.1)	−0.8 (−2.2 to 0.6)	0.25
Serum potassium <lower limit of the normal range	38/800 (4.8)	38/797 (4.8)	−0.0 (−2.2 to 2.1)	0.99
Confirmed elevations of ALT or AST ≥3× ULN	1/800 (0.1)	8/797 (1.0)	−0.9 (−1.9 to −0.2)	0.02
Creatine kinase ≥10× ULN	0/800	2/797 (0.3)	−0.3 (−0.9 to 0.2)	0.16
Any muscle symptom	32/808 (4.0)	28/804 (3.5)	0.5 (−1.4 to 2.4)	0.61

*ALT denotes alanine aminotransferase, AST aspartate aminotransferase, BP blood pressure, CI confidence interval, and ULN upper limit of the normal range.

TABLE 4.—Cardiovascular Events during the Treatment Phase of the Study*

Event	Anacetrapib (N = 808)	Placebo (N = 804)
	number (percent)	
Prespecified, adjudicated cardiovascular safety end point	16 (2.0)	21 (2.6)
Death from cardiovascular causes	4 (0.5)	1 (0.1)
Nonfatal myocardial infarction	6 (0.7)	9 (1.1)
Hospitalization for unstable angina	1 (0.1)	6 (0.7)
Nonfatal stroke	5 (0.6)	5 (0.6)
Death from any cause	11 (1.4)	8 (1.0)
Heart failure	3 (0.4)	4 (0.5)
Revascularization	8 (1.0)	28 (3.5)
PCI	6 (0.7)	25 (3.1)
CABG	2 (0.2)	3 (0.4)

*The duration of the treatment phase of the study was 76 weeks. CABG denotes coronary-artery bypass grafting, and PCI percutaneous coronary intervention.

The Determining the Efficacy and Tolerability of CETP Inhibition with Anacetrapib trial was designed as a safety study. High-risk patients (total of 1623 subjects with either established coronary artery disease or a 10-year Framingham risk ≥20%) were randomized to either anacetrapib or placebo. All patients were concomitantly treated with a statin. Mean baseline LDL-C and HDL-C levels were approximately 81 and 40 mg/dL, respectively. Anacetrapib was stopped in 142 patients because their LDL-C on therapy fell below 25 mg/dL, a prespecified stopping boundary. Compared with placebo, LDL-C decreased by 39.8%, HDL-C increased by 138%, non-HDL-C decreased by 31.7%, and lipoprotein(a) decreased by 36.4% when measured over 24 weeks. Apoprotein (apo) B decreased by 21% and apo A1 increased by 45%. There were no significant differences between groups in adverse events (Table 3) or in cardiovascular events (Table 4) evaluated over 76 weeks of follow-up. Specifically, no differences were seen in blood pressure, serum electrolytes, incidence of myopathy, or adverse events leading to study drug discontinuation. The incidence of transaminase elevations was lower in the anacetrapib group.

Anacetrapib is a safe promising CETP inhibitor and will now be tested in a randomized, prospective, end point-driven trial in high-risk patients. Its capacity to both raise HDL-C by 138% and augment the LDL reduction of statin therapy by 40% is remarkable. Whether these changes promote incremental reduction in risk for cardiovascular is an issue that will be rigorously tested. In the meantime, it is expected that the populations of HDL particles produced by anacetrapib therapy will be exhaustively evaluated for their size, functionality, and biochemical constitution. If proven to be efficacious, CETP inhibition could potentially revolutionize the management of risk attributable to multiple forms of dyslipidemia.

P. P. Toth, MD, PhD

References

1. Vasan RS, Pencina MJ, Robins SJ, et al. Association of circulating cholesteryl ester transfer protein activity with incidence of cardiovascular disease in the community. *Circulation.* 2009;120:2414-2420.
2. Thompson A, Di Angelantonio E, Sarwar N, et al. Association of cholesteryl ester transfer protein genotypes with CETP mass and activity, lipid levels, and coronary risk. *JAMA.* 2008;299:2777-2788.
3. Barter PJ, Caulfield M, Eriksson M, et al. Effects of torcetrapib in patients at high risk for coronary events. *N Engl J Med.* 2007;357:2109-2122.
4. Kastelein JJ, van Leuven SI, Burgess L, et al. Effect of torcetrapib on carotid atherosclerosis in familial hypercholesterolemia. *N Engl J Med.* 2007;356: 1620-1630.
5. Nissen SE, Tardif JC, Nicholls SJ, et al. Effect of torcetrapib on the progression of coronary atherosclerosis. *N Engl J Med.* 2007;356:1304-1316.

Cholesterol Efflux Capacity, High-Density Lipoprotein Function, and Atherosclerosis

Khera AV, Cuchel M, de la Llera-Moya M, et al (Univ of Pennsylvania, Philadelphia; Children's Hosp of Philadelphia, PA; et al)

N Engl J Med 364:127-135, 2011

Background.—High-density lipoprotein (HDL) may provide cardiovascular protection by promoting reverse cholesterol transport from macrophages. We hypothesized that the capacity of HDL to accept cholesterol from macrophages would serve as a predictor of atherosclerotic burden.

Methods.—We measured cholesterol efflux capacity in 203 healthy volunteers who underwent assessment of carotid artery intima—media thickness, 442 patients with angiographically confirmed coronary artery disease, and 351 patients without such angiographically confirmed disease. We quantified efflux capacity by using a validated ex vivo system that involved incubation of macrophages with apolipoprotein B—depleted serum from the study participants.

Results.—The levels of HDL cholesterol and apolipoprotein A-I were significant determinants of cholesterol efflux capacity but accounted for less than 40% of the observed variation. An inverse relationship was noted between efflux capacity and carotid intima-media thickness both before and after adjustment for the HDL cholesterol level. Furthermore, efflux capacity was a strong inverse predictor of coronary disease status (adjusted odds ratio for coronary disease per 1-SD increase in efflux capacity, 0.70; 95% confidence interval [CI], 0.59 to 0.83; P<0.001). This relationship was attenuated, but remained significant, after additional adjustment for the HDL cholesterol level (odds ratio per 1-SD increase, 0.75; 95% CI, 0.63 to 0.90; P=0.002) or apolipoprotein A-I level (odds ratio per 1-SD increase, 0.74; 95% CI, 0.61 to 0.89; P=0.002). Additional studies showed enhanced efflux capacity in patients with the metabolic syndrome and low HDL cholesterol levels who were treated with pioglitazone, but not in patients with hypercholesterolemia who were treated with statins.

Conclusions.—Cholesterol efflux capacity from macrophages, a metric of HDL function, has a strong inverse association with both carotid intima—media thickness and the likelihood of angiographic coronary artery disease, independently of the HDL cholesterol level. (Funded by the National Heart, Lung, and Blood Institute and others.) (Tables 2 and 3).

▶ Although high-density lipoprotein (HDL) particles are believed capable of engaging in a broad range of atheroprotective functions because of their complex proteasome and ability to bind to a number of different cell surface receptors, it is likely that their most important function is to drive reverse

TABLE 2.—Beta Coefficients for the Association between Cholesterol Efflux Capacity and Carotid Intima—Media Thickness

Linear-Regression Covariates*	Beta Coefficient per 1-SD Increase in Efflux Capacity (95% CI)	P Value
Age and sex	−0.02 (−0.04 to −0.003)	0.02
Age, sex, and cardiovascular risk factors	−0.02 (−0.04 to −0.004)	0.02
Age, sex, cardiovascular risk factors, and high-density lipoprotein cholesterol	−0.03 (−0.06 to −0.01)	0.003
Age, sex, cardiovascular risk factors, and apolipoprotein A-I	−0.04 (−0.06 to −0.01)	0.005

*Cardiovascular risk factors were systolic blood pressure, glycated hemoglobin, and low-density lipoprotein cholesterol.

TABLE 3.—Coronary Artery Disease Status According to Quartile of Efflux Capacity

Variable	No. of Patients	Odds Ratio for Coronary Artery Disease (95% CI)*		
		Adjusted for Cardiovascular Risk Factors	Adjusted for Cardiovascular Risk Factors and HDL Cholesterol	Adjusted for Cardiovascular Risk Factors and Apolipoprotein A-I
Quartile 1	198	1.00	1.00	1.00
Quartile 2	198	0.75 (0.48–1.16)	0.79 (0.51–1.24)	0.77 (0.49–1.21)
Quartile 3	198	0.58 (0.37–0.89)	0.64 (0.41–1.00)	0.63 (0.40–0.99)
Quartile 4	199	0.40 (0.25–0.63)	0.48 (0.30–0.78)	0.46 (0.28–0.75)
P value for trend		<0.001	0.002	0.002

*Cardiovascular risk factors included in the logistic-regression model were age, sex, smoking status, presence or absence of diabetes, presence or absence of hypertension, and low-density lipoprotein cholesterol. HDL denotes highdensity lipoprotein.

cholesterol transport (RCT). The concept of RCT was first proposed by Glomset[1] and has been validated in both animal and human models. It has been challenging to establish the contribution of HDL cholesterol (HDL-C) raising to overall cardiovascular risk reduction in clinical trials because observed changes in this lipoprotein fraction tend to be modest,[2] although some studies have certainly found a positive correlation with multivariate regression analysis.[3,4] In recent years, attention has turned to trying to establish the role of measuring HDL functionality and capacity for RCT, as this may better quantify the role of HDL treatment and/or modification in cardiovascular risk reduction.

Khera and coworkers evaluated the relative contributions of HDL-C, apolipoprotein AI (apo AI), and the capacity to efflux cholesterol from macrophages in an ex vivo assay system to atherosclerotic disease burden. Cholesterol efflux capacity was inversely and independently associated with risk for increased carotid intima media thickness (Table 2) and established coronary artery disease (CAD) (Table 3) even after adjusting for HDL-C and apo AI levels. In a logistic regression model adjusted for age and gender, both HDL-C and efflux capacity were inversely associated with risk for CAD (Fig 1 in the original article). For each 1 standard deviation in serum HDL-C, there was a 29% reduction in risk for CAD. Male gender and cigarette smoking were both associated with reduced efflux capacity. Of interest are the observations that statin therapy was not associated with increased efflux capacity, but the treatment of patients with metabolic syndrome with pioglitazone was associated with a significant 11% increase in efflux capacity.

These findings usher in a new era in HDL clinical investigation. This study establishes the feasibility of an ex vivo efflux capacity assay to evaluate the functionality of an individual's HDL particles. It also confirms in human patients that efflux capacity is a legitimate and important determinant of atherosclerotic disease burden, and its importance may exceed such simple measurements as those for HDL-C and apo AI. Assays evaluating the ability of HDLs to antagonize lipoprotein oxidation, reverse endothelial dysfunction, and reduce inflammation may also assume roles. More work will have to be performed to establish the precise positioning and cost-effectiveness of such assays in daily clinical practice. Although meta-analyses suggest that on therapy elevations with statins impact risk for cardiovascular events[5] and rates of disease progression,[6] this study was unable to demonstrate an increase in efflux capacity in patients treated with statins. In contrast, a significant increase in efflux capacity in patients with insulin resistance was shown with pioglitazone. These findings and their clinical implications certainly warrant further study.

P. P. Toth, MD, PhD

References

1. Glomset JA. The plasma lecithins:cholesterol acyltransferase reaction. *J Lipid Res.* 1968;9:155-167.
2. Briel M, Ferreira-Gonzalez I, You JJ, et al. Association between change in high density lipoprotein cholesterol and cardiovascular disease morbidity and mortality: systematic review and meta-regression analysis. *BMJ.* 2009;338:b92.
3. Robins SJ. Targeting low high-density lipoprotein cholesterol for therapy: lessons from the Veterans Affairs High-density Lipoprotein Intervention Trial. *Am J Cardiol.* 2001;88:19N-23N.
4. Cui Y, Watson DJ, Girman CJ, et al. Effects of increasing high-density lipoprotein cholesterol and decreasing low-density lipoprotein cholesterol on the incidence of first acute coronary events (from the Air Force/Texas Coronary Atherosclerosis Prevention Study). *Am J Cardiol.* 2009;104:829-834.
5. Brown BG, Zhao XQ, Cheung MC. Should both HDL-C and LDL-C be targets for lipid therapy? A review of current evidence. *J Clin Lipidol.* 2007;1:88-94.
6. Nicholls SJ, Tuzcu EM, Sipahi I, et al. Statins, high-density lipoprotein cholesterol, and regression of coronary atherosclerosis. *JAMA.* 2007;297:499-508.

Prevention of Atherosclerosis

Anti-Apolipoprotein A-1 auto-antibodies are active mediators of atherosclerotic plaque vulnerability

Montecucco F, Vuilleumier N, Pagano S, et al (Geneva Univ Hosps, Switzerland; et al)

Eur Heart J 32:412-421, 2011

Aims.—Anti-Apolipoprotein A-1 auto-antibodies (anti-ApoA-1 IgG) represent an emerging prognostic cardiovascular marker in patients with myocardial infarction or autoimmune diseases associated with high cardiovascular risk. The potential relationship between anti-ApoA-1 IgG and plaque vulnerability remains elusive. Thus, we aimed to investigate the role of anti-ApoA-1 IgG in plaque vulnerability.

Methods and Results.—Potential relationship between anti-ApoA-1 IgG and features of cardiovascular vulnerability was explored both *in vivo* and *in vitro*. *In vivo*, we investigated anti-ApoA-1 IgG in patients with severe carotid stenosis ($n = 102$) and in ApoE$-/-$ mice infused with polyclonal anti-ApoA-1 IgG. *In vitro*, anti-ApoA-1 IgG effects were assessed on human primary macrophages, monocytes, and neutrophils. Intraplaque collagen was decreased, while neutrophil and matrix metalloprotease (MMP)-9 content were increased in anti-ApoA-1 IgG-positive patients and anti-ApoA-1 IgG-treated mice when compared with corresponding controls. In mouse aortic roots (but not in abdominal aortas), treatment with anti-ApoA-1 IgG was associated with increased lesion size when compared with controls. In humans, serum anti-ApoA-1 IgG levels positively correlated with intraplaque macrophage, neutrophil, and MMP-9 content, and inversely with collagen. *In vitro*, anti-ApoA-1 IgG increased macrophage release of CCL2, CXCL8, and MMP-9, as well as neutrophil migration towards TNF-α or CXCL8.

Conclusion.—These results suggest that anti-ApoA-1 IgG might be associated with increased atherosclerotic plaque vulnerability in humans and mice (Tables 3 and 8).

▶ Recent mechanistic studies have demonstrated that the high-density lipoprotein (HDL) proteasome can be altered, resulting in the formation of particles that are proinflammatory and pro-oxidative.[1,2] Adding an additional layer of complexity

TABLE 3.—Parameters of Intraplaque Vulnerability

Carotid Intraplaque Parameters	Anti-ApoA-1 Negative (n = 82)	Anti-ApoA-1 Positive (n = 20)	P-Value
Plaque size, cm	1.7 (1.5−2)	1.5 (1.3−1.9)	0.38
Plaque stenosis, % of lumen	80 (75−90)	75 (70−80)	0.30
Upstream portion			
% lipid	5.98 (2.86−9.37)	7.11 (3.31−10.81)	0.42
% total collagen	33.58 (26.15−40.06)	33.29 (25.21−39.24)	0.88
% collagen I	11.54 (9.44−16.9)	13.36 (7.69−15.05)	0.25
% collagen III	13.17 (10.03−17.27)	9.82 (7.55−12.42)	0.005
% of smooth muscle cell-rich area	5.39 (3.16−9.37)	3.53 (2.33−5.85)	0.09
% of macrophage-rich area	4.98 (2.73−9.94)	7.95 (5.59−13.95)	0.02
Lymphocytes/mm^2	2.37 (1.12−5.93)	4.03 (1.62−13.67)	0.14
Neutrophils/mm^2	2.35 (1.12−6.01)	3.27 (2.18−8.44)	0.19
MMP-8 mRNA, fold increase	1.23 (0.38−3.00)	2.56 (0.66−3.86)	0.08
% MMP-9	2.99 (1.29−5.87)	6.25 (2.40−12.6)	0.02
TNF-α mRNA, fold increase	1.20 (0.54−1.95)	1.22 (0.49−1.94)	0.72
CCL2 mRNA, fold increase	0.93 (0.64−1.39)	1.17 (0.65−1.67)	0.37
CCL3 mRNA, fold increase	0.91 (0.62−1.72)	1.15 (0.79−1.58)	0.71
CCL4 mRNA, fold increase	0.88 (0.55−1.53)	1.02 (0.51−1.31)	0.65
CXCL8 mRNA, fold increase	0.96 (0.52−1.87)	1.32 (0.82−2.00)	0.39
Downstream portion			
% lipid	3.45 (1.64−8.37)	4.78 (1.36−10.05)	0.57
% total collagen	20.88 (17.20−23.64)	17.90 (12.82−20.49)	0.01
% collagen I	6.40 (4.27−11.29)	5.45 (2.98−7.04)	0.06
% collagen III	6.63 (4.11−10.28)	4.58 (3.27−5.84)	0.03
% of smooth muscle cell-rich area	2.87 (1.62−4.38)	2.69 (1.69−3.88)	0.69
% of macrophage-rich area	6.88 (2.62−16.12)	11.17 (7.44−18.37)	0.04
Lymphocytes/mm^2	2.09 (0.98−5.37)	2.81 (1.24−11.50)	0.34
Neutrophils/mm^2	2.98 (0.66−8.51)	9.85 (3.88−15.12)	0.002
MMP-8 mRNA, fold increase	1.13 (0.34−3.25)	1.19 (0.80−2.28)	0.95
% MMP-9	4.77 (1.94−9.66)	19.37 (6.76−25.69)	<0.0001
TNF-α mRNA, fold increase	1.46 (0.78−2.77)	0.96 (0.62−2.06)	0.08
CCL2 mRNA, fold increase	1.37 (0.78−2.05)	1.95 (1.15−2.38)	0.07
CCL3 mRNA, fold increase	1.37 (0.84−2.14)	1.63 (0.58−2.18)	0.87
CCL4 mRNA, fold increase	1.38 (0.89−2.35)	1.75 (0.64−2.45)	0.91
CXCL8 mRNA, fold increase	1.16 (0.54−2.28)	0.91 (0.41−1.71)	0.32

Data are expressed as median [interquartile range (IQR)].
MMP, matrix metalloprotease.

TABLE 8.—Secretion of Neutrophil and Monocyte Chemoattractants, as Well as MMP-8 and MMP-9 From Human Primary Macrophages

Mediator Released	Cell Culture Assay					
	CTL Medium	LPS (1 ng/mL)	Stimulation CTL IgG (40 mg/mL)	Anti-ApoA-1 IgG (40 mg/mL)	Anti-ApoA-1 IgG-Negative Patients	Anti-ApoA-1 IgG-Positive Patients
CCL2, pg/mL	7 (5–11)	260* (233–2876)	6.9 (4.6–9.5)	291† (225–1047)	10.8 (8–42.9)	173.7§ (134.7–264.7)
CXCL8, pg/mL	131 (62–180)	7158* (6591–16840)	51 (73–228)	4189‡ (4181–11654)	209 (160–313)	1327§ (788–2274)
TNF-α, pg/mL	BDL	320* (225–456)	BDL	74‡ (25–106)	BDL	33§ (12.1–52)
MMP-8, pg/mL	95 (57–168)	326* (54–3635)	1 (1–77)	14.8‡ (1–173)	71 (34–3192)	139$^\|$ (43–28359)
MMP-9, ng/mL	4.2 (0.4–62)	26* (14–32)	8.7 (4–13)	59‡ (45–83)	8.4 (3.7–15.3)	40§ (16.6–59)
Pro-MMP-9 activity, ng/mL	16 (14–18)	50* (37–61)	21 (16–23)	32‡ (27–42)	18 (16–21)	33§ (25–40)

Data are expressed as median and (IQR) ($n = 7$). BDL, below the detection limit of the assay. For statistical analysis, the lower detection limit value was used.

*$P < 0.05$ vs. control medium.

$^\dagger P < 0.05$ vs. control IgG.

$^\ddagger P$: NS (not significant) vs. control IgG.

$^\S P < 0.005$ vs. anti-ApoA-1 IgG-negative patients.

$^\| P$ = NS (not significant) vs. anti-ApoA-1 IgG negative patients.

to this, it has been shown that patients with rheumatoid arthritis or coronary artery disease can develop autoantibodies to apoprotein (apo) AI, the primary apoprotein constituent of HDLs. The presence of immunoglobulins to apo AI in serum is associated with increased levels of oxidized LDL and other markers of unstable atherosclerotic plaque. HDLs localize to the subendothelial space during reverse cholesterol transport. Should antibodies bind to apo AI, this could not only inactivate HDL but also potentially exacerbate host defense—mediated inflammation, resulting in accelerated atherogenesis.

Montecucco and coworkers explored the impact of anti—apo AI IgG antibodies on carotid atherosclerotic plaque dynamics in both in vivo and in vitro models. Compared with patients with negative results for anti—apo AI, patients with positive results for anti—apo AI had reduced content of collagen III and increased activity of matrix metalloproteinase (MMP) 9, a collagenase (Table 1). Patients positive for anti—apo AI also had a higher density of macrophages and neutrophils within the plaque. No other differences in lipid content, inflammatory gene expression, or lymphocyte content were noted. These findings were reproduced reasonably well in an apo E double-knockout mouse model treated with anti—apo AI IgG antibodies. Aortic atherosclerotic lesion size, neutrophil density, and the expression of MMP 8 and MMP 9 were all increased. Consistent with increased MMP expression, plaque collagen content was decreased. When human macrophages were treated with anti—apo AI IgG antibodies, cellular expression of such inflammatory mediators as tumor necrosis factor α, MMP 9, and CXCL8 were all increased (Table 2).

These data certainly expand the complexity surrounding the relationship between HDL particles and atherosclerosis. It is not yet clear why some patients with chronic inflammatory disease and coronary artery disease (CAD; also an inflammatory disease) develop an autoimmune response to the apo AI in their HDL fraction. These studies suggest that anti—apo AI antibodies can potentiate the inflammatory response. This inflammatory nidus appears to be associated with increased macrophage and neutrophil influx, increased inflammatory mediator expression, increased elaboration of MMPs, and augmented collagen proteolysis. All these changes are correlated with reduced plaque stability and increased risk for cardiovascular events. Future studies will have to be designed to further delineate the prevalence of anti—apo AI autoimmunity and whether or not specific threshold levels of such antibodies correlate with increased risk for CAD and CAD-related events. Genetic, metabolic, and environmental triggers for anti—apo AI antibody generation are also yet to be defined.

P. P. Toth, MD, PhD

References

1. Ansell BJ. Targeting the anti-inflammatory effects of high-density lipoprotein. *Am J Cardiol.* 2007;100:n3-n9.
2. Shao B, Oda MN, Vaisar T, Oram JF, Heinecke JW. Pathways for oxidation of high-density lipoprotein in human cardiovascular disease. *Curr Opin Mol Ther.* 2006;8:198-205.

Early Signs of Atherosclerosis in Diabetic Children on Intensive Insulin Treatment: A population-based study

Margeirsdottir HD, Stensaeth KH, Larsen JR, et al (Oslo Univ Hosp, Norway; Oslo Diabetes Res Centre, Norway)
Diabetes Care 33:2043-2048, 2010

Objective.—To evaluate early stages of atherosclerosis and predisposing factors in type 1 diabetic children and adolescents compared with age- and sex-matched healthy control subjects.

Research Design and Methods.—All children and adolescents with type 1 diabetes, aged 8–18 years in Health Region South-East in Norway were invited to participate in the study ($n = 800$). A total of 40% ($n = 314$) agreed to participate and were compared with 118 age-matched healthy control subjects. Carotid artery intima-media thickness (cIMT) and elasticity were measured using standardized methods.

Results.—Mean age of the diabetic patients was 13.7 years, mean diabetes duration was 5.5 years, and mean A1C was 8.4%; 97% were using intensive insulin treatment, and 60% were using insulin pumps. Diabetic patients had more frequently elevated cIMT than healthy control subjects: 19.5% were above the 90th centile of healthy control subjects, and 13.1% were above the 95th centile ($P < 0.001$). Mean cIMT was higher in diabetic boys than in healthy control subjects (0.46 ± 0.06 vs. 0.44 ± 0.05 mm, $P = 0.04$) but not significantly so in girls. There was no significant difference between the groups regarding carotid distensibility, compliance, or wall stress. None of the subjects had atherosclerotic plaque formation. Although within the normal range, the mean values of systolic blood pressure, total cholesterol, LDL cholesterol, and apolipoprotein B were significantly higher in the diabetic patients than in the healthy control subjects.

Conclusions.—Despite short disease duration, intensive insulin treatment, fair glycemic control, and no signs of microvascular complications, children and adolescents with type 1 diabetes had slightly increased cIMT compared with healthy control subjects, and the differences were more prominent in boys (Tables 1 and 3).

▶ The hyperglycemic milieu characteristic of diabetes mellitus (DM) is injurious to arterial vessel walls and promotes atherogenesis. Agonizing receptors of advanced glycosylated end products promote intravascular inflammation and oxidation. In the Diabetes Control and Complications Trial/Epidemiology of Diabetes Interventions and Complications study, tight glycemic control was shown to reduce rates of carotid intima media thickness (CIMT) progression better than less tight control.[1] Atherosclerosis begins early in life, and multiple studies of unfortunate young (18-25 years) men killed in the Korean War and the Vietnam War demonstrated significant coronary atherosclerosis in almost half of the subjects autopsied. Tight glycemic control is well documented for reducing risk of microangiopathy. While we still lack definitive convincing evidence (trends are observed) for significant cardiovascular

TABLE 1.—Clinical Characteristics and Metabolic and Anthropometric Data of the Participants

	Total Diabetes	Total Control	P	Male Diabetes	Male Control	P	Female Diabetes	Female Control	P
n	314	118		155	53		159	65	
Age (years)	13.8 ± 2.8	13.2 ± 2.6	0.73	13.4 ± 2.80	13.3 ± 2.44	0.7	14.1 ± 2.85	13.2 ± 2.7	0.03
Duration of diabetes (years)	5.5 ± 3.4			5.6 ± 3.4	0		5.4 ± 3.4		0
Pubertal stage (Tanner)	3.2 ± 1.5	2.9 ± 1.4	0.36	2.9 ± 1.6	2.8 ± 1.4	0.52	3.5 ± 1.4	3.0 ± 1.4	0.15
Height (cm)	160.4 ± 14.4	156.8 ± 13.6	0.02	160.6 ± 14.7	157.6 ± 16.2	0.24	160.3 ± 12.3	156.2 ± 12.6	0.02
Weight (kg)	54.9 ± 16.7	47.9 ± 13.4	<0.001	53.3 ± 17.4	46.9 ± 12.1	0.004	56.5 ± 14.4	48.7 ± 14.4	0.001
BMI (kg/m²)	20.9 ± 3.939	19.1 ± 0.3	<0.001	20.1 ± 3.6	18.6 ± 2.3	0.001	21.6 ± 4.1	19.5 ± 3.6	0.001
Waist circumference (cm)	71.2 ± 10.0	66.7 ± 6.7	<0.001	70.3 ± 10.0	65.9 ± 6.5	0.001	72.1 ± 9.9	67.4 ± 6.8	<0.001
SBP (mmHg)	101.0 ± 10.1	98.0 ± 10.2	0.006	101.0 ± 9.8	96.8 ± 10.7	0.01	101.0 ± 10.3	99.0 ± 9.6	0.18
DBP (mmHg)	60.5 ± 8.3	58.5 ± 7.8	0.22	59.6 ± 8.4	58.1 ± 9.2	0.29	61.5 ± 8.2	58.8 ± 6.2	0.009
Smoking	11 (3.5)	2 (2)	0.53	2 (1.3)	0 (0)	1	9 (5.7)	2 (3.1)	0.52
Urinary albumin-to-creatinine ratio	1.4 ± 3.7	1.3 ± 1.9	0.72	1.8 ± 4.9	1.1 ± 1.7	0.32	1.0 ± 1.1	1.5 ± 2.0	0.11
S-creatinine (_mol/l)	53.1 ± 10.3	54.5 ± 10.1	0.23	53.7 ± 10.8	55.5 ± 10.2	0.3	52.5 ± 9.7	53.6 ± 9.9	0.43
Fasting blood glucose (mmol/l)	10.9 ± 4.8	4.9 ± 0.4	<0.001	10.1 ± 5.1	4.9 ± 0.4	<0.001	10.8 ± 4.5	4.8 ± 0.5	<0.001
A1C (%)	8.4 ± 1.3	5.3 ± 0.5	<0.001	8.3 ± 1.2	5.3 ± 0.6	<0.001	8.4 ± 1.3	5.3 ± 0.4	<0.001
Mean A1C (%)	8.2 ± 1.0			8.1 ± 1.0			8.2 ± 1.0		
A1 months*	119 ± 104.1			120.8 ± 107.1			117.9 ± 101.5		
Total cholesterol (mmol/l)	4.6 ± 0.9	4.3 ± 0.8	0.002	4.6 ± 0.8	4.3 ± 0.8	0.11	4.7 ± 0.8	4.4 ± 0.7	0.004
HDL cholesterol (mmol/l)	1.8 ± 0.4	1.70 ± 0.4	0.07	1.8 ± 0.4	1.7 ± 0.5	0.8	1.8 ± 0.4	1.7 ± 0.3	0.20
LDL cholesterol (mmol/l)	2.5 ± 0.7	2.3 ± 0.7	0.028	2.5 ± 0.7	2.2 ± 0.7	0.13	2.5 ± 0.7	2.4 ± 0.7	0.09
LDL-to-HDL cholesterol ratio	1.5 ± 0.6	1.5 ± 0.7	0.7	1.5 ± 0.7	1.4 ± 0.7	0.48	1.5 ± 0.6	1.5 ± 0.6	0.99
Total-to-LDL cholesterol ratio	2.7 ± 0.8	2.7 ± 0.8	0.7	2.7 ± 0.8	2.6 ± 0.8	0.48	2.7 ± 0.7	2.7 ± 0.7	0.89
Triglycerides (mmol/l)	0.8 ± 0.4	0.7 ± 0.4	0.32	0.8 ± 0.4	0.7 ± 04	0.35	0.8 ± 0.4	0.8 ± 0.4	0.51
ApoB (g/l)	0.7 ± 0.2	0.7 ± 0.2	<0.001	0.7 ± 0.2	0.7 ± 0.2	0.02	0.8 ± 0.2	0.7 ± 0.2	0.006
ApoA1 (g/l)	1.6 ± 0.3	1.5 ± 0.3	0.003	1.6 ± 0.3	1.5 ± 0.3	0.48	1.6 ± 0.3	1.4 ± 0.3	<0.001
ApoB-to-ApoA1 ratio	0.5 ± 0.2	0.5 ± 0.3	0.75	0.5 ± 1.6	0.5 ± 0.1	0.37	0.5 ± 0.1	0.5 ± 0.3	0.44

(Continued)

TABLE 1. (*continued*)

	Total			Male			Female		
	Diabetes	Control	P	Diabetes	Control	P	Diabetes	Control	P
Insulin dose (U/kg/day)	0.9 ± 0.4			0.9 ± 0.3			0.9 ± 0.4		
Injections per day									
1–2	1 (0.4)			0			1 (0.6)		
3	6 (2.4)			3 (2.5)			3 (2.3)		
≥4	95 (37.5)			45 (37.5)			50 (37.6)		
Insulin pumps	151 (59.7)			72 (60)			79 (59.3)		

Data are means ± SD and n (%).

*The number of months from the diagnosis until the first registered A1C value multiplied by A1C units above the upper normal reference value (6.4%) of the first registered value, plus the number of months from the first to second registration multiplied by A1C units above the upper normal reference value of the second registered value, and so on until the time of cIMT analysis.

TABLE 3.—CIMT and Vessel Elasticity

		Total		Male			Female		
	Diabetes	Control	P	Diabetes	Control	P	Diabetes	Control	P
cIMT (mm)	0.45 ± 0.054	0.44 ± 0.045	0.11	0.46 ± 0.057	0.44 ± 0.057	0.04	0.44 ± 0.050	0.44 ± 0.044	0.94
DC (kPa^{-1})	0.35 ± 0.026	0.36 ± 0.023	0.48	0.35 ± 0.025	0.35 ± 0.020	0.93	0.36 ± 0.027	0.36 ± 0.024	0.42
CC (m^2/kPa^{-1})	9.95 ± 0.657	9.90 ± 0.564	0.48	10.08 ± 0.680	10.06 ± 0.534	0.83	9.82 ± 0.610	9.78 ± 0.560	0.58
Yongs modulus (kPa)	4.17 ± 1.438	4.30 ± 0.951	0.38	4.29 ± 1.075	4.37 ± 1.013	0.62	4.06 ± 1.718	4.24 ± 0.901	0.42

Data are means ± SD.

event reduction in response to intensive glycemic control, there is little question as to the significant long-term risk for cardiovascular disease in children who develop type 1 DM.

In this investigation by Margeirsdottir and coworkers, 314 children with a mean age of 13.7 years, mean A1c level of 8.4%, and mean duration of DM of 5.5 years underwent CIMT screening and were compared with nondiabetic control subjects. A significant percentage of these children (19.5%) were above the 90th percentile for age for CIMT. There was no difference in CIMT between diabetic and nondiabetic girls. The boys did manifest a statistically significant difference in CIMT. Consistent with the fact that at 0.46 mm there is very little lipid accumulation, there were no differences between groups for carotid distensibility, wall stress, or compliance. When comparing diabetic and nondiabetic subjects, diabetic ones had significantly higher total cholesterol and low-density lipoprotein cholesterol. There was also a mean 3/2 mm Hg difference in the systolic/diastolic blood pressure between groups, and diabetic children on average weighed 7 kg more than their nondiabetic counterparts.

For the boys in this study, intensive insulin therapy did not appear to offer adequate protection against the earliest changes underlying carotid atherosclerosis. With a 7-kg difference in weight between groups, over time and with continued weight gain in response to intensive insulin therapy, many of these children could also develop insulin resistance, which could antagonize glucose control and exacerbate blood pressure elevations and dyslipidemia. There is considerable uncertainty and caution about the use of statins in children. There are no long-term safety or outcome studies with statins in children. The role of statins in children with familial hypercholesterolemia is reasonably well defined, with multiple statins having an indication for use in these children from the age of 10 years. Children with type 1 DM pose significant challenges, but the use of statin therapy should be expanded to children with type 1 DM especially if there is evidence of CIMT thickening with or without concomitant dyslipidemia. Statins either alone[2] or in combination with niacin[3] or ezetimibe[4] have been shown to reduce rates of CIMT progression. It is critical that more be done therapeutically in the setting of primordial prevention to reduce risk of both macrovascular and microvascular events in children with type 1 DM.

P. P. Toth, MD, PhD

References

1. Nathan DM, Lachin J, Cleary P, et al. Intensive diabetes therapy and carotid intima-media thickness in type 1 diabetes mellitus. *N Engl J Med.* 2003;348:2294-2303.
2. Crouse JR 3rd, Raichlen JS, Riley WA, et al. Effect of rosuvastatin on progression of carotid intima-media thickness in low-risk individuals with subclinical atherosclerosis: the meteor trial. *JAMA.* 2007;297:1344-1353.
3. Taylor AJ, Lee HJ, Sullenberger LE. The effect of 24 months of combination statin and extended-release niacin on carotid intima-media thickness: ARBITER 3. *Curr Med Res Opin.* 2006;22:2243-2250.
4. Fleg JL, Mete M, Howard BV, et al. Effect of statins alone versus statins plus ezetimibe on carotid atherosclerosis in type 2 diabetes: The SANDS (Stop Atherosclerosis in Native Diabetics Study) trial. *J Am Coll Cardiol.* 2008;52:2198-2205.

Statin Safety

Cardiovascular Event Reduction and Adverse Events Among Subjects Attaining Low-Density Lipoprotein Cholesterol <50 mg/dl With Rosuvastatin: The JUPITER Trial (Justification for the Use of Statins in Prevention: an Intervention Trial Evaluating Rosuvastatin)

Hsia J, MacFadyen JG, Monyak J, et al (AstraZeneca LP, Wilmington, DE; Harvard Med School, Boston, MA)
J Am Coll Cardiol 57:1666-1675, 2011

Objectives.—The purpose of this study was to assess the impact on cardiovascular and adverse events of attaining lowdensity lipoprotein cholesterol (LDL-C) levels <50 mg/dl with rosuvastatin in apparently healthy adults in the JUPITER (Justification for the Use of Statins in Prevention: an Intervention Trial Evaluating Rosuvastatin) trial.

Background.—The safety and magnitude of cardiovascular risk reduction conferred by treatment to LDL-C levels below current recommended targets remain uncertain.

Methods.—A cohort of 17,802 apparently healthy men and women with high-sensitivity C-reactive protein ≥2 mg/l and LDL-C <130 mg/dl were randomly allocated to rosuvastatin 20 mg daily or placebo, and followed up for allcause mortality, major cardiovascular events, and adverse events. In a post-hoc analysis, participants allocated to rosuvastatin were categorized as to whether or not they had a follow-up LDL-C level <50 mg/dl.

Results.—During a median follow-up of 2 years (range up to 5 years), rates of the primary trial endpoint were 1.18, 0.86, and 0.44 per 100 person-years in the placebo group (n = 8,150) and rosuvastatin groups without LDL-C <50 mg/dl (n = 4,000) or with LDL-C <50 mg/dl (n = 4,154), respectively (fully-adjusted hazard ratio: 0.76; 95% confidence interval: 0.57 to 1.00 for subjects with no LDL-C <50 mg/dl vs. placebo and 0.35, 95% confidence interval: 0.25 to 0.49 for subjects attaining LDL-C <50 mg/dl; p for trend <0.0001). For all-cause mortality, corresponding event rates were 0.67, 0.65, and 0.39 (p for trend = 0.004). Rates of myalgia, muscle weakness, neuropsychiatric conditions, cancer, and diabetes mellitus were not significantly different among rosuvastatin-allocated participants with and without LDL-C <50 mg/dl.

Conclusions.—Among adults with LDL-C <130 mg/dl and high-sensitivity C-reactive protein ≥2 mg/l, rosuvastatin-allocated participants attaining LDL-C <50 mg/dl had a lower risk of cardiovascular events without a systematic increase in reported adverse events (Figs 2 and 3).

▶ There are lingering concerns over how low-density lipoprotein cholesterol (LDL-C) can be safely reduced. In addition, as LDL-C gets very low (< 70 mg/dL), the relationship between LDL-C and risk for cardiovascular events becomes more curvilinear with potentially less and less risk reduction per milligram per deciliter decrease in this lipoprotein. In both the Pravastatin

Or atorVastatin Evaluation and Infection Trial[1] and Treating to New Targets trial,[2] lower LDL-C level attainment correlated with improved risk reduction. In the Justification for the Use of Statins in Primary Prevention: An Intervention Trial Evaluating Rosuvastatin trial, a mean attained LDL-C of 55 mg/dL was found to be both safe and efficacious relative to placebo.[3] In this investigation by Hsia et al, a post hoc analysis of event rates was performed among subjects attaining an LDL-C < 50 mg/dL or LDL-C > 50 mg/dL with rosuvastatin compared with placebo. The patients who attained LDL-C < 50 mg/dL clearly had substantially lower risk for cardiovascular events and mortality compared with LDL > 50 mg/dL or placebo (Fig 2). Compared with placebo, LDL-C > 50 mg/dL and < 50 mg/dL were associated with statistically highly significant reductions in the primary composite end point of 24% and 65%, respectively. Compared with both placebo and attained LDL-C > 50 mg/dL, those patients achieving an LDL-C < 50 mg/dL experienced superior benefit in the primary composite end point across all prespecified subgroups (Fig 3). In the group with LDL-C < 50 mg/dL, all-cause mortality was significantly reduced by 46% compared with placebo. When comparing subjects in the LDL-C < 50 mg/dL group with the placebo and LDL-C > 50 mg/dL groups, there was

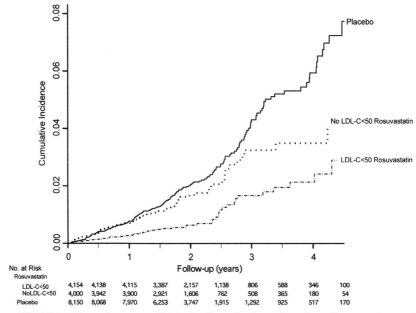

FIGURE 2.—Time to Occurrence of Major Cardiovascular Events According to Treatment Group and Achieved LDL-C Concentrations. Kaplan-Meier curves for the primary study endpoint, time to first occurrence of cardiovascular death, myocardial infarction, stroke, arterial revascularization, or hospitalized unstable angina for subjects allocated to placebo (**solid line**), rosuvastatin with no low-density lipoprotein cholesterol (LDL-C) <50 mg/dl (**dashed line**), and rosuvastatin with LDL-C <50 mg/dl (**dotted line**); p for trend <0.0001. (Reprinted from Hsia J, MacFadyen JG, Monyak J, et al. Cardiovascular event reduction and adverse events among subjects attaining low-density lipoprotein cholesterol <50 mg/dl with rosuvastatin: the JUPITER trial (Justification for the Use of Statins in Prevention: an Intervention Trial Evaluating Rosuvastatin). *J Am Coll Cardiol.* 2011;57:1666-1675, Copyright 2011, with permission from the American College of Cardiology.)

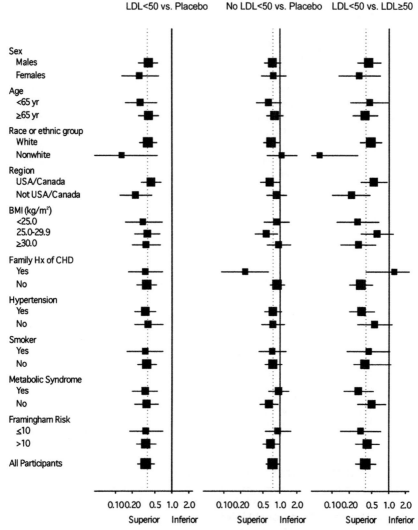

FIGURE 3.—Primary Endpoint in Pre-Specified Subgroups Within JUPITER Trial, Stratified by Achieved LDL-C. Hazard ratios and 95% confidence intervals for the primary endpoint are shown for patients without and with low-density lipoprotein cholesterol (LDL-C) <50 mg/dl compared with placebo and for rosuvastatin-allocated patients with versus without LDL-C <50 mg/dl. Among the 30 subgroups assessed, p values for interaction were all >0.05, except for family history (Hx) of premature coronary heart disease (CHD) in the rosuvastatin-allocated group without LDL <50 mg/dl versus placebo (p for interaction = 0.003) and white versus nonwhite ethnicity for rosuvastatin-allocated patients with versus without LDL-C <50 mg/dl (p for interaction = 0.03). BMI = body mass index. (Reprinted from Hsia J, MacFadyen JG, Monyak J, et al. Cardiovascular event reduction and adverse events among subjects attaining low-density lipoprotein cholesterol <50 mg/dl with rosuvastatin: the JUPITER trial (Justification for the Use of Statins in Prevention: an Intervention Trial Evaluating Rosuvastatin). *J Am Coll Cardiol.* 2011;57:1666-1675, Copyright 2011, with permission from the American College of Cardiology.)

no significant increase in risk for adverse events, including hemorrhagic stroke, new onset diabetes mellitus, myalgia, myopathy, or liver toxicity.

While these analyses are post hoc and must be considered hypothesis generating, they are most certainly consistent with the conclusion that reducing LDL-C even beyond current recommendations for very high risk patients (ie, <70 mg/dL)[4,5] is both efficacious and safe. These findings are consistent with another analysis of PROVE-IT, which showed that among patients who sustained an acute coronary syndrome, the patients with the lowest risk for recurrent events were those with an attained LDL-C of <40 mg/dL on statin therapy.[6] It would be particularly important to investigate this issue further in a prospective randomized trial in patients at highest risk for recurrent events, such as those with a history of unstable angina pectoris and previous myocardial infarction and those who undergo frequent percutaneous coronary stenting despite comprehensive risk factor goal attainment.

P. P. Toth, MD, PhD

References

1. Cannon CP, Braunwald E, McCabe CH, et al. Intensive versus moderate lipid lowering with statins after acute coronary syndromes. *N Engl J Med.* 2004;350: 1495-1504.
2. LaRosa JC, Grundy SM, Waters DD, et al. Intensive lipid lowering with atorvastatin in patients with stable coronary disease. *N Engl J Med.* 2005;352:1425-1435.
3. Ridker PM. The JUPITER trial: results, controversies, and implications for prevention. *Circ Cardiovasc Qual Outcomes.* 2009;2:279-285.
4. Grundy SM, Cleeman JI, Merz CN, et al. Implications of recent clinical trials for the National Cholesterol Education Program Adult Treatment Panel III Guidelines. *Circulation.* 2004;110:227-239.
5. Smith SC Jr, Allen J, Blair SN, et al. AHA/ACC, National Heart, Lung, and Blood Institute. AHA/ACC guidelines for secondary prevention for patients with coronary and other atherosclerotic vascular disease: 2006 update: endorsed by the National Heart, Lung, and Blood Institute. *Circulation.* 2006;113:2363-2372.
6. Wiviott SD, Cannon CP, Morrow DA, Ray KK, Pfeffer MA, Braunwald E. Can low-density lipoprotein be too low? The safety and efficacy of achieving very low low-density lipoprotein with intensive statin therapy: a PROVE it-TIMI 22 substudy. *J Am Coll Cardiol.* 2005;46:1411-1416.

Stroke and Peripheral Artery Disease

Serum Apolipoprotein AI and B Are Stronger Biomarkers of Diabetic Retinopathy Than Traditional Lipids

Sasongko MB, Wong TY, Nguyen TT, et al (Univ of Melbourne, Victoria, Australia; et al)
Diabetes Care 34:474-479, 2011

Objective.—To describe and compare the associations of serum lipoproteins and apolipoproteins with diabetic retinopathy.

Research Design and Methods.—This was a cross-sectional study of 224 diabetic patients (85 type 1 and 139 type 2) from a diabetes clinic. Diabetic retinopathy was graded from fundus photographs according to the Airlie House Classification system and categorized into mild, moderate, and vision-threatening diabetic retinopathy (VTDR). Serum traditional lipids (total, LDL, non—HDL, and HDL cholesterol and triglycerides) and apolipoprotein AI (apoAI), apolipoprotein B (apoB), and the apoB-to-apoAI ratio were assessed.

Results.—Diabetic retinopathy was present in 133 (59.4%) individuals. After adjustment for age, sex, diabetes duration, A1C, systolic blood pressure, and diabetes medications, the HDL cholesterol level was inversely associated with diabetic retinopathy (odds ratio 0.39 [95% CI 0.16—0.94], highest versus lowest quartile; $P_{trend} = 0.017$). The ApoAI level was inversely associated with diabetic retinopathy (per SD increase, 0.76 [95% CI 0.59—0.98]), whereas apoB (per SD increase, 1.31 [1.02—1.68]) and the apoB-to-apoAI ratio (per SD increase, 1.48 [1.13—1.95]) were positively associated with diabetic retinopathy. Results were similar for mild to moderate diabetic retinopathy and VTDR. Traditional lipid levels improved the area under the receiver operating curve by 1.8%, whereas apolipoproteins improved the area by 8.2%.

Conclusions.—ApoAI and apoB and the apoB-to-apoAI ratio were significantly and independently associated with diabetic retinopathy and diabetic retinopathy severity and improved the ability to discriminate diabetic retinopathy by 8%. Serum apolipoprotein levels may therefore be stronger biomarkers of diabetic retinopathy than traditional lipid measures (Table 2).

▶ Diabetic retinopathy is a severe dreaded complication of diabetes mellitus and is the principal cause of adult onset blindness worldwide. It is clear that hyperglycemia, duration of diabetes, and severity of hypertension all affect risk for retinopathy among patients with diabetes. It is well established that controlling glycemic indices and blood pressure are associated with reductions in the development and rate of progression of diabetic retinopathy. It is less clear if the levels of lipids and lipoproteins affect retinopathy development and progression. The Diabetes Control and Complications Trial suggested that such components of the lipid profile as triglycerides and high-density lipoprotein cholesterol (HDL-C) had a weak relationship to retinopathy, although the total cholesterol to HDL-C ratio and low-density lipoprotein cholesterol (LDL-C) levels did correlate with risk for macular edema and hard exudates.[1] In the Fenofibrate Intervention and Event Lowering in Diabetes trial,[2] fenofibrate therapy was associated with a 31% significant reduction in risk of needing laser photocoagulation therapy for proliferative retinopathy. Benefit emerged within 1 year but was not associated with changes in lipid levels. The impact of lipids and lipoproteins on risk for retinopathy among diabetics is an important one and warrants further investigation.

Sasongko and coworkers evaluated the relationship between risk for retinopathy and lipids and apolipoproteins (apos) in 224 patients with type 1 (85) or type 2 (139) diabetes. This was a cross-sectional study of consecutively recruited patients in a diabetes clinic. There were no significant associations between total cholesterol, non-HDL-C, LDL-C, or triglycerides and risk for retinopathy. There were, however, significant associations between HDL-C, apo

TABLE 2.—Associations of Serum Lipids with Any Diabetic Retinopathy

Serum lipids	% of Events	Model 1*	Any Retinopathy P Value	Model 2†	P Value
Cholesterol (mmol/L)					
1st quartile, <3.8	16.4	1.00		1.00	
2nd quartile, 3.8-4.5	12.8	0.91 (0.53−1.57)		0.73 (0.40−1.35)	
3rd quartile, 4.5-5.2	14.6	1.02 (0.59−1.76)		0.88 (0.47−1.66)	
4th quartile, ≥5.2	14.2	1.03 (0.60−1.78)	0.82*	0.90 (0.47−1.74)	0.89*
Per SD increase (1.1)		0.94 (0.78−1.14)	0.54	0.91 (0.72−1.14)	0.40
HDL cholesterol (mmol/L)					
1st quartile, <0.9	21.2	1.00		1.00	
2nd quartile, 0.9-1.3	16.4	0.84 (0.40−1.75)		0.80 (0.34−1.89)	
3rd quartile, 1.3-1.9	13.1	0.46 (0.22−0.95)		0.37 (0.15−0.86)	
4th quartile, ≥1.9	12.0	0.39 (0.19−0.79)	0.003*	0.39 (0.16−0.94)	0.017*
Per SD decrease (0.5)		0.84 (0.66−1.08)	0.182	0.94 (0.71−1.24)	0.44
Non−HDL cholesterol (mmol/L)					
1st quartile, <1.9	16.4	1.00		1.00	
2nd quartile, 1.9-2.4	13.1	0.68 (0.34−1.35)		0.65 (0.30−1.42)	
3rd quartile, 2.4-2.9	16.1	1.13 (0.55−2.32)		0.93 (0.42−2.06)	
4th quartile, ≥2.9	15.0	0.95 (0.47−1.92)	0.75*	0.70 (0.29−1.65)	0.61*
Per SD increase (0.8)		1.00 (0.79−1.29)	0.96	0.87 (0.65−1.18)	0.38
LDL cholesterol (mmol/L)					
1st quartile, <1.9	14.9	1.00		1.00	
2nd quartile, 1.9-2.4	18.2	1.56 (0.77−3.16)		1.20 (0.52−2.76)	
3rd quartile, 2.4-2.9	10.9	0.71 (0.34−1.46)		0.43 (0.18−1.06)	
4th quartile, ≥2.9	14.9	1.31 (0.63−2.71)	0.95*	1.07 (0.45−2.53)	0.67*
Per SD increase (0.8)		1.12 (0.86−1.46)	0.40	1.07 (0.77−1.48)	0.68
Triglyceride (mmol/L)					
1st quartile, <0.9	18.5	1.00		1.00	
2nd quartile, 0.9-1.3	13.1	1.00 (0.59−1.72)		0.91 (0.50−1.66)	
3rd quartile, 1.3-1.9	12.2	0.77 (0.45−1.31)		0.73 (0.38−1.41)	
4th quartile, ≥1.9	14.4	1.03 (0.60−1.76)	0.82*	0.90 (0.47−1.73)	0.65*
Per SD increase (1.1)		0.98 (0.81−1.20)	0.88	0.95 (0.75−1.19)	0.65
ApoAI (g/L)					
1st quartile, <0.9	19.2	1.00		1.00	
2nd quartile, 0.9-1.3	13.9	0.45 (0.25−0.82)		0.37 (0.19−0.72)	
3rd quartile, 1.3-1.9	13.7	0.39 (0.22−0.69)		0.48 (0.24−0.96)	
4th quartile, ≥1.9	10.6	0.26 (0.15−0.48)	<0.001*	0.33 (0.16−0.69)	0.015*
Per SD decrease (0.3)		0.67 (0.54−0.83)	<0.001	0.76 (0.59−0.98)	0.034
ApoB (g/L)					
1st quartile, <0.9	11.3	1.00		1.00	
2nd quartile, 0.9-1.3	15.0	1.90 (1.10−3.27)		2.10 (1.15−3.82)	
3rd quartile, 1.3-1.9	15.0	1.92 (1.14−3.31)		1.89 (1.03−3.43)	
4th quartile, ≥1.9	16.4	2.69 (1.53−4.73)	0.001*	2.69 (1.39−5.20)	0.005*
Per SD increase (0.3)		1.36 (1.10−1.54)	0.004	1.31 (1.02−1.68)	0.035
ApoB-to-apoAI ratio					
1st quartile, <0.9	11.8	1.00		1.00	
2nd quartile, 0.9-1.3	12.7	1.23 (0.72−2.09)		0.99 (0.55−1.80)	
3rd quartile, 1.3-1.9	15.3	1.86 (1.08−3.20)		1.62 (0.88−2.97)	
4th quartile, ≥1.9	17.6	2.84 (1.61−5.00)	<0.001*	2.13 (1.07−4.23)	0.017*
Per SD increase (0.2)		1.60 (1.28−2.00)	<0.001	1.48 (1.13−1.95)	0.005

Data are ORs (95% CI). Each risk factor is in separate models. Model 1: adjusted for age and sex. Model 2: model 1 plus adjusted for duration of diabetes, A1C, SBP, BMI, use of diabetic medications, lipid-lowering agents, and insulin. Age, duration of diabetes, A1C, SBP, and BMI were treated as continuous variables.

*P_{trend}.

A1, apo B, and the ratio of apo B to apo A1 (apo B:apo A). When comparing patients in the first to fourth quartile for HDL-C and apo A1, there is a 61% and 67% lower risk for retinopathy, respectively, after controlling for age, gender, duration of diabetes, hemoglobin A_{1c}, systolic blood pressure, body mass index, use of diabetic medications, lipid-lowering agents, and insulin (Table 2). When comparing patients in the first to fourth quartile for apo B and the apo B:apo A, the hazard ratio for retinopathy increases significantly by 2.69- and 2.84-fold, respectively.

It is urgent to confirm these findings in a larger cohort and to determine whether or not these relationships are valid in both type 1 and type 2 diabetes mellitus. There is also a need to better define whether or not lipid-modifying therapy beneficially affects risk for the development and progression of diabetic retinopathy. Given the finding that HDL-C and apo A1 are protective against the development of retinopathy, it would be important to determine if niacin/statin combination therapy or cholesterol ester transfer protein inhibition reduces risk of retinopathy in patients with diabetes mellitus. Because apo B and ratio of apo B to apo A1 both correlate with risk for retinopathy, it would be of value to perform a prospective clinical trial with statins in diabetics and determine whether or not these agents affect the development or course of this disease. In the meantime, fenofibrate therapy is associated with reduced need for laser photocoagulation in diabetic patients and can be considered in the setting of hypertriglyceridemia and/or low serum levels of HDL-C.

P. P. Toth, MD, PhD

References

1. Miljanovic B, Glynn RJ, Nathan DM, Manson JE, Schaumberg DA. A prospective study of serum lipids and risk of diabetic macular edema in type 1 diabetes. *Diabetes.* 2004;53:2883-2892.
2. Keech A, Simes RJ, Barter P, et al. Effects of long-term fenofibrate therapy on cardiovascular events in 9795 people with type 2 diabetes mellitus (the FIELD study): randomised controlled trial. *Lancet.* 2005;366:1849-1861.

3 Obesity

Introduction

This year, our obesity section documents the progress that has been made in obesity research on all fronts: etiology, comorbidities, medical treatment, surgical treatment, and a new field—metabolic and bariatric surgery—to treat obesity and type 2 diabetes mellitus.

Obesity is a disease and can be considered as a state of chronic low-grade inflammation that can lead to cardiovascular disease, type 2 diabetes, obstructive sleep apnea, and a myriad of other disorders. The inflammation has been localized to the adipose cell and surroundings, heralded by the macrophage crown-like structure (CLS), and it has been shown to be affected positively by treatments including diet, exercise, and surgery.

The etiology of the high prevalence of obesity in the current environment has been the subject of intense scrutiny, and the prevailing yet largely unproven causes include high availability of calorically dense and nutrient-poor food. However, the dramatic increase in childhood obesity prevalence suggests that this environmental interaction has exponential influence in the earliest years of life. Research continues to investigate interactions between the environment and early and even fetal stages of life.

Among some of the purported causes of obesity, ambient temperature, added ingredients to the food supply, and lack of sleep have been among the most intriguing. Those who sleep on average less than others seem to have higher body mass index, and alterations in stress and cortisol production may be the culprits.

There is a dearth of pharmaceutical products for obesity treatment, but the landscape is rich with promise. Harnessing the potential of beneficial enzymes and peptides is one avenue of development, such as alpha lipoic acid. Other avenues include gut hormone manipulation and development of ways to increase fatty acid oxidation at the adipose tissue level.

Surgical procedures such as the Roux-en-Y gastric bypass and the laparoscopic adjustable gastric band are increasing in popularity and continue to exhibit decreases in morbidity and mortality rates as surgeons become more familiar with performing the procedures. The concept of metabolic surgery as a treatment for obesity and type 2 diabetes mellitus is growing in acceptance as evidence continues to mount that the gut is a major organ of glycemic control, not only because of the pancreas but also because of the intestinal secretion of gut hormones that signal satiety and induce pancreatic secretion of insulin. Mimicking the action of these hormones may allow the emergence of a pharmacotherapeutic option for what is becoming known as a "medical gastric bypass." This would most likely take the form of a combination of drugs that could include leptin, a GLP-1 agonist, and an appetite suppressant. It is becoming clear that a single drug treatment will not maintain a lowered body set point and that several pathways to the appetite and satiety centers in the hypothalamus need to be modulated to achieve this goal.

The burden of obesity has become a global problem in developing and developed nations, and the associated comorbidities place an enormous strain on health care resources. The sequelae of type 2 diabetes and cardiovascular disease are the most potent causes of mortality in this society and are directly related to diet and lack of physical activity. It is imperative that we find multidiscipline preventative and treatment strategies for this worldwide epidemic. While it is true that increasing energy expenditure through a more active lifestyle in and out of the work environment would do much to reverse the obesity epidemic and that healthier food such as fresh fruits and vegetables should replace the processed foods we are consuming now for the same reason, this is easier to proclaim than to implement nationally and globally.

We are in dire need of strategies to combat the rising obesity epidemic that is affecting adults and children around the world. Continued efforts to develop preventive measures and treatment modalities should be the focus of research to address the leading cause of morbidity and mortality of the 21st century.

Caroline M. Apovian, MD

Diet and Obesity

Sustained improvement in mild obstructive sleep apnea after a diet- and physical activity–based lifestyle intervention: postinterventional follow-up
Tuomilehto H, for the Kuopio Sleep Apnea Group (Univ of Eastern Finland, Kuopio, Finland; et al)
Am J Clin Nutr 92:688-696, 2010

Background.—Obesity is the most important risk factor for obstructive sleep apnea (OSA). Weight-reduction programs have been observed to represent effective treatment of overweight patients with OSA. However, it is not known whether beneficial changes remain after the end of the intervention.

Objective.—The aim of the study was to assess the long-term efficacy of a lifestyle intervention based on a healthy diet and physical activity in a randomized, controlled, 2-y postintervention follow-up in OSA patients.

Design.—Eighty-one consecutive overweight [body mass index (in kg/m^2): 28–40] adult patients with mild OSA were recruited. The intervention group completed a 1-y lifestyle modification regimen that included an early 12-wk weight-reduction program with a very-lowcalorie diet. The control group received routine lifestyle counseling. During the second year, no dietary counseling was offered. Change in the apnea-hypopnea index (AHI) was the main objective outcome variable, and changes in symptoms were used as a subjective measurement.

Results.—A total of 71 patients completed the 2-y follow-up. The mean (± SD) changes in diet and lifestyle with simultaneous weight reduction (−7.3 ± 6.5 kg) in the intervention group reflected sustained improvements in findings and symptoms of OSA. After 2 y, the reduction in the AHI was significantly greater in the intervention group ($P = 0.049$). The intervention lowered the risk of OSA at follow-up; the adjusted odds ratio for OSA was 0.35 (95% CI: 0.12−0.97; $P = 0.045$).

Conclusion.—Favorable changes achieved by a 1-y lifestyle intervention aimed at weight reduction with a healthy diet and physical activity were sustained in overweight patients with mild OSA after the termination of supervised lifestyle counseling. This trial was registered at clinicaltrials.gov as NCT00486746.

▶ Obstructive sleep apnea (OSA) is characterized by repeated episodes of apnea and hypopnea during sleep. It is associated with insulin resistance, type 2 diabetes mellitus, and cardiovascular morbidity and mortality. Obesity is the most important risk factor predisposing for OSA. OSA perpetuates obesity possibly through hormonal changes because of stress caused by hypoxemia and inflammation.[1,2] Although the increased risk of cardiovascular disease is mainly encountered in patients with more severe OSA, patients with mild OSA (apnea-hypopnea index [AHI] between 5 and 15 events/h) are also at increased risk. Weight loss has been shown to improve OSA, therefore, lifestyle changes are an integral part of therapy in overweight/obese patients with OSA.[3]

Tuomilehto et al investigated whether the beneficial effect of weight loss on OSA persists 1 year after the end of a 1 year lifestyle intervention study. This study reports the 2-year follow-up study of overweight/obese patients with mild OSA initially randomized to 12-week very-low-calorie diet followed by intensive lifestyle changes for 1 year, while the control group received routine dietary counseling. After 1 year no dietary counseling was offered to either group, and the main outcome was change in AHI in both groups. After 2 years, the study group lost 7.3 ± 6.5 kg and the control group lost 2.4 ± 2.1 kg ($P = .09$). The change in body mass index and waist circumference was statistically significant in the intervention group. Although the intervention group gained some of the weight lost through the lifestyle intervention at the follow-up, they still had a 65% reduced risk of OSA and a 50% decrease in the progression of the disease compared with the control group. The beneficial effect of weight loss on OSA was also observed in patients of the control group that succeeded to lose weight.

This study was able to show a sustained beneficial effect of weight loss in patients with OSA 1 year after the cessation of the active intervention. Because obesity is a risk factor not only for OSA but also for type 2 diabetes and cardiovascular disease, weight loss has beneficial effects well beyond improvement in respiratory function. This study emphasizes the value of weight loss also as primary therapy for mild OSA.

R. Ness-Abramof, MD

References

1. Vgontzas AN. Does obesity play a major role in the pathogenesis of sleep apnoea and its associated manifestations via inflammation, visceral adiposity, and insulin resistance? *Arch Physiol Biochem.* 2008;114:211-223.
2. Trakada G, Chrousos G, Pejovic S, Vgontzas A. Sleep Apnea and its association with the Stress System, Inflammation, Insulin Resistance and Visceral Obesity. *Sleep Med Clin.* 2007;2:251-261.
3. Foster GD, Borradaile KE, Sanders MH, et al. Sleep AHEAD Research Group of Look AHEAD Research Group. A randomized study on the effect of weight loss on obstructive sleep apnea among obese patients with type 2 diabetes: the Sleep AHEAD study. *Arch Intern Med.* 2009;169:1619-1626.

Nutrition in infancy and long-term risk of obesity: evidence from 2 randomized controlled trials
Singhal A, Kennedy K, Lanigan J, et al (Univ College London, UK; et al)
Am J Clin Nutr 92:1133-1144, 2010

Background.—Growth acceleration as a consequence of relative over-nutrition in infancy has been suggested to increase the risk of later obesity. However, few studies have investigated this association by using an experimental study design.

Objective.—We investigated the effect of early growth promotion on later body composition in 2 studies of infants born small for gestational age (weight <10th percentile in study 1 and <20th percentile in study 2).

Design.—We reviewed a subset of children ($n = 153$ of 299 in study 1 and 90 of 246 in study 2) randomly assigned at birth to receive either a control formula or a nutrient-enriched formula (which contained 28–43% more protein and 6–12% more energy than the control formula) at 5–8 y of age. Fat mass was measured by using bioelectric impedance analysis in study 1 and deuterium dilution in study 2.

Results.—Fat mass was lower in children assigned to receive the control formula than in children assigned to receive the nutrient-enriched formula in both trials [mean (95% CI) difference for fat mass after adjustment for sex: study 1: -38% (-67%, -10%), $P = 0.009$; study 2: -18% (-36%, -0.3%), $P = 0.04$]. In nonrandomized analyses, faster weight gain in infancy was associated with greater fat mass in childhood.

Conclusions.—In 2 prospective randomized trials, we showed that a nutrient-enriched diet in infancy increased fat mass later in childhood. These experimental data support a causal link between faster early weight gain and a later risk of obesity, have important implications for the management of infants born small for gestational age, and suggest that the primary prevention of obesity could begin in infancy.

▶ Early nutrition and infant growth are purported to influence obesity risk in adolescence and adulthood. Observational studies have reported that early nutrition practices and rapid growth predispose infants to later obesity development and greater adiposity.[1,2] This evidence emphasizes the need for prospective randomized intervention studies to examine the nutritional factors that set the stage for long-term chronic disease risk.

In the present article, Singhal et al report the first causal association that nutrient exposure in infancy directly leads to increased adiposity in later childhood. Two cohorts of term infants that were small for gestational age (< 10th percentile for study 1 and < 20th percentile for study 2) were randomized to receive either standard formula or a nutrient-enriched formula. The initial objective of this study was to improve infant growth and development with the use of a nutrient-enriched formula. However, the authors observed that infants fed the nutrient-enriched formula grew faster and gained more adipose tissue at 5 to 8 years follow-up relative to standard formula. Strikingly, children that received the nutrient-enriched formula had 22% to 38% greater adiposity than standard formula as assessed by direct skin fold measures or bioelectric impedance analysis. This difference held true after adjusting for sex, height in childhood, maternal body mass index, body weight z score, and socioeconomic status. Thus, the authors were able to conclude for the first time that early nutrition and growth contribute to obesity risk independent of genetic factors.

This was a well-designed and controlled prospective randomized study. A few limitations were acknowledged that limit the interpretation of the findings, as well as point to areas that are important for future investigation. The infants in this study were term but small for gestational age, which prevents extrapolation to infants with normal or above-normal birth weights or preterm infants. Although it is likely that similar findings may be observed in these infant populations, future studies should be directed at establishing the effects of infant nutrition on obesity risk. Another limitation of this investigation is that the nutrient-enriched formulas were greater not only in calories but also in protein (28%-48% more), trace elements, minerals, and vitamins relative to the standard formula. This restricts our ability to discern which individual nutrients or calories alone may promote later adiposity development. Nonetheless, Singhal et al clearly demonstrate that a formula designed to facilitate early rapid growth contributes significantly to later increased adiposity.

Strategies to combat obesity in adulthood have proven to be challenging and disappointingly unsuccessful. This article provides persuasive evidence that early nutrition intervention and infant weight gain contribute significantly to later adiposity. Based on the results of this study, the authors suggest that approximately 20% of the population risk of being overweight in childhood in a Western society may be ascribed to early nutrition. Thus, this study underscores the importance of understanding early factors that contribute to obesity risk, particularly given the challenges in treating this disease in later life.

M. R. Ruth, PhD

References

1. Owen CG, Martin RM, Whincup PH, Smith GD, Cook DG. Effect of infant feeding on the risk of obesity across the life course: a quantitative review of published evidence. *Pediatrics.* 2005;115:1367-1377.
2. Dietz WH. Critical periods in childhood for the development of obesity. *Am J Clin Nutr.* 1994;59:955-959.

Insufficient Sleep Undermines Dietary Efforts to Reduce Adiposity
Nedeltcheva AV, Kilkus JM, Imperial J, et al (The Univ of Chicago, IL; Univ of Wisconsin, Madison)
Ann Intern Med 153:435-441, 2010

Background.—Sleep loss can modify energy intake and expenditure.

Objective.—To determine whether sleep restriction attenuates the effect of a reduced-calorie diet on excess adiposity.

Design.—Randomized, 2-period, 2-condition crossover study.

Setting.—University clinical research center and sleep laboratory.

Patients.—10 overweight nonsmoking adults (3 women and 7 men) with a mean age of 41 years (SD, 5) and a mean body mass index of 27.4 kg/m^2 (SD, 2.0).

Intervention.—14 days of moderate caloric restriction with 8.5 or 5.5 hours of nighttime sleep opportunity.

Measurements.—The primary measure was loss of fat and fat-free body mass. Secondary measures were changes in substrate utilization, energy expenditure, hunger, and 24-hour metabolic hormone concentrations.

Results.—Sleep curtailment decreased the proportion of weight lost as fat by 55% (1.4 vs. 0.6 kg with 8.5 vs. 5.5 hours of sleep opportunity, respectively; $P = 0.043$) and increased the loss of fat-free body mass by 60% (1.5 vs. 2.4 kg; $P = 0.002$). This was accompanied by markers of enhanced neuroendocrine adaptation to caloric restriction, increased hunger, and a shift in relative substrate utilization toward oxidation of less fat.

Limitation.—The nature of the study limited its duration and sample size.

Conclusion.—The amount of human sleep contributes to the maintenance of fat-free body mass at times of decreased energy intake. Lack of sufficient sleep may compromise the efficacy of typical dietary interventions for weight loss and related metabolic risk reduction.

▶ Sleep restriction and obesity are both linked to the modern way of living. Epidemiological studies have shown that short sleep duration is associated with obesity in children and adults.[1] Possible mechanism by which sleep deprivation may promote weight gain includes increase in appetite because of changes in orexigenic hormones (increase in ghrelin and decrease of leptin levels)[2] and increased food intake to fight fatigue or cope with stress among other possible mechanisms. The question remains whether short sleep is the cause or correlates with obesity. Short-term studies have shown an increase

Chapter 3—Obesity / **89**

in hunger in adults deprived of sleep, but the effect of sleep deprivation on weight loss has not been well studied.

Nedeltcheva and colleagues investigated whether sleep restriction attenuates the effect of a reduced-calorie diet on adiposity. They recruited 10 overweight adults who had a normal sleep duration (slept between 6.5-8.5 hours per day). The patients were randomly assigned to sleep 5.5 hours or 8.5 hours and caloric restriction (90% of the resting metabolic rate) during 14 days. Sleep deprivation decreased the proportion of weight loss as fat by 55% and increased the loss of fat-free mass by 60% (Fig 2 in the original article). Sleep-deprived patients were hungrier and had less fat oxidation. In this study, sleep restriction was not accompanied by an increase in cortisol, serum triiodothyronine, free thyroxine, and plasma catecholamines. Leptin levels were similar between groups.

The main limitation of the study is the small number of patients and the wide range of total body expenditure between the 2 sleep conditions. The main question is whether sleep-deprived obese subjects will improve fat loss by increasing sleep duration. This study suggests that recommendation for lifestyle changes to induce weight loss should include a good night's sleep.

R. Ness-Abramof, MD

References

1. Cappuccio FP, Taggart FM, Kandala NB, et al. Meta-analysis of short sleep duration and obesity in children and adults. *Sleep.* 2008;31:619-626.
2. Taheri S, Lin L, Austin D, Young T, Mignot E. Short sleep duration is associated with reduced leptin, elevated ghrelin, and increased body mass index. *PLoS Med.* 2004;1:e62.

Effect of Caloric Restriction with and without Exercise on Metabolic Intermediates in Nonobese Men and Women

Redman LM, Huffman KM, Landerman LR, et al (Pennington Biomed Res Ctr, Baton Rouge, LA; Veterans Affairs Med Ctr, Durham, NC; Duke Univ Med Ctr, Durham, NC)

J Clin Endocrinol Metab 96:E312-E321, 2011

Objectives.—The objective of the study was to evaluate whether serum concentrations of metabolic intermediates are related to adiposity and insulin sensitivity (Si) in overweight healthy subjects and compare changes in metabolic intermediates with similar weight loss achieved by diet only or diet plus exercise.

Design.—This was a randomized controlled trial.

Participants and Intervention.—The cross-sectional study included 46 (aged 36.8 ± 1.0 yr) overweight (body mass index 27.8 ± 0.7 kg/m^2) subjects enrolled in a 6-month study of calorie restriction. To determine the effect of diet only or diet plus exercise on metabolic intermediates, 35 subjects were randomized to control (energy intake at 100% of energy requirements); CR (25% calorie restriction), or CR+EX: (12.5% CR plus 12.5% increase in energy expenditure by exercise).

Main Outcome Measures.—Serum concentrations of eight fatty acids, 15 amino acids, and 45 acylcarnitines (ACs) measured by targeted mass spectrometry.

Results.—In overweight subjects, the concentrations of C2 AC and long-chain ACs were positively associated with percent fat ($R^2 = 0.75$, $P = 0.0001$) and Si ($R^2 = 0.12$, $P = 0.05$). The percent fat ($R^2 = 0.77$, $P < 0.0001$), abdominal visceral fat ($R^2 = 0.64$, $P < 0.0001$), and intrahepatic fat ($R^2 = 0.30$, $P = 0.0002$) were positively associated with fatty acid concentrations. There was a significant increase in an AC factor (comprised of C2 and several medium chain ACs) in the CR group ($P = 0.01$).

Conclusion.—In nonobese subjects, fasted serum ACs are associated with Si and fat mass. Despite similar weight loss, serum ACs increase with CR alone but not CR+EX. A greater improvement in Si with weight loss during CR+EX interventions may be related to improved coupling of β-oxidation and tricarboxylic acid cycle flux induced by exercise.

▶ Comprehensive Assessment of the Long-Term Effect of Reducing Intake of Energy (phase 1) is a study designed to evaluate the health benefits of caloric restriction (CR) with and without exercise in sedentary, nonobese, healthy individuals. Patients were randomized to a weight maintenance diet, 25% or 12.5% CR and 12.5% energy expenditure as aerobic exercise.[1] Metabolic changes such as improved insulin sensitivity, an adaptive decrease in metabolic rate, and lowering of the 10-year estimated cardiovascular risk were observed in this study.

CR is associated with longevity.[2] It is not clear what is the mechanism by which CR promotes its beneficial effect. It is possible that it is mediated through improvement in insulin sensitivity, energy metabolism, or neuro-hormonal changes. This study was designed to investigate the mechanism by which CR improved insulin resistance and could prevent diseases of aging. Redman et al measured concentrations of eight fatty acids, 15 amino acids, and 45 acylcarnitines (ACs) before and after the intervention and its correlation to insulin sensitivity. Changes in body weight, abdominal visceral fat, and whole-body fat mass were similar between the CR and CR exercise group, but insulin sensitivity was increased by 66% after CR and exercise compared with an increase of 40% after CR alone. This finding can be explained by a more complete fat oxidation in the exercise group. Another important finding is that in spite of similar weight loss, serum AC increased with CR but not with CR and exercise (Fig 1 in the original aricle), another finding that could be explained by better β-oxidation.

R. Ness-Abramof, MD

References

1. Lefevre M, Redman LM, Heilbronn LK, et al. Caloric restriction alone and with exercise improves CVD risk in healthy non-obese individuals. *Atherosclerosis.* 2009;203:206-213.
2. Mehta LH, Roth GS. Caloric restriction and longevity: the science and the ascetic experience. *Ann N Y Acad Sci.* 2009;1172:28-33.

New Developments in Obesity

Dietary intervention-induced weight loss decreases macrophage content in adipose tissue of obese women

Kováčiková M, Sengenes C, Kováčová Z, et al (Franco-Czech Laboratory for Clinical Res on Obesity, Prague, France; Rangueil Inst of Molecular Medicine, Toulouse, France; et al)
Int J Obes 35:91-98, 2011

Objective.—Accumulation of adipose tissue macrophages (ATMs) is observed in obesity and may participate in the development of insulin resistance and obesity-related complications. The aim of our study was to investigate the effect of long-term dietary intervention on ATM content in human adipose tissue.

Design.—We performed a multi-phase longitudinal study.

Subjects and Measurements.—A total of 27 obese pre-menopausal women (age 39 ± 2 years, body mass index $33.7 \pm 0.5 \, \text{kg m}^{-2}$) underwent a 6-month dietary intervention consisting of two periods: 4 weeks of very low-calorie diet (VLCD) followed by weight stabilization composed of 2 months of low-calorie diet and 3 to 4 months of weight maintenance diet. At baseline and at the end of each dietary period, samples of subcutaneous adipose tissue (SAT) were obtained by needle biopsy and blood samples were drawn. ATMs were determined by flow cytometry using combinations of cell surface markers. Selected cytokine and chemokine plasma levels were measured using enzyme-linked immunosorbent assay. In addition, in a subgroup of 16 subjects, gene expression profiling of macrophage markers in SAT was performed using real-time PCR.

Results.—Dietary intervention led to a significant decrease in body weight, plasma insulin and C-reactive protein levels. After VLCD, ATM content defined by CD45+/14+/206+ did not change, whereas it decreased at the end of the intervention. This decrease was associated with a down-regulation of macrophage marker mRNA levels (CD14, CD163, CD68 and LYVE-1 (lymphatic vessel endothelial hyaluronan receptor-1)) and plasma levels of monocyte-chemoattractant protein-1 (MCP-1) and CXCL5 (chemokine (C-X-C motif) ligand 5). During the whole dietary intervention, the proportion of two ATM subpopulations distinguished by the CD16 marker was not changed.

Conclusion.—A 6-month weight-reducing dietary intervention, but not VLCD, promotes a decrease in the number of the whole ATM population with no change in the relative distribution of ATM subsets.

▶ This article highlights the revisiting of an old technique in obesity research: the sampling of subcutaneous adipose tissue for the purpose of obtaining information on the alteration of cardiovascular risk and inflammation. These authors tested 27 obese women before, during, and after an intervention of diet with biopsy and blood samples obtained. Adipose tissue macrophages (ATMs) have been shown to be present in animal models and human studies of obesity in fat tissue and herald inflammation, which has been correlated with novel inflammatory markers in blood as well as insulin resistance. This group obtained fat tissue before and after dietary intervention to show whether or not this changed ATM population. ATM population was measured by flow cytometry using cell surface markers. This study showed that 4 weeks of a very low-calorie diet did not change the number of ATMs but that a 6-month weight reducing dietary intervention did see a decrease in the number of whole ATMs. This article is important because it is the first time that a specific intervention of diet has been shown to change macrophage number and show a time scale for this occurrence. Therefore, this study provides evidence that ATM number in obese women is *not* changed after a short-term calorie restriction with weight loss but *is* decreased after a longer 6-month period that includes weight maintenance. The study also looked at type of macrophages and found that there was no change in macrophage phenotype after the 2 phases of dietary intervention. Longer studies will likely need to be performed to see if this does change after longer weight maintenance periods. There is still much to be learned about alteration of macrophage number and type after weight loss and weight maintenance. For example, it is unknown whether or not this change after weight loss is accompanied by equally weighted changes in risk factors or whether these macrophage changes are not temporally related to blood risk factors. The larger question is also still unanswered, that is, what stimuli initiate the proliferation of macrophages into adipose tissue. This is the beginning of much literature regarding adipose tissue inflammation in 2011.

C. Apovian, MD

Downregulation of Adipose Tissue Fatty Acid Trafficking in Obesity: A Driver for Ectopic Fat Deposition?

McQuaid SE, Hodson L, Neville MJ, et al (Univ of Oxford, UK)
Diabetes 60:47-55, 2011

Objective.—Lipotoxicity and ectopic fat deposition reduce insulin signaling. It is not clear whether excess fat deposition in nonadipose tissue arises from excessive fatty acid delivery from adipose tissue or from impaired adipose tissue storage of ingested fat.

Research Design and Methods.—To investigate this we used a whole-body integrative physiological approach with multiple and simultaneous stable-isotope fatty acid tracers to assess delivery and transport of endogenous and exogenous fatty acid in adipose tissue over a diurnal cycle in lean ($n = 9$) and abdominally obese men ($n = 10$).

Results.—Abdominally obese men had substantially (2.5-fold) greater adipose tissue mass than lean control subjects, but the rates of delivery of nonesterified fatty acids (NEFA) were downregulated, resulting in normal systemic NEFA concentrations over a 24-h period. However, adipose tissue fat storage after meals was substantially depressed in the obese men. This was especially so for chylomicron-derived fatty acids, representing the direct storage pathway for dietary fat. Adipose tissue from the obese men showed a transcriptional signature consistent with this impaired fat storage function.

Conclusions.—Enlargement of adipose tissue mass leads to an appropriate downregulation of systemic NEFA delivery with maintained plasma NEFA concentrations. However the implicit reduction in adipose tissue fatty acid uptake goes beyond this and shows a maladaptive response with a severely impaired pathway for direct dietary fat storage. This adipose tissue response to obesity may provide the pathophysiological basis for ectopic fat deposition and lipotoxicity.

▶ Ectopic fat deposition or the distribution of fat to nonadipose tissue organs may contribute significantly to the development and onset of cardiometabolic disease, including insulin resistance and cardiovascular disease.[1] Adipose tissue acts as an energy sink during periods of energy excess, and it has been proposed that when this depot is no longer able to efficiently uptake fat, lipid is deposited in nonadipose organs such as the liver and heart. However, the mechanisms leading to ectopic fat deposition are not completely understood.

McQuaid et al conducted an eloquent study investigating the metabolic fate of dietary fat in abdominally obese men to better understand if ectopic fat deposition arises from greater secretion of fatty acids or reduced storage of dietary fat in adipose tissue. The authors observed downregulation of 11 genes involved in fatty acid trafficking in subcutaneous adipose tissue, indicating impairment in the movement of fatty acids into and out of adipose tissue in the obese state. With the use of stable isotope tracer studies, the authors provided more concrete evidence that the movement of fat into adipose tissue is impaired. There was a significant reduction in the movement of dietary triglycerides from the periphery into subcutaneous adipose tissue in response to 3 meals over a 24-hour period. This signifies impairment in the ability to uptake fat, which the authors propose is the process driving ectopic fat deposition, particularly in the liver. The authors noted that fasting plasma concentrations of fatty acids were greater in abdominally obese men. However, there was no overall difference in diurnal levels (following 3 meals in a 24-hour period) relative to lean men, indicating that per gram adipose tissue obese individuals secrete less fatty acids.

This was a well-conducted study; however, there are a few limitations that restrict our interpretation of the findings to the general population. For example, the sample size was relatively small and was limited to men. Because of the recognized differences in adipose tissue distribution and metabolism in men compared with women, future studies should be directed at understanding fatty acid trafficking in women. In addition, although subjects were deemed to be abdominally obese, there was no measurement of subcutaneous and visceral adipose tissue depots. Moreover, adipose tissue was collected from abdominal subcutaneous adipose tissue, and, thus, the trafficking of fatty acids across visceral adipocytes cannot be gleaned from this study.

The partitioning of fat into nonadipose tissues is postulated as a contributor to the metabolic derangements present in obesity. This study presents the first evidence that impaired fatty acid uptake into subcutaneous adipose tissue may be one of the underlying mechanisms driving ectopic fat deposition in obese men. Future studies are necessary to verify these findings in a larger cohort, as well as in women.

M. R. Ruth, PhD

Reference

1. Unger RH, Clark GO, Scherer PE, Orci L. Lipid homeostasis, lipotoxicity and the metabolic syndrome. *Biochim Biophys Acta.* 2010;1801:209-214.

Pharmacological Treatment of Obesity

Effects of Alpha-Lipoic Acid on Body Weight in Obese Subjects

Koh EH, Lee WJ, Lee SA, et al (Univ of Ulsan College of Medicine, Seoul, Republic of Korea; et al)
Am J Med 124:85.e1-85.e8, 2011

Purpose.—Alpha-lipoic acid is an essential cofactor for mitochondrial respiratory enzymes that improves mitochondrial function. We previously reported that alpha-lipoic acid markedly reduced body weight gain in rodents. The purpose of this study was to determine whether alpha-lipoic acid reduces body weight in obese human subjects.

Methods.—In this randomized, double-blind, placebo-controlled, 20-week trial, 360 obese individuals (body mass index [BMI] $\geq$30 kg/m^2 or BMI 27-30 kg/m^2 plus hypertension, diabetes mellitus, or hypercholesterolemia) were randomized to alpha-lipoic acid 1200 or 1800 mg/d or placebo. The primary end point was body weight change from baseline to end point.

Results.—The 1800 mg alpha-lipoic acid group lost significantly more weight than the placebo group (2.1%; 95% confidence interval, 1.4-2.8; $P < .05$). Urticaria and itching sensation were the most common adverse events in the alpha-lipoic acid groups, but these were generally mild and transient.

Conclusion.—Alpha-lipoic acid 1800 mg/d led to a modest weight loss in obese subjects. Alpha-lipoic acid may be considered as adjunctive therapy for obesity (Fig 2).

▶ The prevalence of obesity is rapidly increasing worldwide. Lifestyle changes are the first-line therapy for the treatment of obesity, but, unfortunately, it has not proven effective, with most patients regaining the weight lost through diet. Pharmacotherapy for obesity has been disappointing. The approved medications have a modest effect on weight loss and a problematic safety profile, resulting in the withdrawal of sibutramine from the market because of increased cardiovascular risk and of rimonabant because of depressive symptoms.[1,2] It is not surprising that we are in desperate need of safe pharmacological therapies for obesity. Liraglutide is now being evaluated for the treatment of obesity after its approval as therapy for type 2 diabetes mellitus.[3]

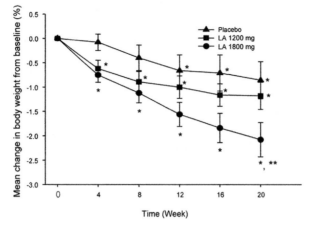

FIGURE 2.—Mean change in body weight from baseline during 20 weeks of treatment with placebo or 1200 or 1800 mg/d alpha-lipoic acid (intent-to-treat subjects). Data are reported as mean ± standard error of the mean. *$P < .05$ vs baseline for that group; **$P < .05$ vs placebo. LA = alpha-lipoic acid. (Reprinted from Koh EH, Lee WJ, Lee SA, et al. Effects of alpha-lipoic acid on body weight in obese subjects. *Am J Med.* 2011;124:85.e1-85.e8, with permission from Elsevier.)

The study by Koh and colleagues evaluated the effect of α-lipoic acid, a natural short-chain fatty acid. α-Lipoic acid is an essential cofactor that improves mitochondrial function. It was shown to reduce symptoms of diabetic neuropathy and is used worldwide. In this study, 360 overweight or obese patients were randomized to placebo, 1200 or 1800 mg/day α-lipoic acid for 20 weeks. The 1800-mg/dL group lost significantly more weight than the placebo group (Fig 2). This effect was not observed on the lower dose of 1200 mg, which is twice higher than the 600-mg dose prescribed for neuropathy in diabetic patients. Although the weight loss was small (2.1%), the relative lack of side effects (mainly urticaria and itching) make it an interesting drug that should be further evaluated for weight loss therapy, particularly in patients with type 2 diabetes mellitus.

R. Ness-Abramof, MD

References

1. James WP, Caterson ID, Coutinho W, et al. Effect of sibutramine on cardiovascular outcomes in overweight and obese subjects. *N Engl J Med.* 2010;363:905-917.
2. Topol EJ, Bousser M-G, Fox KA, et al. Rimonabant for prevention of cardiovascular events (CRESCENDO): a randomised, multicentre, placebo-controlled trial. *Lancet.* 2010;376:517-523.
3. Pratley RE, Nauck M, Bailey T, et al. Liraglutide versus sitagliptin for patients with type 2 diabetes who did not have adequate glycaemic control with metformin: a 26-week, randomised, parallel-group, open-label trial. *Lancet.* 2010;375:1447-1456.

Physical Activity and Obesity

Weight Loss, Exercise, or Both and Physical Function in Obese Older Adults

Villareal DT, Chode S, Parimi N, et al (Washington Univ School of Medicine, St Louis; et al)

N Engl J Med 364:1218-1229, 2011

Background.—Obesity exacerbates the age-related decline in physical function and causes frailty in older adults; however, the appropriate treatment for obese older adults is controversial.

Methods.—In this 1-year, randomized, controlled trial, we evaluated the independent and combined effects of weight loss and exercise in 107 adults who were 65 years of age or older and obese. Participants were randomly assigned to a control group, a weight-management (diet) group, an exercise group, or a weight-management-plus-exercise (diet—exercise) group. The primary outcome was the change in score on the modified Physical Performance Test. Secondary outcomes included other measures of frailty, body composition, bone mineral density, specific physical functions, and quality of life.

Results.—A total of 93 participants (87%) completed the study. In the intention-to-treat analysis, the score on the Physical Performance Test, in which higher scores indicate better physical status, increased more in the diet—exercise group than in the diet group or the exercise group (increases from baseline of 21% vs. 12% and 15%, respectively); the scores in all three of those groups increased more than the scores in the control group (in which the score increased by 1%) ($P<0.001$ for the between-group differences). Moreover, the peak oxygen consumption improved more in the diet-exercise group than in the diet group or the exercise group (increases of 17% vs. 10% and 8%, respectively; $P<0.001$); the score on the Functional Status Questionnaire, in which higher scores indicate better physical function, increased more in the diet—exercise group than in the diet group (increase of 10% vs. 4%, $P<0.001$). Body weight decreased by 10% in the diet group and by 9% in the diet—exercise group, but did not decrease in the exercise group or the control group ($P<0.001$). Lean body mass and bone mineral density at the hip decreased less in the diet—exercise group than in the diet group (reductions of 3% and 1%, respectively, in the diet-exercise group vs. reductions of 5% and 3%, respectively, in the diet group; $P<0.05$ for both comparisons). Strength, balance, and gait improved consistently in the diet—exercise group ($P<0.05$ for all comparisons). Adverse events included a small number of exercise-associated musculoskeletal injuries.

Conclusions.—These findings suggest that a combination of weight loss and exercise provides greater improvement in physical function than either intervention alone. (Funded by the National Institutes of Health; ClinicalTrials.gov number, NCT00146107.)

▶ Obesity is a major health problem worldwide. The prevalence of obesity is around 30% to 35% in middle-aged and older adults (> 60 years). Obesity is known to increase cardiovascular disease, type 2 diabetes, and osteoarthritis, among other diseases. The older population has a high prevalence of these comorbidities, but it is not clear whether weight loss will decrease risk factors or morbidity and mortality.[1] There is evidence that being overweight (body mass index, 25-29.9 kg/m^2) is not associated with a higher mortality rate in older people.[2] Until now, few studies addressed the effect of weight loss and exercise on cardiovascular risk factors, exercise capacity, or quality of life.

This study by Villareal et al evaluated the effect of diet or exercise alone to diet and exercise in 107 obese adults older than 65 years to a control group. The primary outcome was the change in score on the modified Physical Performance Test; secondary outcomes included frailty, bone density, body composition, physical function, and quality of life. The Physical Performance Test score increased more in the diet-and-exercise group compared with the diet-alone and exercise-alone groups. All 3 groups had better results compared with the control group. Peak oxygen consumption increased more in the diet-and-exercise group compared with the diet-alone or exercise-alone groups (Fig 2 in the original article). Weight loss was similar in the diet-and-exercise and diet-alone groups, while subjects in the exercise-alone or control groups did not lose weight (Fig 3 in the original article). Lean body mass and bone mineral density decreased less in the diet-and-exercise and exercise-alone groups. Improvement in physical function was also higher in the diet-and-exercise group.

Sarcopenia is a known risk factor for frailty in the older population. In this study, a decrease in muscle mass was observed in the diet groups; this effect was attenuated in the diet-and-exercise group.

Diet and exercise provided the greatest increase in scores on the Physical Performance Tests and also improvement in balance and strength.

The negative effects observed in this study in the diet subgroups were the reductions in muscle mass and bone density. Although this effect was attenuated by exercise, it needs to be further evaluated and, if possible, prevented.

R. Ness-Abramof, MD

References

1. Witham MD, Avenell A. Inerventions to achieve long-term weight loss in obese older people. a systematic review and meta-analysis. *Age Ageing.* 2010;39: 176-184.
2. Janssen I, Mark AE. Elevated body mass index and mortality risk in the elderly. *Obes Rev.* 2007;8:41-59.

Surgical Treatment of Obesity

Remission of Type 2 Diabetes After Gastric Bypass and Banding: Mechanisms and 2 Year Outcomes

Pournaras DJ, Osborne A, Hawkins SC, et al (Musgrove Park Hosp, Taunton, Somerset, UK; et al)
Ann Surg 252:966-971, 2010

Objective.—To investigate the rate of type 2 diabetes remission after gastric bypass and banding and establish the mechanism leading to remission of type 2 diabetes after bariatric surgery.

Summary Background Data.—Glycemic control in type 2 diabetic patients is improved after bariatric surgery.

Methods.—In study 1, 34 obese type 2 diabetic patients undergoing either gastric bypass or gastric banding were followed up for 36 months. Remission of diabetes was defined as patients not requiring hypoglycemic medication, fasting glucose below 7 mmol/L, 2 hour glucose after oral glucose tolerance test below 11.1 mmol/L, and glycated haemoglobin (HbA1c) <6%. In study 2, 41 obese type 2 diabetic patients undergoing either bypass, banding, or very low calorie diet were followed up for 42 days. Insulin resistance (HOMA-IR), insulin production, and glucagon-like peptide 1 (GLP-1) responses after a standard meal were measured.

Results.—In study 1, HbA1c as a marker of glycemic control improved by 2.9% after gastric bypass and 1.9% after gastric banding at latest follow-up ($P < 0.001$ for both groups). Despite similar weight loss, 72% (16/22) of bypass and 17% (2/12) of banding patients ($P = 0.001$) fulfilled the definition of remission at latest follow-up. In study 2, within days, only bypass patients had improved insulin resistance, insulin production, and GLP-1 responses (all $P < 0.05$).

Conclusions.—With gastric bypass, type 2 diabetes can be improved and even rapidly put into a state of remission irrespective of weight loss. Improved insulin resistance within the first week after surgery remains unexplained, but increased insulin production in the first week after surgery may be explained by the enhanced postprandial GLP-1 responses.

▶ Bariatric surgery is currently the most efficacious treatment option for sustained substantial weight loss in severely and morbidly obese individuals. Roux-en-Y gastric bypass (RYGB) is the most commonly performed bariatric surgery, followed by laparoscopic gastric banding. RYGB is increasingly recognized as a major treatment modality for morbidly obese individuals with diabetes. In fact, the 2010 Diabetes Surgery Summit consensus conference has considered the notion to designate weight loss surgery as a diabetes surgery.[1] The RYGB procedure creates a small gastric pouch that is anastomosed to the small intestine below the proximal jejunum, ultimately bypassing nutrient exposure of the duodenum and proximal jejunum.[2] Drastic immediate improvements in glucose metabolism are observed shortly after RYGB that cannot be explained entirely by caloric restriction and weight loss alone. Hence, studies have been initiated to understand the underlying mechanisms accounting for the rapid improvement in glycemic control following RYGB. It is hypothesized that rapid delivery of nutrients to the distal small bowel increases the secretion of gut hormones, including glucagon-like peptide 1 (GLP-1) and gastric inhibitory peptide. GLP-1 is secreted by the L cells of the distal small intestine, and increased plasma levels have been shown to improve glucose metabolism by increasing the secretion of insulin and reducing the secretion of glucagon.[2]

In this study under review, Pournaras et al attempted to determine the effects of RYGB and gastric banding on diabetes remission and glucose metabolism in obese patients with type 2 diabetes. The first study that was conducted determined glycemic control in bariatric surgery patients with type 2 diabetes. Similar improvements in glycated hemoglobin A_{1c} were reported between subjects with type 2 diabetes who had RYGB and gastric banding at 1-year follow-up. However, a greater proportion of RYGB patients (72%) achieved fasting glucose concentrations < 7 mmol/L compared with gastric banding patients (17%) with similar weight loss after 1 year. In addition, RYGB patients had greater and faster rates of remission of diabetes relative to gastric banding patients (Fig 2 in the original article). This provides persuasive evidence that weight loss alone does not account for the rapid improvement in glycemic control in obese patients with type 2 diabetes following RYGB.

Pournaras et al also examined the mechanisms of improved glycemic control following bariatric surgery compared with caloric restriction. One of the key strengths of this study is that the authors attempted to tease out the effects caloric deprivation induced by surgery by including a nonsurgical caloric-restricted group. However, one criticism of this approach is that the caloric-restricted group was not exposed to a surgical procedure, which limits our interpretation of the findings. Nevertheless, significant improvements in insulin resistance as assessed by homeostatic model assessment of insulin resistance were observed in patients with type 2 diabetes within 7 days of RYGB, whereas no improvements were observed in this short time frame for patients without diabetes or those who underwent gastric banding or caloric restriction (1000 kcal/d). Moreover, increased postprandial GLP-1 secretion was observed as early as 2 days postoperatively in the RYGB group. It should be noted that the authors did not report changes in GLP-1 levels for the patients who underwent gastric banding or caloric restriction. Despite the relatively small sample size (n = 5-17/group), these results suggest that the early improvements in insulin secretion and resistance observed in RYGB patients with type 2 diabetes may be because of increased GLP-1 secretion that was induced by the anatomical rearrangements of the gut.

This study provides compelling evidence that the physical rearrangements of the gut during RYGB induce early (≤7 days postoperatively) improvements in insulin resistance, which may be mediated by increased secretion of postprandial GLP-1. These findings not only improve our understanding of the importance of gut-derived hormones in early improvements in glucose homeostasis after bariatric surgery but also support potential pharmaceutical targets for the medical management of insulin resistance in obesity.

M. R. Ruth, PhD

References

1. Rubino F, Kaplan LM, Schauer PR, Cummings DE. The Diabetes Surgery Summit consensus conference: recommendations for the evaluation and use of gastrointestinal surgery to treat type 2 diabetes mellitus. *Ann Surg.* 2010;251:399-405.
2. Beckman LM, Beckman TR, Earthman CP. Changes in gastrointestinal hormones and leptin after Roux-en-Y gastric bypass procedure: a review. *J Am Diet Assoc.* 2010;110:571-584.

Diet and Gastrointestinal Bypass–Induced Weight Loss: The Roles of Ghrelin and Peptide YY

Chandarana K, Gelegen C, Karra E, et al (Univ College London, UK; et al)
Diabetes 60:810-818, 2011

Objective.—Bariatric surgery causes durable weight loss. Gut hormones are implicated in obesity pathogenesis, dietary failure, and mediating gastrointestinal bypass (GIBP) surgery weight loss. In mice, we determined the effects of diet-induced obesity (DIO), subsequent dieting, and GIBP surgery on ghrelin, peptide YY (PYY), and glucagon-like peptide-1 (GLP-1). To evaluate PYY's role in mediating weight loss post-GIBP, we undertook GIBP surgery in *PyyKO* mice.

Research Design and Methods.—Male C57BL/6 mice randomized to a high-fat diet or control diet were killed at 4-week intervals. DIO mice underwent switch to ad libitum low-fat diet (DIO-switch) or caloric restriction (CR) for 4 weeks before being killed. *PyyKO* mice and their DIO wild-type (WT) littermates underwent GIBP or sham surgery and were culled 10 days post-operatively. Fasting acyl-ghrelin, total PYY, active GLP-1 concentrations, stomach *ghrelin* expression, and colonic *Pyy* and *glucagon* expression were determined. Fasting and postprandial PYY and GLP-1 concentrations were assessed 30 days postsurgery in GIBP and sham pair-fed (sham.PF) groups.

Results.—DIO progressively reduced circulating fasting acylghrelin, PYY, and GLP-1 levels. CR and DIO-switch caused weight loss but failed to restore circulating PYY to weight-appropriate levels. After GIBP, WT mice lost weight and exhibited increased circulating fasting PYY and colonic *Pyy* and *glucagon* expression. In contrast, the acute effects of GIBP on body weight were lost in *PyyKO* mice. Fasting PYY and postprandial PYY and GLP-1 levels were increased in GIBP mice compared with sham.PF mice.

Conclusions.—PYY plays a key role in mediating the early weight loss observed post-GIBP, whereas relative PYY deficiency during dieting may compromise weight-loss attempts.

▶ Gastric bypass surgery (GBS) induces immediate and substantial weight loss in morbidly obese individuals. Caloric deprivation caused by the physical restrictions of the gut accounts for a significant proportion of the initial weight loss; however, additional factors are likely involved. A hypothesis currently under investigation suggests that changes induced by the anatomical rearrangement of the gut modify key appetite regulatory gut-derived hormones, including anorectic hormone peptide YY (PYY), ghrelin, and glucagonlike peptide 1. Batterham et al, the laboratory from which this study was produced, first established that PYY3-36 (main circulating form of PYY) reduces food intake in normal-weight and obese human subjects.[1,2] Other researchers have demonstrated that this gut hormone is also likely involved in long-term body weight regulation.[3] Higher fasting and postprandial systemic levels have been reported after Roux-en-Y GBS suggesting that PYY may contribute to surgery-induced weight loss.[3]

In the study reviewed here, Chandarana et al provide the first evidence that the anorectic hormone PYY may be directly involved in facilitating weight loss immediately following GBS. A diet-induced (high fat) obese PYY knockout (KO) mouse model was utilized to directly determine the role of PYY on surgically induced weight loss. The authors observed that wild-type obese mice that underwent enterogastro anastomosis (EGA) had higher circulating PYY levels and lost significantly more weight than PYY KO mice. Moreover, 10 days postoperatively, PYY KO mice that had EGA lost similar body weight relative to sham surgery PYY KO mice. This signifies that PYY is an essential mediator in early weight loss following GBS.

The authors clearly demonstrated, through the use of a pair-fed sham (no gut anatomical changes) group, that food restriction alone does not account for the changes in PYY observed after bypass surgery. Thus, this study presents key evidence that GBS itself modifies gut hormones, evidence that we would not be able to easily glean from human studies. Moreover, mice that underwent caloric restriction after a period of high-fat feeding had lower-than-expected PYY levels for their body weight. This implies that PYY may act against weight loss and weight loss maintenance during caloric deprivation.

One of the main limitations of the study is that it is difficult to extrapolate the results directly to humans that undergo Roux-en-Y GBS because different anatomical changes were used in the mouse model. Unlike Roux-en-Y GBS the EGA performed in animals does not bypass the stomach. Rather, nutrient passage was blocked to the duodenum by pyloric ligation, and the stomach was anastomosed to the midjejunum. Thus, as the authors recognize, the hormonal changes induced by this surgical procedure may differ from GBS in humans.

Overall, this study provides crucial insight into mechanisms of early weight loss following GBS which are distinct from caloric restriction alone. In addition to improving our knowledge of surgery-induced weight loss, this study provides evidence that PYY may be a promising therapeutic target in the treatment of obesity.

M. R. Ruth, PhD

References

1. Batterham RL, Cowley MA, Small CJ, et al. Gut hormone PYY(3-36) physiologically inhibits food intake. *Nature.* 2002;418:650-654.

2. Batterham RL, Cohen MA, Ellis SM, et al. Inhibition of food intake in obese subjects by peptide YY3—36. *N Engl J Med.* 2003;349:941-948.
3. Karra E, Batterham RL. The role of gut hormones in the regulation of body weight and energy homeostasis. *Mol Cell Endocrinol.* 2010;316:120-128.

4 Thyroid

Introduction

Many studies I have selected for the 2011 YEAR BOOK are likely to have an important impact for the practice in endocrinology but also for future research in this field. In my eyes, the following 2 articles are of major importance.

One study, published by Neumann and coworkers, described a new small-molecule antagonist that inhibits Graves' disease (GD) antibody activation of the TSH receptor. GD is caused by persistent, unregulated stimulation of thyroid cells by thyroid-stimulating antibodies (TSAbs) that activate the TSH receptor (TSHR). TSAbs, like TSH, bind primarily to the large amino-terminal ectodomain of TSHR. The authors of the present study formerly reported the first small molecule TSHR antagonist, which inhibited TSH-stimulated signaling, and the first TSHR inverse agonist, which is an antagonist that inhibits basal (or constitutive or agonist-independent) TSHR signaling in addition to TSH-stimulated signaling. In the present study, the authors optimized small-molecule TSHR ligands. They developed a better inverse agonist. This study has a major clinical implication. None of the therapies applied thus far in GD patients is pathogenesis-based. All therapies do not inhibit the production of TSAbs or TSAb activation of TSHR signaling. This type of therapy with a small molecule might be more easily titrated to achieve a euthyroid state and might be used to treat recurrences associated with antithyroid drugs and radioactive iodine.

Another important publication was that of Lam and coworkers, who investigated the role of sorafenib for the treatment of metastasized medullary thyroid cancer (MTC). In this study, MTC patients received sorafenib, a multikinase inhibitor. Of 16 patients with sporadic MTC, one achieved partial response, 87% had stable disease. The median progression-free survival was 17.9 months. Even though the response rate was quite low, sorafenib is a reasonably well-tolerated oral therapy that offers clinical benefit and may be an option for patients with sporadic metastatic MTC who are not able to participate in clinical trials.

These are just a couple examples of brilliant studies published in 2010. I hope you enjoy reading these and the other articles.

Matthias Schott, MD, PhD

Miscellaneous

A New Small-Molecule Antagonist Inhibits Graves' Disease Antibody Activation of the TSH Receptor

Neumann S, Eliseeva E, McCoy JG, et al (Natl Insts of Health, Bethesda, MD; et al)
J Clin Endocrinol Metab 96:548-554, 2011

Context.—Graves' disease (GD) is caused by persistent, unregulated stimulation of thyrocytes by thyroid-stimulating antibodies (TSAbs) that activate the TSH receptor (TSHR). We previously reported the first small-molecule antagonist of human TSHR and showed that it inhibited receptor signaling stimulated by sera from four patients with GD.

Objective.—Our objective was to develop a better TSHR antagonist and use it to determine whether inhibition of TSAb activation of TSHR is a general phenomenon.

Design.—We aimed to chemically modify a previously reported small-molecule TSHR ligand to develop a better antagonist and determine whether it inhibits TSHR signaling by 30 GD sera. TSHR signaling was measured in two *in vitro* systems: model HEK-EM293 cells stably overexpressing human TSHRs and primary cultures of human thyrocytes. TSHR signaling was measured as cAMP production and by effects on thyroid peroxidase mRNA.

Results.—We tested analogs of a previously reported small-molecule TSHR inverse agonist and selected the best NCGC00229600 for further study. In the model system, NCGC00229600 inhibited basal and TSH-stimulated cAMP production. NCGC00229600 inhibition of TSH signaling was competitive even though it did not compete for TSH binding; that is, NCGC00229600 is an allosteric inverse agonist. NCGC00229600 inhibited cAMP production by 39 ± 2.6% by all 30 GD sera tested. In primary cultures of human thyrocytes, NCGC00229600 inhibited TSHR-mediated basal and GD sera up-regulation of thyroperoxidase mRNA levels by 65 ± 2.0%.

Conclusion.—NCGC00229600, a small-molecule allosteric inverse agonist of TSHR, is a general antagonist of TSH receptor activation by TSAbs in GD patient sera.

▶ Graves disease (GD) is caused by persistent unregulated stimulation of thyroid cells by thyroid-stimulating antibodies (TSAbs) that activate the thyrotropin (TSH) receptor (TSHR). TSAbs, like TSH, bind primarily to the large aminoterminal ectodomain of TSHR. For most antibodies tested, TSAbs and TSH compete for binding to TSHR. The authors of this study previously reported the first small molecule TSHR antagonist (NIDDK/CEB-52),[1] which inhibited TSH-stimulated signaling, and the first TSHR inverse agonist (NCGC00161856),[2] which is an antagonist that inhibits basal (or constitutive or agonist independent) TSHR signaling in addition to TSH-stimulated signaling. TSHR is one of the minority of G protein—coupled receptors that exhibit easily measurable basal signaling activity in vitro. In previous reports of this group, they provided compelling evidence that these drug-like compounds bind to TSHR in its serpentine region at what is termed an allosteric site and do not compete for binding with TSH. In this study the authors optimized small molecule TSHR ligands. They developed a better inverse agonist (NCGC00229600), which is an analog of NCGC00161856. The structure of this new compound is shown in Fig 1 in the original article (right panel). It clearly shows a dose-depending decrease in TSH signaling. Importantly, the authors could also demonstrate an inhibition of thyroid peroxidase messenger RNA expression (Fig 5 in the original article).

This study has a major clinical implication. None of the therapies applied thus far in patients with GD is pathogenesis based. All therapies do not inhibit the production of TSAbs or TSAb activation of TSHR signaling. This type of therapy with a small molecule might be more easily titrated to achieve a euthyroid state and might be used to treat recurrences associated with antithyroid drugs and radioactive iodine. In the next step, studies in animal models should be initiated to show clinical effectiveness. After finishing this study and after exclusion of major side effects, a phase 1 trial could be initiated in patients with GD.

M. Schott, MD, PhD

References

1. Neumann S, Kleinau G, Costanzi S, et al. A low-molecular-weight antagonist for the human thyrotropin receptor with therapeutic potential for hyperthyroidism. *Endocrinology.* 2008;149:5945-5950.
2. Neumann S, Huang W, Eliseeva E, Titus S, Thomas CJ, Gershengorn MC. A small molecule inverse agonist for the human thyroid-stimulating hormone receptor. *Endocrinology.* 2010;151:3454-3459.

CXCL9 and CXCL11 Chemokines Modulation by Peroxisome Proliferator-Activated Receptor-α Agonists Secretion in Graves' and Normal Thyrocytes

Antonelli A, Ferrari SM, Frascerra S, et al (Univ of Pisa, School of Medicine, Italy; et al)
J Clin Endocrinol Metab 95:E413-E420, 2010

Context.—Peroxisome proliferator-activated receptor (PPAR)-α has been shown to exert immunomodulatory effects in autoimmune disorders. However, until now, no data were present in the literature about the effect of PPARα activation on CXCL9 and CXCL11 chemokines in general or on secretion of these chemokines in thyroid cells.

Objective and Design.—The presence of PPARα and PPARγ has been evaluated by real-time-PCR in Graves' disease (GD) and control cells in primary culture. Furthermore, we have tested the role of PPARα and PPARγ activation on CXCL9 and CXCL11 secretion in GD and control cells after stimulation of these chemokines secretion with IFNγ and TNFα.

Results.—This study shows the presence of PPARα and PPARγ in GD and control cells. A potent dose-dependent inhibition by PPARα-agonists was observed on the cytokines-stimulated secretion of CXCL9 and CXCL11 in GD and control cells. The potency of the PPARα agonists used was maximum on the secretion of CXCL9, reaching about 90% of inhibition by fenofibrate and 85% by ciprofibrate. The relative potency of the compounds was different with each chemokine; for example, gemfibrozil exerted a 55% inhibition on CXCL11, whereas it had a weaker activity on CXCL9 (40% inhibition). PPARα agonists were stronger (ANOVA, $P < 0.001$) inhibitors of CXCL9 and CXCL11 secretion in thyrocytes than PPARγ agonists.

Conclusions.—Our study shows the presence of PPARα in GD and control thyrocytes. PPARα activators are potent inhibitors of the secretion of CXCL9 and CXCL11, suggesting that PPARα may be involved in the modulation of the immune response in the thyroid.

▶ The peroxisome proliferator—activated receptors (PPARs) (PPARα and PPARγ) are ligand-activated nuclear receptors with a wide range of effects on metabolism, cellular proliferation, differentiation, and immune response. Irrespective of that, CXC α-chemokines (helper T-cell subtype 1 [T_H1]), especially CXCL9, CXCL10, and CXCL11, play an important role in the initial phases of autoimmune thyroid disorders. Serum CXCL10 levels are increased in Graves disease (GD), especially in patients with active disease, and the CXCL10 decrease after thyroidectomy or after radioiodine shows that it is more likely to have been produced inside the thyroid gland. PPARα has already been shown to be expressed in thyroid cells. In this article, the authors have tested the possible modulatory role of PPARα activation on the CXC chemokines CXCL9 and CXCL11 secretion in GD and control thyrocytes in primary culture. The presence of PPARα in the thyroid cells and the immunomodulatory effect of PPARα agonists on the production of T_H1 chemokines (Fig 1 in the original article) suggest that PPARα may be involved in the modulation of the immune response both in control and in GD cells, probably by interaction with endogenous ligands. A therapeutic use of PPARα ligands in thyroid autoimmunity remains to be explored, but it is suggested by the fact that their effect on chemokines has been exerted at near-therapeutic doses. If the immunomodulatory role of PPARα ligands will be confirmed in orbital fibroblasts and preadipocytes, a therapeutic use of PPARα ligands in Graves orbitopathy might be hypothesized. In conclusion, this study shows the presence of PPARα in primary normal thyrocytes such as in those from patients with GD. PPARα activators are able to inhibit the secretion of the CXCL9 and CXCL11 chemokines, suggesting that PPARα may be involved in the modulation of the immune response in the thyroid.

M. Schott, MD, PhD

Thyroid Function within the Upper Normal Range Is Associated with Reduced Bone Mineral Density and an Increased Risk of Nonvertebral Fractures in Healthy Euthyroid Postmenopausal Women
Murphy E, Glüer CC, Reid DM, et al (Imperial College London, UK; Universitätsklinikum Schleswig-Holstein, Kiel, Germany; Univ of Aberdeen, UK; et al)
J Clin Endocrinol Metab 95:3173-3181, 2010

Context.—The relationship between thyroid function and bone mineral density (BMD) is controversial. Existing studies are conflicting and confounded by differences in study design, small patient numbers, and sparse prospective data.

Objective.—We hypothesized that variation across the normal range of thyroid status in healthy postmenopausal women is associated with differences in BMD and fracture susceptibility.

Design.—The Osteoporosis and Ultrasound Study (OPUS) is a 6-yr prospective study of fracture-related factors.

Setting.—We studied a population-based cohort from five European cities.

Participants.—A total of 2374 postmenopausal women participated. Subjects with thyroid disease and nonthyroidal illness and those receiving drugs affecting thyroid status or bone metabolism were excluded, leaving a study population of 1278 healthy euthyroid postmenopausal women.

Interventions.—There were no interventions.

Main Outcome Measures.—We measured free T_4 (fT4) (picomoles/liter), free T_3 (fT3) (picomoles/liter), TSH (milliunits/liter), bone turnover markers, BMD, and vertebral, hip, and nonvertebral fractures.

Results.—Higher fT4 ($\beta = -0.091$; $P = 0.004$) and fT3 ($\beta = -0.087$; $P = 0.005$) were associated with lower BMD at the hip, and higher fT4 was associated with increasing bone loss at the hip ($\beta = -0.09$; $P = 0.015$). After adjustment for age, body mass index, and BMD, the risk of nonvertebral fracture was increased by 20% ($P = 0.002$) and 33%($P = 0.006$) in women with higher fT4 or fT3, respectively, whereas higher TSH was protective and the risk was reduced by 35% ($P = 0.028$). There were independent associations between fT3 and pulse rate ($\beta = 0.080$; $P = 0.006$), increased grip strength ($\beta = 0.171$; $P < 0.001$), and better balance ($\beta = 0.099$; $P < 0.001$), indicating that the relationship between thyroid status and fracture risk is complex.

Conclusions.—Physiological variation in normal thyroid status is related to BMD and nonvertebral fracture (Fig 2).

▶ Low bone mineral density (BMD), prior or parental history of fracture, low body mass index (BMI), use of glucocorticoids, smoking, excessive alcohol consumption, untreated thyrotoxicosis, and other factors increase susceptibility to osteoporosis. Even subclinical hyperthyroidism, defined by a suppressed thyrotropin (TSH) level in the presence of normal thyroid hormone concentrations, is associated with fracture, and treatment with T4 at doses that suppress

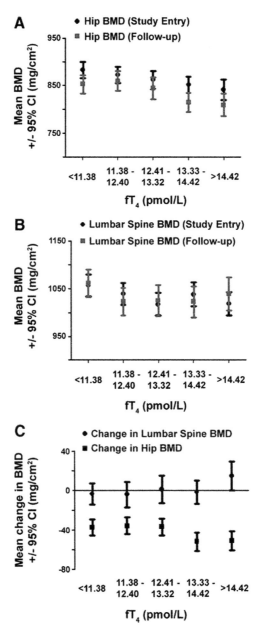

FIGURE 2.—Graphs showing hip (A) and lumbar spine (B) mean BMD ± 95% confidence interval (CI) at the time of entry into the study and after 6-yr follow-up in relation to quintiles of fT4 concentration. (C) Mean change in BMD ± 95% CI in relation to fT4. (Reprinted from Murphy E, Glüer CC, Reid DM, et al. Thyroid function within the upper normal range is associated with reduced bone mineral density and an increased risk of nonvertebral fractures in healthy euthyroid postmenopausal women. *J Clin Endocrinol Metab*. 2010;95:3173-3181, Copyright © 2010, with permission from The Endocrine Society.)

TSH is associated with increased bone turnover and low BMD in postmeno-pausal women. The prevalence of thyroid disease increases with age: 3% of women older than 50 years receive T4, and more than 20% are overtreated. Subclinical hyperthyroidism affects a further 1.5% of women older than 60 years, and its prevalence increases with age. Nevertheless, the role of thyroid hormones in the pathogenesis of osteoporosis remains uncertain. The aim of this study by Murphy et al was to investigate the correlation between the thyroid status in healthy euthyroid postmenopausal women and differences in BMD and fracture susceptibility.

The authors enrolled 566 premenopausal and 2374 postmenopausal women. In 44 cases a spine fracture was detected. As shown in Fig 2, there was no correlation between thyroid function and fracture risk of the spine. In contrast, there was an increased risk in regard to hip fractures (+20% if free T4 (fT4) was within the upper quintile and +33% if free T3 (fT3) was within the upper quintile). In contrast, a relatively high TSH level was somehow protective. These data clearly show that the effect of thyroid hormones on the bone is complex. Nonetheless, fT3 and fT4 levels within the upper normal range may already influence BMD.

M. Schott, MD, PhD

Thyroid Autoimmunity

Induction of Murine Neonatal Tolerance Against Graves' Disease Using Recombinant Adenovirus Expressing the TSH Receptor A-Subunit

Wu L, Xun L, Yang J, et al (The First Affiliated Hosp of Xi'an Jiaotong Univ School of Medicine, People's Republic of China)
Endocrinology 152:1165-1171, 2011

Graves' disease is a common organ-specific autoimmune disease. The identity of its autoantigen, the TSH receptor (TSHR), was established and used to induce a typical animal model. A-subunit, the shed portion of TSHR, either initiates or amplifies the autoimmune response of the thyroid gland, thereby causing Graves' disease in humans. In the present study, we investigate the effect of the TSHR A-subunit on the induction of murine neonatal tolerance for the development of Graves' disease. Female BALB/c mice were pretreated with different doses of adenovirus expressing the A-subunit of TSHR (Ad-TSHR289) by either ip or im injection within the first 24 h after their birth. Graves' disease was induced after the animals reached adulthood. Nearly all mice pretreated with the high dose of Ad-TSHR289 failed to develop TSHR antibodies, detected by the TSH-binding inhibition assay, hyperthyroidism, and thyroid follicular hyperplasia. The mice preimmunized im with the lower doses of Ad-TSHR289 developed a relatively low level of TSH-binding inhibition and the low incidence of hyperthyroidism. Accordingly, the percentages of splenic CD4+CD25+/CD4+ and CD25+Foxp3+/CD4+ Treg cells were increased in mice pretreated with the high dose of Ad-TSHR289. Taken together, our data strongly indicate that the immunotolerance against

Graves' disease could be induced in neonatal mice using a specific TSHR antigen in a high dose either by ip or im injection, preventing the development of Graves' disease.

▶ The thyrotropin (TSH) receptor is the main autoantigen in the development of Graves disease (GD). However, several lines of evidence indicate that the TSH receptor (TSHR) A-subunit, comprising most of the ectodomain component rather than the entire molecule, serves as the autoantigen. An improved murine model of GD was generated by repeated intramuscular (IM) injection with an adenovirus vector expressing TSHR, producing hyperthyroidism in approximately 30% to 50% of the immunized animals.[1] The aim of this study was to investigate the effect of an immunization using the TSHR A-subunit on the induction of murine neonatal tolerance for the development of GD. Female BALB/c mice were pretreated with different doses of adenovirus expressing the A-subunit of TSHR (Ad-TSHR289) by either intraperitoneal or IM injection within the first 24 hours after their birth. GD was induced after the animals reached adulthood. Nearly all mice pretreated with the high dose of Ad-TSHR289 failed to develop TSHR antibodies, detected by the TSH-binding inhibition assay, hyperthyroidism, and thyroid follicular hyperplasia. Thyroid histology is shown in Fig 4 in the original article. Importantly, this immunization regime also resulted in an induction of regulatory T cells (Fig 5B in the original article). This could be one explanation for the induction of immune tolerance in these mice. Another possibility could be that proteins encoded by a DNA vaccine is produced endogenously and expressed in the context of self-major histocompatibility complex, and therefore is recognized as self resulting in tolerance rather than immunity. This immune tolerance mouse model may help to develop a tolerogenic therapy in humans.

M. Schott, MD, PhD

Reference

1. Nagayama Y, Kita-Furuyama M, Ando T, et al. A novel murine model of Graves' hyperthyroidism with intramuscular injection of adenovirus expressing the thyrotropin receptor. *J Immunol.* 2002;168:2789-2794.

Neutral Antibodies to the TSH Receptor Are Present in Graves' Disease and Regulate Selective Signaling Cascades
Morshed SA, Ando T, Latif R, et al (James J. Peters Veterans Affairs Med Ctr, NY)
Endocrinology 151:5537-5549, 2010

TSH receptor (TSHR) antibodies (Abs) may be stimulating, blocking, or neutral in their functional influences and are found in patients with autoimmune thyroid disease, especially Graves' disease (GD). Stimulators are known to activate the thyroid epithelial cells via both Gs- and Gq-coupled signaling pathways, whereas blockers inhibit the action of

TSH and may act as weak agonists. However, TSHR neutral Abs do not block TSH binding and are unable to induce cAMP via Gsα. The importance of such neutral Abs in GD remains unclear because their functional consequence has been assumed to be zero. We hypothesized that: 1) neutral TSHR Abs are more common to GD than generally recognized; 2) they may induce distinct signaling imprints at the TSHR not seen with TSH itself; and 3) these signaling events may alter cellular function. To evaluate these hypotheses, we first confirmed the presence of neutral TSHR Abs in sera from patients with GD and then, using mouse and hamster neutral TSHR monoclonal Abs (N-mAbs) performed detailed signaling studies, including a proteomic Ab array, with rat thyrocytes (FRTL-5) as targets. This allowed us to examine a battery of signaling cascades and their downstream effectors. Neutral TSHR Abs were indeed frequently present in sera from patients with GD. Sixteen of 27 patients (59%) had detectable neutral TSHR Abs by competition assay with N-mAbs. On examining signaling cascades, we found that N-mAbs induced signal transduction, primarily via the protein kinase A II cascade. In addition to the activation of phosphatidylinositol 3K/Akt, N-mAbs, unlike TSH, had the ability to exclusively activate the mammalian target of rapamycin/p70 S6K, nuclear factor-κB, and MAPK-ERK1/2/p38α signaling cascades and their downstream effectors p90 ribosomal kinase/MAPK-interacting kinase-1/mitogen and stress-activated kinase-1 and N-mAbs activated all forms of protein kinase C isozymes. To define the downstream effector mechanisms produced by these signaling cascades, cytokine production, proliferation, and apoptosis in thyrocytes were investigated. Although N-mAbs produced less cytokines and proliferation compared with TSH, they had the distinction of inducing thyroid cell apoptosis under the experimental conditions used. When dissecting out possible mechanisms of apoptosis, we found that activation of multiple oxidative stress markers was the primary mechanism orchestrating the death signals. Therefore, using oxidative stress-induced apoptosis, N-mAbs may be capable of exacerbating the autoimmune response in GD via apoptotic cells inducing antigen-driven mechanisms. This may help explain the inflammatory nature of this common disorder.

▶ Autoantibodies to the thyrotropin receptor (TSHR) are keys to the disease process in autoimmune thyroid disease, particularly Graves disease (GD). The repertoire of TSHR antibodies (Abs) includes stimulating, blocking, and neutral varieties. Both stimulating and many blocking Abs are conformational and exert variable effects on thyrocyte growth.[1] A recent study from the same group clearly indicated, using monoclonal hamster TSHR Abs of the neutral variety, that they induced certain signaling cascades with unclear downstream effectors.[1] This study was undertaken to confirm the existence of such Abs in Graves sera and to further characterize signaling events relating to downstream effector mechanisms. These data confirmed and extended the earlier observations[1] that neutral Abs are indeed present in human GD using 3 independent immunoassays. In this article, the authors could also demonstrate that neutral TSHR Abs can induce via oxidative stress signaling mechanisms in thyrocytes

(Fig 4 in the original article). Thus, Abs directed against TSHR linear epitopes in autoimmune thyroid disease may initiate an inflammatory process by the activation of selective signaling pathways and subsequent oxidative stress—induced thyrocyte death, which may result in a chronic inflammation within the thyroid gland.

M. Schott, MD, PhD

Reference

1. Morshed SA, Latif R, Davies TF. Characterization of thyrotropin receptor antibody-induced signaling cascades. *Endocrinology.* 2009;150:519-529.

Thyrotropin Receptor-Stimulating Graves' Disease Immunoglobulins Induce Hyaluronan Synthesis by Differentiated Orbital Fibroblasts from Patients with Graves' Ophthalmopathy Not Only Via Cyclic Adenosine Monophosphate Signaling Pathways

van Zeijl CJJ, Fliers E, van Koppen CJ, et al (Univ of Amsterdam, The Netherlands; Schering-Plough Res Inst, Oss, The Netherlands)
Thyroid 21:169-176, 2011

Background.—Both expression of the thyrotropin receptor (TSHR) and the production of hyaluronan (HA) by orbital fibroblasts (OF) have been proposed to be implicated in the pathogenesis of Graves' ophthalmopathy (GO). HA is synthesized by three types of HA synthase. We hypothesized that TSHR activation by recombinant human TSH (rhTSH) and TSHR-stimulating Graves' disease immunoglobulins (GD-IgGs) via induced cyclic adenosine monophosphate (cAMP) signaling increases HA synthesis in differentiated OF from GO patients.

Methods.—Cultured human OF, obtained during decompression surgery from 17 patients with severe GO, were stimulated *in vitro* to differentiate into adipocytes. Differentiation was evaluated by phase-contrast microscopy. The differentiated OF were stimulated by rhTSH or by TSHR-stimulating GD-IgG. We measured cAMP using a biochemical assay, HA synthase mRNA expression by quantitative polymerase chain reaction, and HA in the supernatant by enzyme-linked immunosorbent assay.

Results.—All differentiated OF cultures expressed higher levels of *TSHR* mRNA than nondifferentiated OF cultures. Stimulation by rhTSH induced a marked cAMP response in 11 of 12 differentiated OF cultures, but no measurable HA response in all but one differentiated OF cultures. By contrast, stimulation by GD-IgG induced a moderate cAMP response in a number of differentiated OF cultures, but a marked HA response in the majority of differentiated OF cultures.

Conclusion.—Stimulation of differentiated OF by GD-IgG, but not by rhTSH, induces HA synthesis in the majority of patients, suggesting that in most patients TSHR-mediated cAMP signaling does not play a pivotal role in GD-IgG-induced HA synthesis in differentiated OF cultures.

▶ Orbital fibroblasts (OFs) are assumed to play a major role in the pathogenesis of Graves ophthalmopathy (GO). The aim of this study was to evaluate the effect of recombinant human thyrotropin (rhTSH) and Graves disease (GD) IgG on adenosine monophosphate (cAMP) signaling and hyaluronan (HA) synthesis in differentiated OF from patients with GO. The authors cultured human OFs that were obtained from decompression operations of 17 patients with severe GO. They could demonstrate that all differentiated OF cultures expressed higher levels of TSH receptor (TSHR) messenger RNA than nondifferentiated OF cultures. Stimulation by rhTSH induced a marked cAMP response in 11 of 12 differentiated OF cultures, but no measurable HA response in all but one differentiated OF cultures. By contrast, stimulation by GD-IgG induced a moderate cAMP response in a number of differentiated OF cultures, but a marked HA response in most differentiated OF cultures (Fig 3 in the original article). The finding that GD-IgG induces HA synthesis, despite lower GD-IgG—induced cAMP production compared with rhTSH-induced cAMP production, suggests that the TSHR-mediated cAMP response does not play a major role in GD-IgG—induced HA synthesis in differentiated GO OF. Hence, additional signaling pathways must be involved in GD-IgG—induced HA synthesis. It is possible that increased expression of TSHR in differentiated cultures is responsible for the effect of TSHR-stimulating GD-IgG on HA synthesis via activation of alternative downstream signaling pathways. In agreement with this notion is a recent study by Morshed et al showing that 3 potent stimulating TSHR-antibodies influence the intracellular extracellular signal—regulated kinases (ERK1/2) pathway in primary thyrocytes.[1] It is also possible that activation of the insulinlike growth factor 1 receptor by GD-IgG is involved in GD-IgG—induced HA synthesis, which has been suggested from other authors.

M. Schott, MD, PhD

Reference

1. Morshed SA, Latif R, Davies TF. Characterization of thyrotropin receptor antibody-induced signaling cascades. *Endocrinology.* 2009;150:519-529.

Prevalence of Parietal Cell Antibodies in a Large Cohort of Patients with Autoimmune Thyroiditis
Checchi S, Montanaro A, Ciuoli C, et al (Univ of Siena, Italy)
Thyroid 20:1385-1389, 2010

Background.—Autoimmune thyroiditis (AIT) may be associated with other organ-specific autoimmune disorders, including autoimmune gastritis, but the prevalence of this association is not entirely quantified. The aim of this study was to investigate the prevalence of parietal cell antibodies (PCA) in a large cohort of consecutive patients with AIT.

Methods.—We retrospectively studied 2016 consecutive women and 258 men with AIT seen at our referral center in the period from 2004 to 2008. All patients were screened for the presence of PCA in the serum.

Results.—The prevalence of serum PCA in female patients was 29.7% and progressively increased from 13% in the first-second decade of life to peak at 42% in the ninth decade. During follow up, 21.1% of the PCA-positive patients converted to PCA-negative status. Mean (± standard deviation) basal PCA levels in this group were significantly lower (32 ± 28 U/mL) compared with those remaining PCA positive (129 ± 200 U/mL). A similar prevalence (29.8%) with a similar age-dependency was found in male patients.

Conclusions.—In conclusion, our study demonstrates a high, age-dependent prevalence of PCA in an unselected large population of patients with AIT.

▶ Autoimmune thyroiditis (AIT) is frequently associated with other organ-specific autoimmune disorders, including autoimmune gastritis, but the prevalence of this association is not entirely quantified. The aim of this study was to investigate the prevalence of parietal cell antibodies (PCAs) in a large cohort of consecutive patients with AIT. Within a retrospective analysis the authors investigated more than 2000 patients with AIT. There was a clear age-dependent increase of PCA-positive AIT patients (Fig 2 in the original article). An interesting observation of this study is that PCA-positive patients had lower thyroid volume, higher levels of thyroperoxidase antibodies (correlated with PCA levels), and higher rate of overt or subclinical hypothyroidism, suggesting the presence of a more severe form of thyroiditis. Another important point is that nearly 20% of PCA-positive patients converted to PCA-negative status during follow-up. The reasons for this are not evident, but the observation that this subgroup of patients was the one with the lowest positive levels of PCA (compared with PCA-positive patients not converting to PCA negative) may lead to speculation that such low positive levels of PCA are not significant and may be probably considered as normal, thus increasing the cutoff between PCA-positive and PCA-negative status.

M. Schott, MD, PhD

High Rate of Persistent Hypothyroidism in a Large-Scale Prospective Study of Postpartum Thyroiditis in Southern Italy

Stagnaro-Green A, Schwartz A, Gismondi R, et al (George Washington Univ School of Medicine and Health Sciences, DC; Univ of Illinois, Chicago; Casa di Cura "Salus," Brindisi, Italy; et al)
J Clin Endocrinol Metab 96:652-657, 2011

Context.—The incidence of postpartum thyroiditis (PPT) varies widely in the literature. Limited data exist concerning the hormonal status of women with PPT at the end of the first postpartum year.

Objective.—Our aim was to conduct a large prospective study of the incidence and clinical course of PPT.

Design.—A total of 4394 women were screened for thyroid function and thyroid autoantibodies at 6 and 12 months postpartum. Women were classified as being at high or low risk of having thyroid disease before any thyroid testing.

Setting.—The study was conducted at two ambulatory clinics in southern Italy, an area of mild iodine deficiency.

Patients.—A total of 4394 pregnant women were studied.

Intervention.—There was no intervention.

Main Outcome Measures.—We measured incidence, clinical presentation, and course of postpartum thyroiditis.

Results.—The incidence of postpartum thyroiditis was 3.9% (169 of 4384). Women classified as being at high risk for thyroid disease had a higher incidence of PPT than women classified as low risk (11.1 *vs.* 1.9%; odds ratio, 6.69; 95% confidence interval, 4.63, 9.68). Eighty-two percent of the 169 women with PPT had a hypothyroid phase during the first postpartum year. At the end of the first postpartum year, 54% of the 169 women had persistent hypothyroidism.

Conclusions.—One of every 25 women in southern Italy developed PPT. Women at high risk for thyroid disease have an increased rate of PPT. The high rate of permanent hypothyroidism at 1 yr should result in a reevaluation of the widely held belief that most women with PPT are euthyroid at the end of the first postpartum year (Table 2).

▶ Postpartum thyroiditis (PPT) is the occurrence of transient thyroid hormonal abnormalities in the first year after delivery in women who were euthyroid before pregnancy. The aim of this study was to investigate the prevalence, clinical presentation, and course of PPT in a prospective cohort of patients. In this study, the incidence of PPT was 3.9%. Women classified as being at high risk

TABLE 2.—Clinical Progressions of PPT and Associated Thyroid Function Test Values at 6 and 12 Months

	Euthyroid at 6 Months		Hyperthyroid at 6 Months		Hypothyroid at 6 Months	
	Hypothyroid at 12 Months	Hyperthyroid at 12 Months	Hypothyroid at 12 Months	Euthyroid at 12 Months	Hypothyroid at 12 Months	Euthyroid at 12 Months
TSH at 6 months (median, IQR)	2.15 (1.58)	1.35 (1.88)	0.02 (0.04)	0.03 (0.05)	6.7 (1.8)[a]	5.2 (0.77)[a]
TSH at 12 months (median, IQR)	7.25 (5.5)[a]	0.04 (0.10)[a]	7.4 (6.0)[a]	2.0 (1.3)[a]	7.9 (3.8)[a]	3.05 (1.2)[a]
FT4 at 6 months	11.5 (2.3)	13.0 (1.8)	27.3 (6.3)	23.7 (4.9)	8.3 (0.69)	9.1 (0.65)
FT4 at 12 months	8.4 (0.85)[a]	17.8 (10.2)[a]	8.0 (0.93)[a]	12.8 (1.4)[a]	8.2 (0.82)[a]	10.9 (1.7)[a]
No. (%) of women with PPT with this progression	38 (22.5%)	4 (2.4%)	23 (13.6%)	27 (16.0%)	31 (18.3%)	46 (27.2%)

Values of thyroid function tests are given as means (SD), except where noted. IQR, Interquartile range.
[a]Values significantly different in paired comparisons between clinical progressions with a common 6-month thyroid status, based on Scheffé tests (for FT4) or Mann-Whitney U tests (for TSH).

for thyroid disease had a higher incidence of PPT than women classified as low risk. Of the 169 women with PPT, 82% had a hypothyroid phase during the first postpartum year. At the end of the first postpartum year, 54% of the 169 women had persistent hypothyroidism. Detailed data are given in Table 2. This study is the largest prospective cohort to evaluate the incidence, clinical presentation, and course of PPT. The most unexpected finding in this study was that slightly over 50% of all women who developed PPT remained hypothyroid at the end of the first postpartum year. Thyroid peroxidase titer in the first trimester of pregnancy in women who developed PPT was not predictive of persistent hypothyroidism at 1 year. Similar findings were noted by other authors before. It is well documented that the prevalence of permanent hypothyroidism 5 to 10 years after an episode of PPT is between 20% and 60%. Similarly, it is generally accepted that the vast majority of women with PPT are euthyroid at the end of the first postpartum year. Although there are limited data on this subject (because most PPT studies did not follow patients until 1 year postpartum), these data do not support this contention. In summary, the high prevalence of hypothyroidism at the end of the first postpartum year is noteworthy because it is a novel finding with significant clinical implications. Specifically, it will be important to evaluate thyroid function tests at 1 year postpartum in all women with PPT to identify individuals with ongoing hypothyroidism who require levothyroxine treatment.

M. Schott, MD, PhD

T. Baehring, PhD

Hypothyroidism and Thyroid Autoimmune Disease

Outcome of Very Long-Term Treatment with Antithyroid Drugs in Graves' Hyperthyroidism Associated with Graves' Orbitopathy

Elbers L, Mourits M, Wiersinga W (Univ of Amsterdam, The Netherlands)
Thyroid 21:279-283, 2011

Background.—It is still debated which treatment modality for Graves' hyperthyroidism (GH) is most appropriate when Graves' orbitopathy (GO) is present. The preference in our center has been always to continue antithyroid drugs for GH (as the block-and-replace [B-R] regimen) until all medical and/or surgical treatments for GO are concluded and the eye disease does not require any further therapy (except prescription of lubricants). This usually takes more than 2 years. The aim of this study was to evaluate the outcome of long-term B-R regimen for GH in GO patients by assessment (after discontinuation of B-R) of (a) the recurrence rate of GH and (b) the relapse rate of GO and its association with recurrent GH and/or ^{131}I therapy.

Methods.—A retrospective follow-up study was done among all patients referred to the Academic Medical Center in Amsterdam between 1995 and 2005 for GO. The inclusion criteria for the study were a history of GH and GO and a history of treatment for GH with a B-R regimen for more than 2 years. The exclusion criteria were a history of ^{131}I therapy or thyroidectomy before the end of GO treatment. A questionnaire was sent to 255 patients and returned by 114. Of these patients, 73 qualified for the study. Recurrences of GH and/or GO as indicated by returned questionnaires were checked with treating physicians.

Results.—Patients were treated with B-R for a median of 41 months (range: 24—132). The median follow-up after discontinuation of the B-R regimen was 57 months (range: 12—170). Recurrent GH occurred in 27 of the 73 study patients (37%) at a median of 3 months (range: 1—65) after withdrawal of antithyroid drug therapy. Nineteen of the 27 patients with recurrent hyperthyroidism were treated with ^{131}I therapy. A relapse of GO was not encountered in any of the 73 patients.

Conclusion.—The study suggests that long-term B-R treatment of GH in GO patients is associated with a recurrence rate of hyperthyroidism of about 37%. With the regimen employed, recurrence of hyperthyroidism and recurrence of hyperthyroidism followed by treatment with ^{131}I appears not to be a likely cause of relapse of GO. The data suggest that B-R treatment of GH until GO has become inactive and does not require any further treatment is a feasible option and does not jeopardize the improvement that occurred in GO.

▶ There is much debate on the most appropriate way to treat Graves hyperthy-roidism (GH) in the presence of moderate to severe Graves orbitopathy (GO). Each of the 3 available treatment modalities has its own advantages and disad-vantages in this setting. Treatment with antithyroid drugs appears rather neutral with respect to the course of the eye changes, but its disadvantage is the risk on recurrent hyperthyroidism and an associated flare-up of the ophthalmopathy. [131]I therapy is associated with a small but definite risk of worsening of GO; the risk is greater when the eye disease is still active. The risk of developing or worsening of eye changes after ^{131}I therapy in patients with GH with no or mild GO can be greatly diminished by a course of prednisone (eg, 0.25 mg/kg per day for 12 weeks, or even lower doses for a shorter period of time) (3,5). There is, however, no good data on the effectiveness of these rather low doses of prednisone in preventing worsening of eye changes when ^{131}I therapy is given in patients with moderate to severe and active GO. Much higher doses are likely required, and one could opt for ^{131}I therapy immediately followed by weekly intravenous methylprednisolone pulses for 3 months. The aim of this study was to investigate the outcome of GO if patients receive a block-and-replace (B-R) regimen. The authors assessed the recurrence rate of GH after withdrawal of antithyroid drugs, the treatment of recurrences, and whether this affected the course of the ophthalmopathy. Within this study, none of the patients did, in fact, require further orbital therapy, which confirms the expertise of this group. Although patient questionnaires were initially used, the responses were confirmed by contacting the specialists treating the patients if the patients were no longer being followed at the Orbital Center. Nonetheless, only about one-third of patients invited to participate were finally included. Some were excluded because their thyroid disease had been prematurely treated with radioactive iodine or thyroidectomy; presumably, none of these cases was resistant to the antithyroid drug regimen. Despite these potential drawbacks to the study, several facts support the concept that prolonged anti-thyroid treatment can reduce recurrences: (1) Graves disease will eventually burn out in many patients, (2) thyroid-stimulating immunoglobulin levels do tend to drop following treatment with antithyroid drugs (or surgery), (3) certain thionamides appear to have immunosuppressive properties, and (4) some of the risk factors for a relapse of GH are also associated with increased risk of progression of Graves ophthalmopathy (eg, smoking and goiter size). If more specific thyrotropin receptor antibodies correlate consistently with the activity of orbitopathy (1), they could prove useful in determining when to perform reconstructive orbital surgery and/or discontinue antithyroid drug therapy.

M. Schott, MD, PhD

Type 1 and type 2 iodothyronine deiodinases in the thyroid gland of patients with 3,5,3'-triiodothyronine-predominant Graves' disease

Ito M, Toyoda N, Nomura E, et al (Kuma Hosp, Kobe, Hyogo, Japan; Kansai Med Univ, Shinmachi, Hirakata City, Japan; et al)
Eur J Endocrinol 164:95-100, 2011

Objective.—3,5,3'-triiodothyronine-predominant Graves' disease (T_3-P-GD) is characterized by a persistently high serum T_3 level and normal or even lower serum thyroxine (T_4) level during antithyroid drug therapy. The source of this high serum T_3 level has not been clarified. Our objective was to evaluate the contribution of type 1 and type 2 iodothyronine deiodinase (D1 (or DIO1) and D2 (or DIO2) respectively) in the thyroid gland to the high serum T_3 level in T_3-P-GD.

Methods.—We measured the activity and mRNA level of both D1 and D2 in the thyroid tissues of patients with T_3-P-GD ($n=13$) and common-type GD (CT-GD) ($n=18$) who had been treated with methimazole up until thyroidectomy.

Results.—Thyroidal D1 activity in patients with T_3-P-GD (492.7 ± 201.3 pmol/mg prot per h) was significantly higher ($P<0.05$) than that in patients with CT-GD (320.7 ± 151.9 pmol/mg prot per h). On the other hand, thyroidal D2 activity in patients with T_3-P-GD (823.9 ± 596.4 fmol/mg prot per h) was markedly higher ($P<0.005$) than that in patients with CT-GD (194.8 ± 131.6 fmol/mg prot per h). There was a significant correlation between the thyroidal D1 activity in patients with T_3-PGD and CT-GD and the serum FT_3-to-FT_4 ratio ($r=0.370$, $P<0.05$). Moreover, there was a strong correlation between the thyroidal D2 activity in those patients and the serum FT_3-to-FT_4 ratio ($r=0.676$, $P<0.001$).

Conclusions.—Our results suggest that the increment of thyroidal deiodinase activity, namely D1 and especially D2 activities, may be responsible for the higher serum FT_3-to-FT_4 ratio in T_3-P-GD (Fig 1).

▶ The monodeiodination of thyroxine (T_4) to 3,5,3'-triiodothyronine (T_3) activates the major secretory product of the iodine-sufficient human thyroid gland,

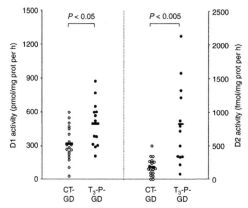

FIGURE 1.—D1 and D2 activities in thyroid tissues. Open circles represent CT-GD patients; closed circles represent T_3-P-GD patients; solid squares represent mean value levels. (Reprinted from Ito M, Toyoda N, Nomura E, et al. Type 1 and type 2 iodothyronine deiodinases in the thyroid gland of patients with 3,5,3'-triiodothyronine-predominant Graves' disease. *Eur J Endocrinol.* 2011;164:95-100, with permission from European Society of Endocrinology.)

producing 80% of the circulating T_3 in humans. Type 1 and type 2 iodothyronine deiodinase (D1 [or DIO1] and D2 [or DIO2], respectively) catalyze this reaction. The roles of D1 and D2 in the production of circulating T_3 in humans are unknown. Both D1 and D2 activities are demonstrated in the human thyroid, and Salvatore et al[1] reported that intrathyroidal T_4 to T_3 conversion by D2 may contribute to the relative increase in thyroidal T_3 production in patients with Graves disease (GD). On the other hand, Laurberg et al[2] estimated by an indirect method using propylthiouracil (PTU) that D1-generated T_3 in the thyroid gland is the major source of plasma T_3 in hyperthyroid humans. Recently, some cases of relatively high serum T_3 levels were reported in patients with follicular thyroid carcinoma, GD during PTU treatment, thyroglobulin gene mutations, and McCune-Albright syndrome. In these cases, D2 activity in the thyroid tissues was increased, and the T_4 to T_3 conversion catalyzed by D2 was assumed to be responsible for the T_3 toxicosis. In this study, the authors evaluated thyroidal activities and messenger RNA levels of both D1 and D2 in patients with T_3-predominant GD (T_3-P-GD) and common-type GD. This study explains the pathogenesis based on advances in our understanding of the 2 activating deiodinase enzymes that convert T_4 to T_3 (Fig 1). However, gaps in our knowledge remain. D1 in peripheral tissues is stimulated by high levels of T_3, but this may contribute little to serum T_3 in this situation because free T_4 is normal or low in T_3-P-GD. The transcriptional regulation of D2 is stimulated by cyclic adenosine monophosphate that is generated in the thyroid by the thyrotropin-receptor antibody.[3] However, T_3 causes downregulation of D2 by a posttranslational mechanism involving ubiquitin-mediated proteasomal degradation.[3] The half-life of D2 is only 40 minutes; it is rapidly activated or suppressed. In hyperthyroidism, the activity of D2 is suppressed. The relative contribution of D1 and D2 to the thyroid's secretion of T_3 in hyperthyroidism is still unclear, and the relative contributions in this rare variant of GD still remain to be clarified. Nevertheless, the data of this recent contribution provide good evidence to show that thyroidal 5'-deiodinases are responsible for the elevated serum T_3 in T_3-P-GD.

M. Schott, MD, PhD

References

1. Salvatore D, Tu H, Harney JW, Larsen PR. Type 2 iodothyronine deiodinase is highly expressed in human thyroid. *J Clin Invest.* 1996;98:962-968.
2. Laurberg P, Vestergaard H, Nielsen S, et al. Sources of circulating 3,5,3'-triiodothyronine in hyperthyroidism estimated after blocking of type 1 and type 2 iodothyronine deiodinases. *J Clin Endocrinol Metab.* 2007;92:2149-2156.
3. Gereben B, Zavacki AM, Ribich S, et al. Cellular and molecular basis of deiodinase-regulated thyroid hormone signaling. *Endocr Rev.* 2008;29:898-938.

Hypothyroidism

CD8+ T Cells Induce Thyroid Epithelial Cell Hyperplasia and Fibrosis

Yu S, Fang Y, Sharav T, et al (Dept of Veterans Affairs Res Service, Columbia, MO; et al)
J Immunol 186:2655-2662, 2011

CD8+ T cells can be important effector cells in autoimmune inflammation, generally because they can damage target cells by cytotoxicity. This study shows that activated CD8+ T cells induce thyroid epithelial cell hyperplasia and proliferation and fibrosis in IFN-$\gamma^{-/-}$ NOD.H-2h4 SCID mice in the absence of CD4+ T cells. Because CD8+ T cells induce proliferation rather than cytotoxicity of target cells, these results describe a novel function for CD8+ T cells in autoimmune disease. In contrast to the ability of purified CD8+ T cells to induce thyrocyte proliferation, CD4+ T cells or CD8 T cell-depleted splenocytes induced only mild thyroid lesions in SCID recipients. T cells in both spleens and thyroids highly produce TNF-α. TNF-α promotes proliferation of thyrocytes in vitro, and anti-TNF-α inhibits development of thyroid epithelial cell hyperplasia and proliferation in SCID recipients of IFN-$\gamma^{-/-}$ splenocytes. This suggests that targeting CD8+ T cells and/or TNF-α may be effective for treating epithelial cell hyperplasia and fibrosis.

▶ Autoimmune thyroiditis is a very common, cell-mediated, organ-specific, autoimmune disease that is characterized by the infiltration of the thyroid gland by (especially) CD8+ cytotoxic T cells. Using cell purification and adoptive transfer, the authors of this study demonstrated a novel function for CD8+ T cells in autoimmunity, where CD8+ T cells function to promote proliferation of target cells in an organ-specific autoimmune disease model. Inhibiting inflammation induced during development of thyroid epithelial cell hyperplasia and proliferation (TEC H/P) by targeting a proinflammatory cytokine was effective in inhibiting fibrosis and reducing the abnormal proliferation induced by chronic inflammation. Because anti—tumor necrosis factor (TNF)-α inhibits TEC H/P and fibrosis, the function of TNF-α in this model of TEC H/P is consistent with the role of TNF-α shown in other models (Fig 4 in the original article).

Although this model is not physiologic because the hyperplasia and fibrosis described in this study develops only if interferon-γ is absent, results obtained using this model can still provide important information relative to understanding the mechanisms by which autoreactive CD8$^+$ T cells promote proliferation of epithelial cells instead of killing their targets as they do in some other autoimmune diseases, such as diabetes. Information derived from studies with this model should increase our understanding of mechanisms underlying development of epithelial cell hyperplasia and fibrosis in any organ or tissue.

M. Schott, MD, PhD

Subclinical Thyroid Disease

The Thyroid Epidemiology, Audit, and Research Study (TEARS): The Natural History of Endogenous Subclinical Hyperthyroidism
Vadiveloo T, Donnan PT, Cochrane L, et al (Univ of Dundee, Scotland, UK)
J Clin Endocrinol Metab 96:E1-E8, 2011

Objective.—For patients with subclinical hyperthyroidism (SH), the objective of the study was to define the rates of progression to frank hyperthyroidism and normal thyroid function.

Design.—Record-linkage technology was used retrospectively to identify patients with SH in the general population of Tayside, Scotland, from January 1, 1993, to December 31, 2009.

Patients.—All Tayside residents with at least two measurements of TSH below the reference range for at least 4 months from baseline and normal free T$_4$/total T$_4$ and total T$_3$ concentrations at baseline were included as potential cases. Using a unique patient identifier, data linkage enabled a cohort of SH cases to be identified from prescription, admission, and radioactive iodine treatment records. Cases younger than 18 yr of age were also excluded from the study.

Outcome Measures.—The status of patients was investigated at 2, 5, and 7 yr after diagnosis.

Results.—We identified 2024 cases with SH, a prevalence of 0.63% and an incidence of 29 per 100,000 in 2008. Most SH cases without thyroid treatment remained as SH at 2 (81.8%), 5 (67.5%), and 7 yr (63.0%) after diagnosis. Few patients (0.5–0.7%) developed hyperthyroidism at 2, 5, and 7 yr. The percentage of SH cases reverting to normal increased with time: 17.2% (2 yr), 31.5% (5 yr), and 35.6% (7 yr), and this was more common in SH patients with baseline TSH between 0.1 and 0.4 mU/liter.

Conclusion.—Very few SH patients develop frank hyperthyroidism, whereas a much larger proportion revert to normal, and many remain with SH (Table 5).

▶ Patients with subclinical hyperthyroidism have few or no symptoms of thyroid dysfunction. In the general population, the prevalence of subclinical hyperthyroidism has been reported to range from 0.7% to 12.4%. Recently, it

TABLE 5.—Clinical Outcomes and Transition of Subclinical Cases that were Excluded After 1 yr

n (%)	SH (TSH 0.1–0.4)	SH (TSH < 0.1)	Normal	Hyperthyroid
SH (TSH 0.1–0.4)	1929 (70.0)	536 (19.4)	105 (3.8)	130 (4.7)
SH (TSH < 0.1)	302 (15.9)	1261 (66.2)	89 (4.7)	194 (10.2)

SH, Subclinical hyperthyroidism.

has been recognized that patients with a suppressed thyrotropin (TSH) may have more profound disease than those with a low but unsuppressed TSH.[1] Low TSH concentration is defined as TSH level between 0.1 and 0.4 mU/L, and suppressed TSH is defined as a TSH concentration less than 0.1 mU/L. Some studies have suggested that patients with subclinical hyperthyroidism may develop overt hyperthyroidism at a rate of 1% to 5% per year.[2] However, some other studies have suggested that patients with subclinical hyperthyroidism revert to normal after diagnosis.[3] It has previously been assumed that more patients with a low but unsuppressed TSH revert to normality, and more patients with a suppressed TSH develop overt hyperthyroidism.[1] The aim of the study by Vadiveloo et al was to define the rates of conversion to frank hyperthyroidism and rates in which patients' results normalize.

The study by Vadiveloo et al is the largest study published thus far on the natural history of subclinical hyperthyroidism. The study classifies these patients into 2 groups. The authors conclude that the rate of development of overt hyperthyroidism, 10%, is small in those with a TSH of < 0.1 mU/L, but they ignore the even higher proportion in this category who were given therapy for hyperthyroidism (Table 5). They base the diagnosis of hyperthyroidism on raised free thyroxine and free triiodothyronine levels, but it is likely that the physicians caring for these patients decided that the TSH of < 0.1 mU/L together with whatever thyroid hormone levels the patients had was a sufficient basis for the initiation of therapy. When the authors ignored those under therapy, the progression to overt hyperthyroidism was 6.1% of all patients at 1 year. They consider these patients as having incipient hyperthyroidism and differentiate them from those with stable subclinical hyperthyroidism. The authors tend to emphasize that most patients remain subclinically hyperthyroid or revert to normal, but the take-home message is that in 10% hyperthyroidism will develop within 1 year and that clinical judgment will dictate an intervention in an even higher proportion of patients as they are followed. Clearly, most of those who have slightly subnormal serum TSH levels make up the 2.5% of subjects below the lower 95% confidence interval limit and will probably not require intervention, but this study provides good evidence that those with serum TSH < 0.1 mU/L must be followed carefully. The results support the recommendations of the Task Force on subclinical thyroid disease some years ago in the *Journal of the American Medical Association*.[4]

M. Schott, MD, PhD

References

1. Mitchell AL, Pearce SH. How should we treat patients with low serum thyrotropin concentrations? *Clin Endocrinol (Oxf).* 2010;72:292-296.
2. Sawin CT, Geller A, Wolf PA, et al. Low serum thyrotropin concentrations as a risk factor for atrial fibrillation in older persons. *N Engl J Med.* 1994;331:1249-1252.
3. Parle JV, Franklyn JA, Cross KW, Jones SC, Sheppard MC. Prevalence and follow-up of abnormal thyrotrophin (TSH) concentrations in the elderly in the United Kingdom. *Clin Endocrinol (Oxf).* 1991;34:77-83.
4. Surks MI, Ortiz E, Daniels GH, et al. Subclinical thyroid disease: scientific review and guidelines for diagnosis and management. *JAMA.* 2004;291:228-238.

Thyroid Cancer

Phase II Clinical Trial of Sorafenib in Metastatic Medullary Thyroid Cancer

Lam ET, Ringel MD, Kloos RT, et al (The Ohio State Univ, Columbus; Uniformed Services Univ of the Health Sciences, Bethesda, MD; Natl Cancer Inst, Rockville, MD; et al)

J Clin Oncol 28:2323-2330, 2010

Purpose.—Mutations in the *RET* proto-oncogene and vascular endothelial growth factor receptor (VEGFR) activity are critical in the pathogenesis of medullary thyroid cancer (MTC). Sorafenib, a multikinase inhibitor targeting Ret and VEGFR, showed antitumor activity in preclinical studies of MTC.

Patients and Methods.—In this phase II trial of sorafenib in patients with advanced MTC, the primary end point was objective response. Secondary end points included toxicity assessment and response correlation with tumor markers, functional imaging, and RET mutations. Using a two-stage design, 16 or 25 patients were to be enrolled onto arms A (hereditary) and B (sporadic). Patients received sorafenib 400 mg orally twice daily.

Results.—Of 16 patients treated in arm B, one achieved partial response (PR; 6.3%; 95% CI, 0.2% to 30.2%), 14 had stable disease (SD; 87.5%; 95% CI, 61.7% to 99.5%), and one was nonevaluable. In a post hoc analysis of 10 arm B patients with progressive disease (PD) before study, one patient had PR of 21+ months, four patients had SD ≥15 months, four patients had SD ≤6 months, and one patient had clinical PD. Median progression-free survival was 17.9 months. Arm A was prematurely terminated because of slow accrual. Common adverse events (AEs) included diarrhea, hand-foot-skin reaction, rash, and hypertension. Although serious AEs were rare, one death was seen. Tumor markers decreased in the majority of patients, and *RET* mutations were detected in 10 of 12 sporadic MTCs analyzed.

Conclusion.—Sorafenib is reasonably well tolerated, with suggestion of clinical benefit for patients with sporadic MTC. Caution should be taken because of the rare but fatal toxicity potentially associated with sorafenib.

▶ In the past, some data[1] were already published for the treatment of advanced, iodine-refractory thyroid cancers with the multityrosine kinase inhibitor sorafenib with multiple targets, including BRAF and vascular endothelial growth factor receptor (VEGFR) 1 and 2. The aim of this article was to investigate the role of sorafenib for the treatment of metastasized medullary thyroid cancer (MTC). In this study patients received sorafenib 400 mg orally twice daily. Of 16 patients with sporadic MTC, one achieved partial response (PR), 14 had stable disease (standard deviation [SD], 87.5%), and median progression-free survival was 17.9 months (Fig 2 in the original article). The low PR rate but high rate of SD in this study was also observed in former phase II studies of motesanib, a VEGFR inhibitor, in patients with sporadic MTC and vandetanib, an inhibitor of Ret, epidermal growth factor receptor, and VEGFR, in patients with hereditary MTC. This low PR response rate might also be because of limitations of Response Evaluation Criteria for Solid Tumors for assessing response. PR may not be the most accurate way to assess response to such therapies. Nonetheless, sorafenib is a reasonably well-tolerated oral therapy that offers clinical benefit and may be an option for patients with sporadic metastatic MTC who are not able to participate in clinical trials.

M. Schott, MD, PhD

Reference

1. Sherman SI, Wirth LJ, Droz JP, et al. Motesanib diphosphate in progressive differentiated thyroid cancer. N Engl J Med. 2008;359:31-42.

A novel RET inhibitor with potent efficacy against medullary thyroid cancer in vivo

Samadi AK, Mukerji R, Shah A, et al (The Univ of Kansas Med Ctr)
Surgery 148:1228-1236, 2010

Background.—Most medullary thyroid carcinomas (MTC) recur or progress despite curative resection. Current targeted therapies show promise but lack durable efficacy and tolerability. The purpose of this study was to build on previous in vitro work and evaluate withaferin A (WA), a novel RET inhibitor, in a metastatic murine model of MTC.

Methods.—A total of 5 million DRO-81-1 human MTC cells injected in the left posterior neck of nu/nu mice generated metastases uniformly to the liver, spleen, and/or lungs. Treatment with WA (8 mg/kg/day, intraperitoneally, for 21 days) was started for neoplasms >100 mm^3. Endpoints were survival, neoplasm >15,00 mm^3, decreased body weight, or body score (all measured three times/wk).

Results.—All controls (saline; $n = 5$) died or deteriorated from metastatic disease by 7 weeks postinjection. All treated animals were alive (WA; $n = 5$), having tumor regression and growth delay without toxicity or weight loss at 6 weeks posttreatment ($P < .01$). Tumor cells treated with WA demonstrated inhibition of total and phospho-RET levels by Western blot analysis in a dose-dependent manner (almost complete

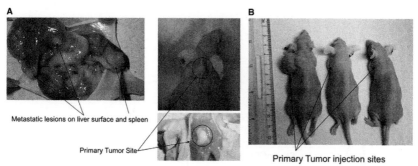

FIGURE 1.—Neck xenografts of DRO81-1 medullary thyroid carcinoma (MTC) cells in nu/nu mice develop metastatic disease similar to human MTCs. MTC xenografts in nu/nu mice were created by injection in the left posterior neck with 5 million DRO81-1 cells. All control animals ($n = 5$) developed progressively enlarging tumor masses with increased disease burden resulting in deterioration of body weight (>10% loss from baseline) as well as decline in body score within 6 to 7 weeks postinjection leading to natural death or euthanized per standard animal protocol monitoring (A) A representative control animal at autopsy is shown, with a view of the primary tumor implant and the intraabdominal metastases (B) A gross comparison of 3 of these animals at 3 week posttreatment (5-weeks postinjection of tumor cells). The control animal on the left has a large primary tumor with evidence of weight loss (eg, the spine is more prominent), while the treated animals (2 on the right) have almost completely regressed neoplasms with no clinical toxicity as evidenced by normal weight, body score, and activity levels. (Reprinted from Samadi AK, Mukerji R, Shah A, et al. A novel RET inhibitor with potent efficacy against medullary thyroid cancer in vivo. *Surgery.* 2010;148:1228-1236, Copyright 2010, with permission from Mosby, Inc.)

inhibition with treatment of 5 μM WA) as well as potent inhibition of phospho-ERK and phospho-Akt levels.

Conclusion.—WA is a novel natural-product RET-inhibitor with efficacy in a metastatic murine model of MTC. Further long-term efficacy/toxicity studies are warranted to evaluate this compound for clinical translation (Figs 1 and 2).

▶ The purpose of this study was to evaluate the efficacy and toxicity of withaferin A (WA) in an in vivo murine xenograft model of medullary thyroid cancer (MTC) using human medullary cancer DRO-81-1 cells that metastasize spontaneously to the lung, liver, and spleen. DRO-81-1 is a true medullary cancer cell line not shown to exhibit potential genetic cross-contamination with melanoma or colon cancer cells. This cell line also produces the hormone calcitonin, allowing for biochemically quantitative assessment of in vivo disease to supplement visible tumor volume measurements. WA has been shown from the same group to inhibit human MTC cell proliferation (TT cells and DRO81-1) in vitro. This inhibition occurred at a greater potency than drugs like 17-AAG, a popular heat shock protein 90 inhibitor that is currently in phase 1/2 clinical trials in patients including patients with MTC. All animals treated with WA showed a tumor regression (Figs 1 and 2). Moreover, tumor cells treated with WA demonstrated inhibition of total and phospho-RET levels by Western blot analysis in a dose-dependent manner as well as potent inhibition of phospho-ERK and phospho-Akt levels. Even though WA has promising efficacy without apparent clinical toxicity thus far, future formal toxicology testing will be

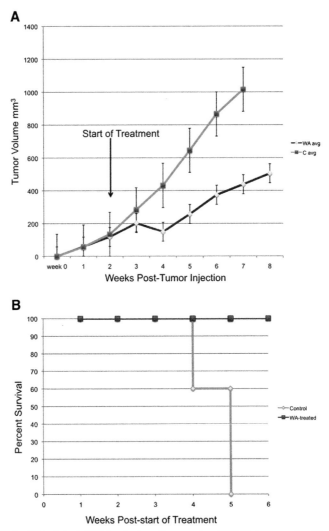

FIGURE 2.—Withaferin A (WA) has in vivo efficacy against DRO 81-1 xenografts without toxicity. Drug efficacy analysis is plotted out for 8 weeks after initial tumor injection (because all control animals [*n* = 5] died by 7 weeks postinjection and all treated animals [*n* = 5] were alive with tumor). Treated animals demonstrated a survival advantage at this time point over controls ($P < .01$) (A) Tumor growth progression is depicted as an average tumor volume (±SEM) for each group by week (average of all 5 animals per group) (B) Survival times are depicted using a Kaplan-Meier curve. The treated animals demonstrated a uniform delay in growth of tumors, with 80% of animals demonstrating an initial regression in tumor volume at 2 weeks into therapy (week 4 after tumor implantation), which was followed by eventual disease progression, albeit at a 3- to 4-week growth delay compared to controls and at a lesser growth trajectory. (Reprinted from Samadi AK, Mukerji R, Shah A, et al. A novel RET inhibitor with potent efficacy against medullary thyroid cancer in vivo. *Surgery.* 2010;148:1228-1236, Copyright 2010, with permission from Mosby, Inc.)

necessary to better evaluate its safety profile in vivo. Overall, these early in vivo data provide evidence to support further development and translation of this compound toward a potential clinical application for patients with metastatic MTC.

M. Schott, MD, PhD

The Prevalence of Occult Medullary Thyroid Carcinoma at Autopsy
Valle LA, Kloos RT (The Ohio State Univ Med Ctr, Columbus)
J Clin Endocrinol Metab 96:E109-E113, 2011

Context.—The prevalence of occult medullary thyroid carcinoma (MTC) in the general population is unknown but may be important when considering strategies to diagnose clinically relevant MTC in nodular goiter or other populations.

Objective.—Our objective was to determine the prevalence of occult MTC in a series of autopsies.

Design.—We conducted a systematic review of autopsy series from 1970 to present using a PubMed search.

Patients.—The patients came from 21 countries, ages ranged from 6—95 yr, both genders were represented, and none had clinical evidence of thyroid disease before autopsy.

Intervention.—Three series were excluded based on tumor size less than 500 µm, non-English language, or insufficient information.

Main Outcome Measure.—Prevalence of occult MTC was calculated.

Results.—An average prevalence of 0.14 and 7.6% for occult MTC and papillary thyroid carcinoma, respectively, was found among 7897 autopsies from 24 published series. Greater than 75% of patients with MTC were more than 60 yr old, and male to female ratio was comparable. Tumor size was virtually all subcentimeter, and there was no lymph node spread, extrathyroidal extension, or distant metastases reported.

Conclusions.—A small number of people in the general population, who do not have known thyroid disease, have occult MTC and die of other causes. This finding of untreated occult MTC without morbidity or mortality should be considered in population prevalence studies, when strategies to detect thyroid neoplasia are considered (e.g. serum calcitonin or ultrasound), and included in cost-effectiveness models of routine serum calcitonin screening for nodular thyroid disease.

▶ Medullary thyroid carcinoma (MTC) is a neuroendocrine tumor originating from the parafollicular C cells of the thyroid. C cells secrete calcitonin (Ct). Serum Ct levels are elevated in C cell disorders, thus making it a sensitive clinical marker for MTC. The prevalence of occult MTC in the general population is not well established. The purpose of this study by Valle and Kloos was to better estimate the prevalence of occult MTC in the general population by analyzing published autopsy series. The autopsy series that were combined for this article spanned 35 years and came from many nations with different prevalences of nodular thyroid diseases (Table 1 in the original article). Diet and other environmental factors have changed, as have the ways that minor thyroid nodules are detected and assessed, from 1971 when thyroid ultrasonography was in its infancy until 2006 when thyroid incidentalomas had burgeoned following the widespread use of MRI, positron emission tomography, and CT scans. It is important to note that in these studies three-fourths of the patients autopsied were older than 60 years, which may bias the data toward benign disease, because sporadic MCT commonly presents in patients in their 40s and 50s and familial MCT tends to present even earlier, while benign thyroid nodularity increases progressively with age. Clearly, occult subcentimeter MCTs are not always benign, even though the ones detected in these autopsies were asymptomatic up to the time of death. Even the so-called benign C-cell hyperplasia (>50 C cells per 3 low-power fields) is considered to be carcinoma in situ for patients with familial MCT or multiple endocrine neoplasia type 2, especially those with certain *RET* mutations.[1] There is a clear need for up-to-date information on the behavior of occult MCT to conduct meaningful risk-benefit and cost-benefit analyses. Unless country- and age-specific data on the incidence and behavior of occult MCT miraculously do become available, it seems that amalgamated temporal and global data will have to do, despite questions about its applicability, particularly to younger patients.

M. Schott, MD, PhD

Reference

1. Kloos RT, Eng C, Evans DB, et al. Medullary thyroid cancer: management guidelines of the American Thyroid Association. *Thyroid.* 2009;19:565-612.

A Decrease of Calcitonin Serum Concentrations Less Than 50 Percent 30 Minutes after Thyroid Surgery Suggests Incomplete C-Cell Tumor Tissue Removal

Faggiano A, Milone F, Ramundo V, et al (Azienda Sanitaria Locale Napoli 1 Centro, Italy; Federico II Univ, Napoli, Italy; et al)
J Clin Endocrinol Metab 95:E32-E36, 2010

Context and Objectives.—The prognosis of medullary thyroid carcinoma (MTC) depends on the completeness of the first surgical treatment. To date, it is not possible to predict whether the tumor has been completely removed after surgery. The aim of this study was to evaluate the reliability of an intraoperative calcitonin monitoring as a predictor of the final outcome after surgery in patients with MTC.

Patients and Methods.—Twenty patients underwent total thyroidectomy and central lymph node dissection on the basis of a positive pentagastrin test. In six cases a preoperative diagnosis of MTC was achieved at the cytological examination. During the surgical intervention, calcitonin was measured at the time of anesthesia, at the time of manipulation, and

10 and 30 min after surgical excision. At the histological examination, 10 patients had MTC and 10 had C cell hyperplasia.

Results.—As compared with calcitonin levels before thyroidectomy, a decrease of calcitonin greater than 50% 30 min after surgery was able to significantly distinguish patients who were cured from those who experienced persistence of disease. It was not possible to find a similar result when the decrease of calcitonin 10 min after surgery was considered.

Conclusions.—A rate of calcitonin decrease less than 50% 30 min after thyroidectomy plus central neck lymph node dissection suggests the persistence of tumor tissue in patients operated for MTC. These results indicate that intraoperative calcitonin monitoring may be a useful tool to predict the completeness of surgery in patients with MTC.

▶ Medullary thyroid carcinoma (MTC) originates from the parafollicular cells of the thyroid. These cells produce calcitonin, which is a highly sensitive and specific marker of MTC for both diagnosis and follow-up. The definitive cure of the tumor is strongly dependent on the completeness of the first surgical treatment. If total thyroidectomy and central neck lymph node dissection are performed in all cases of MTC, it is a matter of debate whether to perform lateral lymph node dissection in any case or to limit this radical approach only to patients with metastases in the central neck compartment or palpable lateral neck lymph nodes. For this purpose, it should be considered that the risk of metastases in the contralateral neck compartment and the mediastinum depends on the size of the primary tumor, the number of central lymph node metastases, and tumor multicentricity. If the first surgical treatment is so crucial for the final outcome of the patient, on the other hand, there are no clear criteria that can indicate to the surgeon whether the tumor has been completely removed after total thyroidectomy plus central lymph node dissection. In a previous study evaluating the usefulness of intraoperative pentagastrin (PG) test in predicting lymph node involvement in patients with MTC who underwent total thyroidectomy plus central lymph node dissection, 80% of subjects were correctly recognized to have postoperative tumor remnants, and this procedure failed to detect tumor remnant in 20% of uncured subjects.[1] In this study by Faggiano et al, intraoperative calcitonin monitoring was performed in patients who were recommended for surgery on the basis of the detection of high basal and PG-stimulated calcitonin levels consistent with a diagnosis of MTC to evaluate the reliability of this intraoperative procedure in predicting the completeness of surgery. This study demonstrates that intraoperative monitoring of calcitonin 10 minutes after surgery is a reliable way to determine whether a patient can be considered free of disease after surgery (Figs 1 and 2 in the original article). The authors suggest that intraoperative calcitonin monitoring seems to be more cost effective than intraoperative PG testing in the recognition of patients with incomplete surgery. The study shows that the main difference is that the sensitivity and negative predictive value of the intraoperative calcitonin monitoring was 100% with no false-negative results, whereas the sensitivity of intraoperative PG testing was 80% and the test had a negative predictive value of 91%, meaning that PG testing did not recognize 20% of the patients who had persistent disease after surgery. The results of this study clearly demonstrate that a decrease of calcitonin serum concentrations greater than 50% 30 minutes after surgery indicates that all the calcitonin-producing tumor tissues have been removed, while a calcitonin decrease of less than 50% suggests that an incomplete surgery has been performed, giving the surgeon an opportunity to perform another lymph node compartment dissection. The data of this study need, however, to be reproduced by other scientists.

M. Schott, MD, PhD

Reference

1. Scheuba C, Bieglmayer C, Asari R, et al. The value of intraoperative pentagastrin testing in medullary thyroid cancer. *Surgery.* 2007;141:166-171.

Prognostic Factors of Disease-Free Survival after Thyroidectomy in 170 Young Patients with a RET Germline Mutation: A Multicenter Study of the Groupe Français d'Etude des Tumeurs Endocrines

Rohmer V, for the Groupe Français des Tumeurs Endocrines (Université Angers, France; et al)

J Clin Endocrinol Metab 96:E509-E518, 2011

Background.—In hereditary medullary thyroid carcinoma (HMTC), prophylactic surgery is the only curative option, which should be properly defined both in time and extent.

Objectives.—To identify and characterize prognostic factors associated with disease-free survival (DFS) in children from HMTC families.

Design.—We conducted a retrospective analysis of a multi-center cohort of 170 patients below age 21 at surgery. Demographic, clinical, genetic, biological data [basal and pentagastrine-stimulated calcitonin (CT and CT/Pg, respectively)], and tumor node metastasis (TNM) status were collected. DFS was assessed based on basal CT levels. Kaplan—Meier curves, Cox regression, and logistic regression models were used to determine factors associated with DFS and TNM staging.

Results.—No patients with a preoperative basal CT <31 ng/ml had persistent or recurrent disease. Medullary thyroid carcinoma defined by a diameter $\geq$10 mm [hazard ratio (HR): 6.0; 95% confidence interval (95%CI): 1.8—19.8] and N1 status (HR: 20.8;95%CI: 3.9—109.8) were independently associated with DFS. Class D genotype [odds ratio (OR): 48.5, 95% CI: 10.6—225.1], preoperative basal CT >30 ng/liter (OR: 43.4, 95% CI: 5.2—359.8), and age >10 (OR: 5.5, 95% CI: 1.4—21.8) were associated with medullary thyroid carcinoma $\geq$10 mm. No patient with a preoperative basal CT <31 ng/ml had a N1 status. Class D genotype (OR: 48.6, 95% CI: 8.6—274.1), and age >10 (OR: 4.6, 95% CI: 1.1—19.0) were associated with N1 status.

Conclusion.—In HMTC patients, DFS is best predicted by TNM staging and preoperative basal CT level below 30 pg/ml. Basal CT, class D genotype, and age constitute key determinants to decide preoperatively timely surgery.

▶ The authors performed a retrospective multicenter study of 170 patients with medullary thyroid carcinoma (MTC) with a germline ret proto-oncogene mutation who were younger than 21 years at the time of thyroid surgery to identify prognostic factors of disease-free survival. Outcomes were best predicted by primary tumor/lymph node (pTN) staging (Fig 2 in the original article). Interestingly, both the T and the N status were independent prognostic parameters. This result allows a prognostic pTNM-based determination of a timely surgical approach, defined by a surgery performed before MTC exceeds 10 mm in diameter or lymph node metastases develop. However, the pTN classification carries limitations because it requires surgery, while the preoperative evaluation of pTN remains an issue to address patients to surgeons in a timely manner. Indeed, current imaging is not sensitive and specific enough to depict lymph node metastases. Therefore, there is a need to highlight parameters closely related to the pTN status to refer such patients to surgeons in a timely manner and define the type of follow-up, according to the surgery performed. Another preoperative marker for persistent disease is the basal serum calcitonin level (Fig 3 in the original article). The authors defined a cutoff of 30 pg/mL as a predictive for not being cured after surgery.

M. Schott, MD, PhD

The Use of Preoperative Routine Measurement of Basal Serum Thyrocalcitonin in Candidates for Thyroidectomy due to Nodular Thyroid Disorders: Results from 2733 Consecutive Patients

Chambon G, Alovisetti C, Idoux-Louche C, et al (Centre Hospitalier Universitaire de Nîmes, France; Hôpital Privé les Franciscaines, Nîmes, France; et al)
J Clin Endocrinol Metab 96:75-81, 2011

Context.—The preoperative routine measurement of basal serum thyrocalcitonin (CT) in candidates for thyroidectomy due to thyroid nodules is currently a subject of debate.

Objective.—The objective of this study was to evaluate the role of systematic basal serum CT measurement in improving the diagnosis and surgical treatment of medullary thyroid carcinoma (MTC) in patients undergoing thyroidectomy for nodular thyroid disorders, regardless of preoperative CT levels.

Design.—We determined basal serum CT levels in 2733 consecutive patients before thyroid surgery and performed a pentagastrin test in patients with hypercalcitoninemia. We correlated basal and stimulated CT levels with intraoperative and definitive histopathological findings, and we analyzed the impact of these results on surgical procedures.

Results.—Twelve MTCs were found among the 43 patients with basal serum CT level of 10 pg/ml or greater. Two MTCs were present among the 2690 patients with normal CT levels. MTC was always present in patients with a basal CT of 60 pg/ml or greater. For CT levels ranging from 10 to 59 pg/ml, MTC was diagnosed in 11% of patients. When preoperative hypercalcitoninemia was present, total thyroidectomy associated with comprehensive intraoperative histopathological analysis allowed the intraoperative diagnosis of five latent, subclinical MTCs. The pentagastrin test gave no additional diagnostic information for the management of patients with elevated preoperative basal serum CT level.

Conclusion.—Routine measurement of CT in the preoperative work-up of nodular thyroid disorders is useful. This procedure improves intraoperative diagnosis of MTC and enables adapted initial surgery, the most determinant factor of treatment success (Table 1).

▶ Medullary thyroid carcinoma (MTC) is an uncommon cancer that results from the neoplastic transformation of the parafollicular C cells of the thyroid gland. MTC is primarily sporadic but also arises in the context of a genetic pathology called multiple endocrine neoplasia type 2. MTC is a differentiated thyroid tumor that maintains the secreting function of C cells, that is, the production of thyrocalcitonin (CT). This small polypeptide hormone is used as a tumor marker for MTC, which is suspected in cases of elevated basal serum CT levels. In patients with nodular thyroid, the measurement of basal serum CT levels has been proposed as a systematic screening method for MTC because its prevalence is about 1% in this population. However, this screening, which is recommended by the European Thyroid Association, has remained controversial for decades. Proponents of the screening find that it allows for an earlier diagnosis of MTC and adapted surgical procedures that finally improve the cure and prognosis of patients. For detractors, this screening is not cost effective, mainly because the incidence of MTC is too low in the nodular thyroid population and because basal serum CT is not sufficiently MTC specific. Indeed, benign C cell hyperplasia (CCH) represents the most frequent cause of CT elevation. The pentagastrin (PG) test has been widely used to improve the specificity of CT as a tumor marker, but this method also lacks specificity and is in any case no longer feasible because of the recent worldwide halt in PG commercialization. Throughout this long debate on the relevance of CT measurement as a screening method of MTC in the workup of nodular thyroid disease, some practical issues of major importance for doctors have been poorly addressed so far. First, should doctors carry out a routine preoperative basal serum CT measurement before the surgical procedure, when a thyroidectomy is already proposed because of nodular thyroid disease? Second, as concerns preoperative hypercalcitoninemia, how should surgical and histopathological procedures be adapted and for which CT values? Finally, it is unclear how the recent unavailability of the PG test modifies these issues.

In this study, the authors report on their experience with 2733 consecutive routine preoperative basal serum CT measurements and PG stimulation tests for the detection of MTC in patients undergoing thyroidectomy for nodular

TABLE 1.—Basal CT Levels, Stimulated CT Levels, Histological Findings, and Characteristics of MTC in the 43 Patients Referred for Surgical Treatment of Nodular Thyroid Diseases and for whom Preoperative Basal Serum CT levels were Greater than 10 pg/ml

Patient no.	Sex	Age (yr)	Basal Serum CT Level (pg/ml)	Stimulated Serum CT Peak (pg/ml)	MTC TN Stage/Size	CCH	Other Histopathologicals Findings
1	F	45	12	—	pT1 pN0/1.5 mm	No	Benign nodular goiter
2	F	54	14	53	pT1 pNX/5 mm	No	Benign nodular goiter, lymphocytic thyroiditis foci
3	H	66	17	—	pT1pNx/3 mm	No	Benign nodular goiter
4	F	54	45	—	pT1pN0/6 mm	Yes	Papillary carcinoma
5	F	58	85	—	pT1pN1b/6 mm	Yes	Toxic benign nodular goiter
6	H	54	206	7,510	pT1pN0/16 mm	No	None
7	F	81	580	—	pT1pN0/11 mm	No	None
8	F	83	655	14,000	pT1pN0/19 mm	No	None
9	H	63	1,900	—	pT2 pN1b/22 mm	No	None
10	F	82	4,419	—	pT3 pN1b/39 mm	No	Papillary microcarcinoma
11	F	61	5,654	—	pT2 pN0/30 mm	No	None
12	F	81	13,000	—	pT3 pN1b/27 mm	No	Lymphocytic thyroiditis foci
13	F	61	12	53	No	Yes	Solitary benign adenoma
14	H	51	12	126	No	Yes	Multifocal papillary microcarcinoma
15	H	67	13	63	No	No	Benign nodular goiter
16	H	57	13	74	No	Yes	Solitary benign adenoma
17	F	45	13	80	No	Yes	Benign nodular goiter
18	H	55	13	203	No	No	Papillary microcarcinoma
19	F	45	14	40	No	Yes	Solitary benign adenoma
20	H	30	14	213	No	Yes	Benign nodular goiter
21	F	70	15	38	No	Yes	Benign nodular goiter
22	H	70	15	38	No	Yes	Thyroiditis, papillary microcarcinoma
23	F	33	15	60	No	Yes	Benign nodular goiter
24	H	59	16	159	No	Yes	Benign nodular goiter
25	H	53	16	159	No	Yes	Solitary benign adenoma
26	F	30	17	38	No	Yes	Benign nodular goiter
27	H	50	18	163	No	Yes	Benign nodular goiter, lymphocytic thyroiditis foci
28	F	43	20	45	No	Yes	Benign nodular goiter
29	H	47	20	56	No	Yes	Benign nodular goiter, lymphocytic thyroiditis foci
30	F	28	20	59	No	Yes	Benign nodular goiter
31	H	64	20	70	No	Yes	Solitary benign adenoma
32	H	52	20	112	No	Yes	Benign nodular goiter
33	H	62	20	161	No	Yes	Solitary benign adenoma
34	H	50	21	450	No	Yes	Benign nodular goiter
35	H	52	22	79	No	Yes	Benign nodular goiter
36	H	64	25	244	No	Yes	Benign nodular goiter
37	H	48	26	100	No	Yes	Solitary benign adenoma
38	H	54	27	249	No	Yes	Benign nodular goiter
39	H	50	28	112	No	Yes	Solitary benign adenoma
40	H	52	34	—	No	Yes	Solitary benign adenoma
41	H	54	35	268	No	Yes	Benign nodular goiter
42	H	61	36	—	No	Yes	Benign nodular goiter
43	F	58	59	—	No	Yes	Benign nodular goiter

F, Female; —, no data available.

disorders regardless of preoperative CT values. Similar to a number of previous studies that have used basal CT determination to screen all patients with nodules, medullary carcinoma of the thyroid (MCT) was found in ∼0.5% of cases (patient details are given in Table 1). The positive predictive value of the CT screening was only about 25%. The American Thyroid Association has not taken a position for or against routine screening,[1] based on the total associated costs and in view of the large fraction of false-positive tests, which do have associated risk (note that approximately three-fourths of the patients with elevated CT levels in this study underwent total thyroidectomy for an apparently benign disease). Still, the central compartment nodes of one patient with subclinical latent micro-MCT probably would have been missed if the screening CT had not been performed. In another 3 cases, the nodule was not on the side where the MCT was found, so the simple lobectomy that probably would have been performed would have missed the MCT, if the high CT level had not been recognized preoperatively. However, data are lacking to support the idea that CCH without germline mutation or subclinical latent MCT develops with time into macro-MTC. In other words, it is not clear whether those latter 3 cases would ever have developed clinical symptoms.

M. Schott, MD, PhD

Reference

1. Cooper DS, Doherty GM, Haugen BR, et al. Revised American Thyroid Association management guidelines for patients with thyroid nodules and differentiated thyroid cancer. *Thyroid.* 2009;19:1167-1214.

Mitochondrial Localization and Regulation of BRAF^{V600E} in Thyroid Cancer: A Clinically Used RAF Inhibitor Is Unable to Block the Mitochondrial Activities of BRAF^{V600E}

Lee MH, Lee SE, Kim DW, et al (Chungnam Natl Univ School of Medicine, Jung-gu Daejeon, Korea; et al)
J Clin Endocrinol Metab 96:E19-E30, 2011

Context.—The oncogenic BRAF^{V600E} mutation results in an active structural conformation characterized by greatly elevated ERK activity. However, additional cellular effects caused by subcellular action of BRAF^{V600E} remain to be identified.

Objective.—To explore these effects, differences in the subcellular localization of wild-type and mutant BRAF in thyroid cancer were investigated.

Results.—A significant proportion of endogenous and exogenous BRAF^{V600E}, but not wild-type BRAF, was detected in the mitochondrial fraction, similar to other BRAF mutants including BRAF^{V600D}, BRAF^{V600K}, BRAF^{V600R}, and BRAF^{G469A}, which showed elevated kinase activity and mitochondrial localization. Induced expression of BRAF^{V600E} suppressed the apoptotic responses against staurosporine and TNFα/cycloheximide. Interestingly, the mitochondrial localization and antiapoptotic activities of BRAF^{V600E}

were unaffected by sorafenib and U0126 suppression of MAPK kinase (MEK) and ERK activities. Similarly, although the RAF inhibitor sorafenib effectively inhibited MEK/ERK activation, it did not block the mitochondrial localization of BRAF^{V600E}. In addition, inducible expression of BRAF^{V600E} increased the glucose uptake rate and decreased O_2 consumption, suggesting that BRAF^{V600E} reduces mitochondrial oxidative phosphorylation, a signature feature of cancer cells. Again, these metabolic alterations resulted by BRAF^{V600E} expression were not affected by the treatment of thyroid cells by sorafenib. Therefore, RAF and MEK inhibitors are unable to block the antiapoptotic activity of BRAF ^{V600E} or correct the high glucose uptake rate and glycolytic activity and suppressed mitochondrial oxidative phosphorylation induced by BRAF ^{V600E}.

Conclusions.—The mitochondrial localization observed in oncogenic BRAF mutants might be related to their altered responses to apoptotic stimuli and characteristic metabolic phenotypes found in thyroid cancer. The inability of MEK and RAF inhibitors, U0126 and sorafenib, respectively, to block the mitochondrial localization of BRAF^{V600E} has additional therapeutic implications for BRAF^{V600E}-positive thyroid cancers.

▶ The findings of this study show that BRAF^{V600E} interacts with mitochondria via an extracellular signal-regulated kinase—independent mutation-specific mitochondrial localization. The mitochondrial localization of BRAF^{V600E} generated antiapoptotic effects and metabolic changes characterized by decreased oxygen consumption and an increased rate of glucose uptake, suggesting reduced mitochondrial oxidative phosphorylation. Surprisingly, clinically used and well-known RAF inhibitor had no effect on the mitochondrial interactions or activities of BRAF^{V600E} (Fig 5 in the original article). These new insights into the mutation-specific roles played by BRAF^{V600E} may be important for the development of future therapeutics.

M. Schott, MD, PhD

Identification and Optimal Postsurgical Follow-Up of Patients with Very Low-Risk Papillary Thyroid Microcarcinomas
Durante C, on behalf of the Papillary Thyroid Cancer Study Group (Università di Roma Sapienza, Italy; et al)
J Clin Endocrinol Metab 95:4882-4888, 2010

Context.—Most papillary thyroid microcarcinomas (PTMCs; $\leq$ 1 cm diameter) are indolent low-risk tumors, but some cases behave more aggressively. Controversies have thus arisen over the optimum postoperative surveillance of PTMC patients.

Objectives.—We tested the hypothesis that clinical criteria could be used to identify PTMC patients with very low mortality/recurrence risks and attempted to define the best strategy for their management and long-term surveillance.

Design.—We retrospectively analyzed data from 312 consecutively diagnosed PTMC patients with T1N0M0 stage disease, no family history of thyroid cancer, no history of head-neck irradiation, unifocal PTMC, no extracapsular involvement, and classic papillary histotypes. Additional inclusion criteria were complete follow-up data from surgery to at least 5 yr after diagnosis. All 312 had undergone (near) total thyroidectomy [with radioactive iodine (RAI) remnant ablation in 137 (44%) — RAI group] and were followed up yearly with cervical ultrasonography and serum thyroglobulin, TSH, and thyroglobulin antibody assays.

Results.—During follow-up (5–23 yr, median 6.7 yr), there were no deaths due to thyroid cancer or reoperations. The first (6–12 months after surgery) and last postoperative cervical sonograms were negative in all cases. Final serum thyroglobulin levels were undetectable (<1 ng/ml) in all RAI patients and almost all (93%) of non-RAI patients.

Conclusion.—Accurate risk stratification can allow safe follow-up of most PTMC patients with a less intensive, more cost-effective protocol. Cervical ultrasonography is the mainstay of this protocol, and negative findings at the first postoperative examination are highly predictive of positive outcomes.

▶ The increasing prevalence of papillary thyroid carcinomas less than 1 cm in diameter (ie, papillary thyroid microcarcinomas [PTMCs]) is a worldwide phenomenon that poses continuous management challenges. Many of these tumors are diagnosed incidentally after surgery for benign thyroid nodular disease; others are discovered by chance during cervical imaging studies performed for various reasons. As noted in the recently published American Thyroid Association (ATA) guidelines for differentiated thyroid cancer,[1] the optimal surveillance protocol for this group of patients has yet to be defined. On the whole, PTMCs have an excellent prognosis and carry a low risk for mortality. Most of these tumors display very indolent behavior, and cure rates as high as 100% have been reported, but in a minority of cases the tumor phenotype is more aggressive with lymph node and distant metastases at the time of diagnosis or during the early postoperative follow-up. For these reasons, controversies have arisen about the most effective management strategy for PTMCs. This retrospective study by Durante and coworkers found that papillary thyroid cancer (PTC) <1 cm without risk factors indicative of more aggressive disease that are treated by thyroidectomy did not recur, regardless of whether radioiodine ablation had been used. The authors recommend that postoperative surveillance of these patients can be based exclusively on ultrasonography and that this can be discontinued after 5 years. It is interesting that they did not use recombinant thyrotropin as a basis for prognosis. They do not recommend radioactive iodine ablation for these patients, and this is consistent with the recent ATA guideline for low-risk PTMC. It should be emphasized that the conditions to be included in the study, as noted above, excluded all of the factors that might contribute to more aggressive disease. In contrast with these conclusions and the data from this study, there are reports of patients with PTMC who have recurrent disease. Arora et al compared 66 patients with PTMC and 136 patients with larger PTC.[2] Recurrence was found in 17% of the patients with PTMC and in 21% with larger PTC; this was not a significant difference. PTMC recurred in 11 patients. Eleven of those with PTMC had recurrence, but 8 had multifocal tumors, 6 had lymph node metastases, 3 had angiolymphatic invasion, and 2 had distant metastases. Patients with these features would have been excluded from the Italian study. Tzvetov et al reported a series of 225 patients with differentiated thyroid carcinomas < 1 cm (98% PTMC)[3]; the median size was 7 mm. Multifocal disease was found in 50%, bilateral disease in 32%, extrathyroidal extension in 16%, lymph node metastases in 26%, and distant metastases in 2.4%; 96% were treated by total thyroidectomy. Not surprisingly, 11% had recurrent disease, as compared with 32% of 543 patients with macroscopic differentiated thyroid cancer at the same institutions. In conclusion, it is certainly correct that the follow-up recommended by Durante et al is appropriate for patients with PTMC with no features of aggressive disease. In patients with PTMC who have findings indicative of more aggressive disease, the follow-up should be much more intensive.

M. Schott, MD, PhD

References

1. Cooper DS, Doherty GM, Haugen BR, et al. Revised American Thyroid Association management guidelines for patients with thyroid nodules and differentiated thyroid cancer. *Thyroid.* 2009;19:1167-1214.
2. Arora N, Scognamiglio T, Lubitz CC, et al. Identification of borderline thyroid tumors by gene expression array analysis. *Cancer.* 2009;115:5421-5431.
3. Tzvetov G, Hirsch D, Shraga-Slutzky I, et al. Well-differentiated thyroid carcinoma: comparison of microscopic and macroscopic disease. *Thyroid.* 2009;19:487-494.

Long-Term Efficacy of Lymph Node Reoperation for Persistent Papillary Thyroid Cancer
Al-Saif O, Farrar WB, Bloomston M, et al (The Ohio State Univ, Columbus)
J Clin Endocrinol Metab 95:2187-2194, 2010

Objective.—The objective of the study was to determine the outcome of surgical resection of metastatic papillary thyroid cancer (PTC) in cervical lymph nodes after failure of initial surgery and I[131] therapy.

Design.—This was a retrospective clinical study.

Setting.—The study was conducted at a university-based tertiary cancer hospital.

Patients.—A cohort of 95 consecutive patients with recurrent/persistent PTC in the neck underwent initial reoperation during 1999–2005. All had previous thyroidectomy (±nodal dissection) and I[131] therapy. Twenty-five patients with antithyroglobulin (Tg) antibodies were subsequently excluded.

Main Outcome Measures.—Biochemical complete remission (BCR) was stringently defined as undetectable TSH-stimulated serum Tg.

Results.—A total of 107 lymphadenectomies were undertaken in these 70 patients through January 2010. BCR was initially achieved in 12 patients (17%). Of the 58 patients with detectable postoperative Tg, 28 had a second reoperation and BCR was achieved in five (18%), seven had a third reoperation, and none achieved BCR. No patient achieving BCR had a subsequent recurrence after a mean follow-up of 60 months (range 4—116 months). In addition, two more patients achieved BCR during long-term follow-up without further intervention. In total, 19 patients (27%) achieved BCR and 32 patients (46%) achieved a TSH-stimulated Tg less than 2.0 ng/ml. Patients who did not achieve BCR had significant reduction in Tg after the first ($P < 0.001$) and second ($P = 0.008$) operations. No patient developed detectable distant metastases or died from PTC.

Conclusions.—Surgical resection of persistent PTC in cervical lymph nodes achieves BCR, when most stringently defined, in 27% of patients, sometimes requiring several surgeries. No biochemical or clinical recurrences occurred during follow-up. In patients who do not achieve BCR, Tg levels were significantly reduced. The long-term durability and impact of this intervention will require further investigation.

▶ Papillary thyroid cancer (PTC), the most common of the well-differentiated thyroid cancers, accounts for about 80% to 85% of follicular cell—derived thyroid cancers in developed countries in which sufficient iodine is present in the diet. Local recurrences are found in 5% to 20% of patients with PTC, two-thirds of which are localized to cervical lymph nodes. The 10-year relative survival rate for individuals with PTC in the United States is about 90%. Still, more than half of the deaths from thyroid cancer are caused by PTC because of its comparatively high frequency. The object of this study was to determine the outcome of patients who underwent potentially curable surgery, the durability of the response, and whether any criteria could predict which patients would benefit from an aggressive surgical approach to locoregional recurrence after failure of initial therapy, including thyroidectomy and radioactive iodine ablation. This study provides important information concerning the outcome of lymphadenectomy in 58 patients with cervical recurrent/persistent PTC. Biochemically complete remission was achieved in 12 patients (17%), using the most stringent definition for no evidence of disease, which is that of the European Thyroid Association and American Thyroid Association; they recommend the following criteria for no evidence of disease: (1) no clinical evidence of tumor, (2) no imaging evidence of tumor (no uptake outside the thyroid bed on the initial posttreatment whole-body scan or, if uptake outside the thyroid bed had been present, no imaging evidence of tumor on a recent diagnostic scan and neck ultrasound), and (3) undetectable serum thyroglobulin (Tg) levels during thyrotropin suppression and stimulation in the absence of interfering antibodies. After a mean follow-up of 60 months, no patient had a relapse. Still, patients who did not achieve a remission had a reduction in serum Tg after the first and second operations ($P < .001$ and $P = .008$, respectively). Moreover, no patient had distant metastases or died of disease. Among the patients who did not experience a remission, Tg levels were significantly reduced, and the authors acknowledge that further follow-up will be necessary for this group of patients. Lastly, the multiple surgeries were performed without long-term hypoparathyroidism or recurrent laryngeal nerve injury. In summary, this study shows the significance of ongoing surveillance and the careful selection of patients for repeated surgery. The validation of retreating patients with persistent lymph node metastases rests on a unique study by Links and coworkers[1] in which survival rates were transformed into standardized survival time to adjust for the baseline mortality rate in the general population. The outcome of the study was that disease-free patients had a normal residual life span, whereas life expectancy was reduced to 60% in patients with persistent disease. Because of this, residual disease should be treated carefully.

M. Schott, MD, PhD

Reference

1. Links TP, van Tol KM, Jager PL, et al. Life expectancy in differentiated thyroid cancer: a novel approach to survival analysis. *Endocr Relat Cancer.* 2005;12: 273-280.

Estimating Risk of Recurrence in Differentiated Thyroid Cancer After Total Thyroidectomy and Radioactive Iodine Remnant Ablation: Using Response to Therapy Variables to Modify the Initial Risk Estimates Predicted by the New American Thyroid Association Staging System
Tuttle RM, Tala H, Shah J, et al (Memorial Sloan-Kettering Cancer Ctr, NY)
Thyroid 20:1341-1349, 2010

Background.—A risk-adapted approach to management of thyroid cancer requires risk estimates that change over time based on response to therapy and the course of the disease. The objective of this study was to validate the American Thyroid Association (ATA) risk of recurrence staging system and determine if an assessment of response to therapy during the first 2 years of follow-up can modify these initial risk estimates.

Methods.—This retrospective review identified 588 adult follicular cell-derived thyroid cancer patients followed for a median of 7 years (range 1—15 years) after total thyroidectomy and radioactive iodine remnant ablation. Patients were stratified according to ATA risk categories (low, intermediate, or high) as part of initial staging. Clinical data obtained during the first 2 years of follow-up (suppressed thyroglobulin [Tg], stimulated Tg, and imaging studies) were used to re-stage each patient based on response to initial therapy (excellent, acceptable, or incomplete). Clinical outcomes predicted by initial ATA risk categories were compared with revised risk estimates obtained after response to therapy variables were used to modify the initial ATA risk estimates.

Results.—Persistent structural disease or recurrence was identified in 3% of the low-risk, 21% of the intermediate-risk, and 68% of the high-risk patients ($p < 0.001$). Re-stratification during the first 2 years of follow-up reduced the likelihood of finding persistent structural disease or recurrence to 2% in low-risk, 2% in intermediate-risk, and 14% in high-risk patients, demonstrating an excellent response to therapy (stimulated Tg < 1 ng/mL without structural evidence of disease). Conversely, an incomplete response to initial therapy (suppressed Tg > 1 ng/mL, stimulated Tg > 10 ng/mL, rising Tg values, or structural disease identification within the first 2 years of follow-up) increased the likelihood of persistent structural disease or recurrence to 13% in low-risk, 41% in intermediate-risk, and 79% in high-risk patients.

Conclusions.—Our data confirm that the newly proposed ATA recurrence staging system effectively predicts the risk of recurrence and persistent disease. Further, these initial ATA risk estimates can be significantly refined based on the assessment of response to initial therapy, thereby providing a dynamic risk assessment that can be used to more effectively tailor ongoing follow-up recommendations (Tables 1 and 5).

▶ The aim of the article by Tuttle et al was to validate the newly proposed American Thyroid Association risk stratification system for prediction of early recurrence of disease and to proceed to demonstrate how these initial risk estimates can be refined by incorporating response to therapy variables in a retrospective review of 588 consecutive thyroid cancer patients followed up for a median of 7 years at a single tertiary care referral center. Of the patients in the high-risk category (Table 1), 14% had no evidence of disease during follow-up, but, unfortunately, 86% of patients in this category had persistent or recurrent disease. Detailed data are given in Table 5. Although the study does not describe the efficacy of various treatments, it is clear that many

TABLE 1.—Initial American Thyroid Association Risk of Recurrence Classification

Low Risk	Intermediate Risk	High Risk
All the following are present	Any of the following is present	Any of the following is present
No local or distant metastases	Microscopic invasion into the perithyroidal soft tissues	Macroscopic tumor invasion
All macroscopic tumor has been resected	Cervical lymph node metastases or ^{131}I uptake outside the thyroid bed on the post-treatment scan done after thyroid remnant ablation	Incomplete tumor resection with gross residual disease
No invasion of locoregional tissues		Distant metastases
Tumor does not have aggressive histology (e.g., tall cell, insular, columnar cell carcinoma, Hurthle cell carcinoma, follicular thyroid cancer).	Tumor with aggressive histology or vascular invasion (e.g., tall cell, insular, columnar cell carcinoma, Hurthle cell carcinoma, follicular thyroid cancer)	
No vascular invasion		
No ^{131}I uptake outside the thyroid bed on the post-treatment scan, if done		

TABLE 5.—Clinical Outcomes Following Initial Therapy for American Thyroid Association Risk Categories

Clinical Outcome Following Initial Therapy	Low (n = 136)	n = 588 Intermediate (n = 291)	High (n = 161)
No evidence of disease (n = 305)	86% (117)	57% (166)	14% (22)
Persistent disease, biochemical evidence (n = 108)	11% (15)	22% (64)	18% (29)
Persistent disease, structurally identifiable (n = 167)	2% (3)	19% (56)	67% (108)
Recurrent disease (n = 8)	1% (1)	2% (5)	1% (2)

patients were moved to lower-risk categories. Nevertheless, current therapeutic modalities are not optimally effective. For example, neck dissection for recurrence in cervical lymph nodes cures only about one-fourth of patients when strict criteria for cure are applied. Cure of metastatic disease by ^{131}I therapy is even less effective, although it is a time-honored tool.

M. Schott, MD, PhD

Total Thyroidectomy Followed by Postsurgical Remnant Ablation May Improve Cancer Specific Survival in Differentiated Thyroid Carcinoma

Doi SAR, Engel JM, Onitilo AA (Univ of Queensland, Brisbane, Australia; Marshfield Clinic — Marshfield Campus, WI; Marshfield Clinic — Weston Ctr, WI)
Clin Nucl Med 35:396-399, 2010

Purpose.—To determine the effect of the extent of thyroidectomy and additional postsurgical radioiodine remnant ablation (RRA) on the survival of patients with differentiated thyroid carcinoma (DTC) after adjustment for risk stage.

Methods.—We electronically identified 614 cases of DTC at our institution between 1987 and 2006. Two treatment variables were created, surgical extent dichotomized to total versus other and a composite of surgery and radioactive iodine ablation. The odds of cancer specific survival and disease-free survival (DFS) were determined using Cox proportional hazards model with adjustment for quantitative tumor-node-metastasis risk score.

Results.—Of 614 patients with DTC during our period, 504 (83%) underwent total thyroidectomy and 104 (17%) underwent lesser surgery. Radioiodine administration was reported for 394 patients who underwent total thyroidectomy with a dose range of 24 to 297 mCi (mean of 116 mCi). Ten-year survival was higher for patients with total thyroidectomy compared with lobectomy: 96% versus 84% ($P < 0.001$, Gehan's Wilcoxon test). Ten-year survival for complete versus incomplete surgery for tumor stages 1 and 2 was 99% versus 96%, and for stages 3 and 4 was 88% versus 52%. Cancer specific death tended to occur earlier in those without RRA postsurgery. There was no overall relationship between DFS and RRA or surgery, but in the higher risk categories surgery retained significance.

Conclusion.—Our data support the routine use of both total or near-total thyroidectomy followed by RRA over all risk categories in DTC. Although the effect of surgery is clear, there is also a trend toward improvement in outcome with RRA for cancer specific survival.

▶ Prognostic indices have been generated that stratify patients with differentiated thyroid carcinoma (DTC) into low- and high-risk prognostic groups. Most patients with DTC are low risk and have an excellent prognosis; the small proportion of patients who are high risk has a relatively worse survival. The extent of thyroidectomy that provides optimal survival for low- and high-risk patients is unknown because no randomized trial has compared outcomes after total thyroidectomy with those after an operation of lesser extent. Nevertheless, retrospective studies demonstrate that total thyroidectomy results in lower recurrence rates and improved survival for papillary thyroid carcinoma of size ≥1 cm compared with lobectomy.[1] One approach that has, therefore, been suggested is to use a less extensive thyroidectomy, such as thyroid lobectomy and isthmusectomy, on patients with a good prognosis, rather than routinely performing total thyroidectomy on all patients. However, total thyroidectomy has been proposed as the optimal operation for all patients with DTC because it provides advantages such as clearing microscopic contralateral disease, allowing accurate postoperative thyroglobulin surveillance, and, possibly, providing better survival.[2] More importantly, however, it enables the use of radioactive iodine as an adjuvant therapy. This hospital-based study was performed to determine the effect of the extent of thyroidectomy and additional postsurgical remnant ablation on the survival of patients with DTC after adjustment for risk stage. The hypothesis of this study was that patients will have better survival with both, regardless of the stage of disease.

I think that several conclusions in this study are troublesome. The use of radioiodine remnant ablation (RRA) in this group of low-risk patients showed a trend in the improvement of cancer-specific mortality. Although total thyroidectomy has a positive effect on cancer-specific mortality, RRA is of only borderline significance for the end point, although hazard ratios for RRA are indicative of improved cancer-specific survival. Moreover, the study could not verify an effect of disease-free survival. The authors suggest that the potential for recurrent disease is more strongly associated with risk score than with the therapeutic interventions, implying that low-risk patients have better disease-free survival, regardless of the use of therapeutic interventions, but suggest that if these interventions are used, cancer-specific survival is probably related to the initial tumor and is improved even in low-risk patients. As a consequence, the authors advocate total thyroidectomy at initial diagnosis along with RRA, which they opine confers the best possible prognosis for the patient. Yet the authors were unable to run analyses on the low-risk group alone, as there were few outcomes in this group and a stratified analysis was not possible. Lastly, tumor size was unknown in 54 patients (8.8%), suggesting that the tumor staging in this study may have not been fully responsive to tumor size, which has a well-described effect on cancer-specific mortality and disease-free survival.

There are a few robust studies that have found total thyroidectomy to significantly decrease cancer-specific mortality in patients with DTC, including some older studies that find a decrease in mortality and recurrence rates with iodine 131 (^{131}I) therapy.[3] All of these studies have been tightly linked to tumor features, patient age, and histology. Two meta-analyses by Sawka et al[4,5] failed to find an effect of RRA on thyroid cancer—specific mortality; however, a pooled analysis of 10-year outcomes found that locoregional recurrence was 4% in ^{131}I-treated patients and 10% in controls (relative risk, 0.31) and the rate of distant metastases was 2% in ^{131}I-treated patients and 4% in controls and was associated with an absolute decrease in distant metastases in ^{131}I-RRA—treated patients. Still, papillary thyroid microcarcinoma (PTMC) fails to show a significant response to ^{131}I RRA, whereas patients with PTMC may be responsive to RRA in tumors invading surrounding tissues or organs, but this occurs rarely.

M. Schott, MD, PhD

References

1. Bilimoria KY, Bentrem DJ, Ko CY, et al. Extent of surgery affects survival for papillary thyroid cancer. *Ann Surg.* 2007;246:375-381.
2. Sosa JA, Udelsman R. Total thyroidectomy for differentiated thyroid cancer. *J Surg Oncol.* 2006;94:701-707.
3. Chow SM, Law SC, Mendenhall WM, et al. Papillary thyroid carcinoma: prognostic factors and the role of radioiodine and external radiotherapy. *Int J Radiat Oncol Biol Phys.* 2002;52:784-795.
4. Sawka AM, Brierley JD, Tsang RW, et al. An updated systematic review and commentary examining the effectiveness of radioactive iodine remnant ablation in well-differentiated thyroid cancer. *Endocrinol Metab Clin North Am.* 2008; 37:457-480.
5. Sawka AM, Thephamongkhol K, Brouwers M, Thabane L, Browman G, Gerstein HC. Clinical review 170: a systematic review and metaanalysis of the effectiveness of radioactive iodine remnant ablation for well-differentiated thyroid cancer. *J Clin Endocrinol Metab.* 2004;89:3668-3676.

Thyroid Cancer Recurrence in Patients Clinically Free of Disease with Undetectable or Very Low Serum Thyroglobulin Values

Kloos RT (The Ohio State Univ Med Ctr, Columbus)
J Clin Endocrinol Metab 95:5241-5248, 2010

Design.—This was a retrospective clinical study.

Setting.—The study was conducted at a university-based tertiary cancer hospital.

Patients.—One hundred seven patients had initial thyroid cancer surgery and subsequent remnant radioiodine ablation. Patients underwent recombinant human TSH (rhTSH)-mediated diagnostic whole-body scan and rhTSH-stimulated thyroglobulin (Tg) measurement before April 2001 if they had no antithyroglobulin antibodies, were clinically free of disease, and had one or more undetectable (≤0.5 ng/ml) or low (0.6−1 ng/ml) basal Tg measurements on levothyroxine. Patients were stratified according to their rhTSH-Tg responses: group 1, Tg 0.5 ng/ml or less (68 patients); group 2, Tg from 0.6 to 2.0 ng/ml (19 patients); and group 3, Tg greater than 2 ng/ml (20 patients).

Main Outcome Measures.—Tumor recurrence was measured.

Results.—In group 1, two of 62 patients (3%) with follow-up recurred. In group 2, 63% converted to group 1, whereas two of 19 (11%) converted to group 3 and then recurred. Sixteen of the initial 20 group 3 patients (80%) recurred, including recurrence rates of 69 and 100% for those with an initial rhTSH-Tg greater than 2.0 ng/ml but 5.0 ng/ml or less, and 4.6 ng/ml or greater, respectively. One group 3 patient died of distant metastases. rhTSH-Tg more accurately predicted tumor recurrence than basal Tg. An rhTSH-Tg threshold of 2.5 ng/ml or greater optimally predicted future recurrence with sensitivity, specificity, and negative and positive predictive values of 80, 97, 95, and 84%, respectively.

Conclusions.—The prevalence of postablation thyroid cancer recurrence is predicted by the rhTSH-Tg response with an optimal Tg threshold of 2.5 ng/ml. Still, recurrent disease occurs in some patients with an initial rhTSH-Tg of 0.5 ng/ml or less (Fig 1).

▶ In the past, surveillance to detect persistent or recurrent differentiated thyroid carcinoma did not include sensitive serum thyroglobulin (Tg) assays or neck

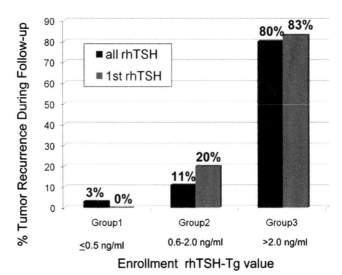

FIGURE 1.—Percentage of patients after thyroidectomy and radioiodine therapy with tumor recurrence during follow-up after an enrollment rhTSH stimulated Tg value was 0.5 ng/ml or less (group 1), 0.6−2.0 ng/ml (group 2), and greater than 2.0 ng/ml (group 3). *Gray bars*, Patients whose enrollment rhTSH testing was their first stimulation after remnant ablation, and the testing was within 2 yr (730 d) of their first thyroid cancer surgery; *black bars*, all patients. (Reprinted from Kloos RT. Thyroid cancer recurrence in patients clinically free of disease with undetectable or very low serum thyroglobulin values. *J Clin Endocrinol Metab*. 2010;95:5241-5248, Copyright © 2010, with permission from The Endocrine Society.)

ultrasonography by experienced thyroid cancer observers. Thus, many patients appeared to be cured by initial therapy of total thyroidectomy (with or without lymph node dissection) and radioiodine remnant ablation only to have recurrent disease discovered years later. The aim of this study by Kloos was to investigate the outcome of patients with thyroid cancer depending on the first stimulated serum Tg levels. The results also show that 3% of those who would be predicted to have no recurrence based on recombinant human thyrotropin (rhTSH)-Tg levels < 0.5 ng/mL do indeed have recurrences of thyroid cancer (Fig 1). The report does not provide data on the pathology of these tumors that might also have predictive value because follicular and Hürthle-cell and tall-cell papillary carcinomas are known to be more aggressive and recurrent.[1] The report also shows that 7 additional patients in the group with rhTSH-Tg levels > 2 ng/mL had recurrence after the first follow-up of this cohort, which was published in the year 2005.[2] When patients with stage 1 thyroid cancer have an undetectable rhTSH-Tg level during 9 to 12 months of follow-up after thyroidectomy, the European Thyroid Association guidelines recommend that serum thyrotropin (TSH) levels should subsequently be maintained in the normal range.[3] However, the 3% recurrence rate found in this study suggests that this might be unwise. One advantage of allowing the serum TSH levels to be in the normal range, rather than suppressed to prevent recurrence, is that subsequent Tg measurements on replacement will be more sensitive for the detection of recurrence.

M. Schott, MD, PhD

References

1. Hundahl SA, Fleming ID, Fremgen AM, Menck HR. A National Cancer Data Base report on 53,856 cases of thyroid carcinoma treated in the U.S., 1985–1995. *Cancer.* 1998;83:2638-2648.
2. Kloos RT, Mazzaferri EL. A single recombinant human thyrotropin-stimulated serum thyroglobulin measurement predicts differentiated thyroid carcinoma metastases three to five years later. *J Clin Endocrinol Metab.* 2005;90:5047-5057.
3. Pacini F, Schlumberger M, Dralle H, Elisei R, Smit JW, Wiersinga W. European consensus for the management of patients with differentiated thyroid carcinoma of the follicular epithelium. *Eur J Endocrinol.* 2006;154:787-803.

Thyroid Cancer Recurrence in Patients Clinically Free of Disease with Undetectable or Very Low Serum Thyroglobulin Values
Kloos RT (The Ohio State Univ Med Ctr, Columbus)
J Clin Endocrinol Metab 95:5241-5248, 2010

Design.—This was a retrospective clinical study.
Setting.—The study was conducted at a university-based tertiary cancer hospital.
Patients.—One hundred seven patients had initial thyroid cancer surgery and subsequent remnant radioiodine ablation. Patients underwent recombinant human TSH (rhTSH)-mediated diagnostic whole-body scan and rhTSH-stimulated thyroglobulin (Tg) measurement before April 2001 if

they had no antithyroglobulin antibodies, were clinically free of disease, and had one or more undetectable (≤0.5 ng/ml) or low (0.6–1 ng/ml) basal Tg measurements on levothyroxine. Patients were stratified according to their rhTSH-Tg responses: group 1, Tg 0.5 ng/ml or less (68 patients); group 2, Tg from 0.6 to 2.0 ng/ml (19 patients); and group 3, Tg greater than 2 ng/ml (20 patients).

Main Outcome Measures.—Tumor recurrence was measured.

Results.—In group 1, two of 62 patients (3%) with follow-up recurred. In group 2, 63% converted to group 1, whereas two of 19 (11%) converted to group 3 and then recurred. Sixteen of the initial 20 group 3 patients (80%) recurred, including recurrence rates of 69 and 100% for those with an initial rhTSH-Tg greater than 2.0 ng/ml but 5.0 ng/ml or less, and 4.6 ng/ml or greater, respectively. One group 3 patient died of distant metastases. rhTSH-Tg more accurately predicted tumor recurrence than basal Tg. An rhTSH-Tg threshold of 2.5 ng/ml or greater optimally predicted future recurrence with sensitivity, specificity, and negative and positive predictive values of 80, 97, 95, and 84%, respectively.

Conclusions.—The prevalence of postablation thyroid cancer recurrence is predicted by the rhTSH-Tg response with an optimal Tg threshold of 2.5 ng/ml. Still, recurrent disease occurs in some patients with an initial rhTSH-Tg of 0.5 ng/ml or less.

▶ The aim of this study was to investigate the outcome of patients with differentiated thyroid cancer with undetectable or very low serum thyroglobulin values. One hundred seven patients were enrolled in the study. They were divided into 3 groups of patients according to their recombinant human thyrotropin (rhTSsH) transgenic insertion (Tg) responses (group 1, Tg 0.5 ng/mL or less [68 patients]; group 2, Tg 0.6-2.0 ng/mL [19 patients]; and group 3, Tg greater than 2 ng/mL [20 patients]). Fig 1 in the original article shows the tumor recurrence rate of all patients. As expected, patients of group 3 showed the highest recurrence rate around 80%. Importantly, however, some patients of the groups 1 and 2 also had tumor recurrence, and this could also be predicted after the first rhTSH stimulation. The 2009 American Thyroid Association guidelines state that the clinical significance of minimally detectable Tg levels is unclear, especially if detected only after thyrotropin stimulation.[1] It is suggested that the Tg trend over time will typically identify patients with clinically significant residual disease. Regarding low-level detectable Tg levels during levothyroxine therapy, the specificity for eventual tumor recurrence in this series when the initial Tg measurements on thyroid hormone replacement (Tg-on) was 0.6 to 1.0 ng/mL was 98% with a positive predictive value of 75%. This finding is in agreement with Schlumberger et al[2] whose findings suggest that detectable Tg values above 0.3 to 0.5 ng/mL indicate the presence residual disease. Regarding low-level detectable stimulated serum Tg (stim-Tg) levels, 63% of group 2 patients converted spontaneously to group 1, a finding previously reported by others. In this series, this was demonstrated a mean of 3.8 years after the initial rhTSH (range, 1.7-8.4 years). This finding supports that group 2 patients typically require only careful neck ultrasound (US) to find obvious residual disease in the minority and, in the majority, continued observation because they will likely spontaneously convert to group 1 without further therapy. However, 11% of group 2 patients eventually demonstrated tumor recurrence. Their recurrent disease was preceded by a rise in stim-Tg over time and eventual conversion to group 3 in both patients despite undetectable Tg-on values in both and a negative neck US in one. This suggests that periodic stim-Tg testing in group 2 may help clarify which patients become group 1 and require less -intensive therapy and follow-up versus identifying those patients with rising stim-Tg values who are likely to manifest tumor recurrence. Still, there are no compelling data that identifying such patients earlier when the Tg-on is still undetectable will translate into a better long-term outcome. In summary, this is an important study that will help identify patients who have a higher risk of tumor recurrence in differentiated thyroid carcinoma.

M. Schott, MD, PhD

References

1. Cooper DS, Doherty GM, Haugen BR, et al. Revised American Thyroid Association management guidelines for patients with thyroid nodules and differentiated thyroid cancer. *Thyroid.* 2009;19:1167-1214.
2. Schlumberger M, Hitzel A, Toubert ME, et al. Comparison of seven serum thyroglobulin assays in the follow-up of papillary and follicular thyroid cancer patients. *J Clin Endocrinol Metab.* 2007;92:2487-2495.

Does an undetectable rhTSH-stimulated Tg level 12 months after initial treatment of thyroid cancer indicate remission?
Klubo-Gwiezdzinska J, Burman KD, Van Nostrand D, et al (Washington Hosp Ctr, DC)
Clin Endocrinol 74:111-117, 2011

Objectives.—Routine monitoring after the initial treatment of differentiated thyroid cancer (DTC) includes periodic cervical ultrasonography (US) and measurement of serum thyroglobulin (Tg) during thyrotrophin (TSH) suppression and after recombinant human TSH (rhTSH) stimulation. The aim of our study was to evaluate the utility of repeated rhTSH-stimulated Tg measurements in patients with DTC who have had no evidence of disease at their initial rhTSH stimulation test performed 1 year after the treatment.

Material and Methods.—A retrospective chart review of 278 patients with DTC who had repeated rhTSH stimulation testing after an initial undetectable rhTSH-stimulated serum Tg level.

Results.—The number of rhTSH stimulation tests performed on individual patients during the follow-up period (3−12 years, mean 6·3) varied from two to seven. Biochemical and/or cytological evidence of potential persistent/recurrent disease based on detectable second or third rhTSH-stimulated Tg values and US findings was observed in 11 (4%) patients. Subsequent follow-up data revealed that in five cases, the results of the second stimulation were false positive, in one case − false negative.

Combined with the negative neck US, the negative predictive value for disease-free survival was 98% after the first undetectable rhTSH-stimulated Tg and 100% after the second one.

Conclusions.—In patients with DTC, the intensity of follow-up should be adjusted to new risk estimates evolving with time. The first rhTSH-stimulated Tg is an excellent predictor for remission, independent of clinical stage at presentation. Second negative rhTSH-Tg stimulation is additionally reassuring and can guide less aggressive follow-up by the measurement of nonstimulated Tg and neck US every few years (Fig 1, Table 3).

▶ The goal of this study was to evaluate the utility of repeated recombinant human thyrotropin (rhTSH)-stimulated thyroglobulin (Tg) measurements in patients with differentiated thyroid cancer who had no evidence of disease at an initial rhTSH stimulation test performed approximately 1 year after thyroidectomy and iodine 131 therapy. Altogether, 278 patients were enrolled into the study. The number of patients tested over a period of more than 6 years are shown in Fig 1. Biochemical and/or cytological evidence of potential persistent/recurrent disease based on detectable second or third rhTSH-stimulated Tg values and ultrasound (US) findings was observed in 11 (4%) patients. Combined with the negative neck US, the negative predictive value for disease-free survival was 98% after the first undetectable rhTSH-stimulated Tg and 100% after the second one (Table 3). Recommendation 77 of the recently modified guidelines for thyroid

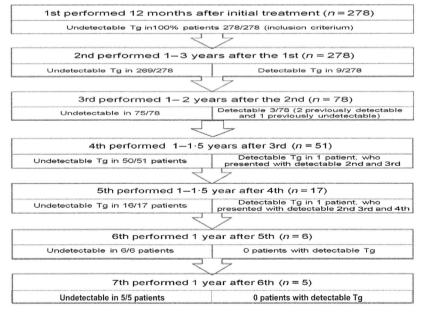

FIGURE 1.—The number of repeated rhTSH stimulation tests during the follow-up period. (Reprinted from Klubo-Gwiezdzinska J, Burman KD, Van Nostrand D, et al. Does an undetectable rhTSH-stimulated Tg level 12 months after initial treatment of thyroid cancer indicate remission?. *Clin Endocrinol.* 2011;74:111-117, with permission from Blackwell Publishing Ltd.)

TABLE 3.—Negative (NPV) and Positive (PPV) Predictive Values, Sensitivity and Specificity of Subsequent Stimulated Tg Levels

	TP	FP	TN	FN	NPV (%)	PPV (%)	Sensitivity (%)	Specificity (%)
Tg1	0	0	272	6	97·8	NA	NA	100
Tg2	5	4	268	1	99·6	55·5	83·3	98·5
Tg3	2	1	75	0	100	66·6	100	98·7
Tg4	1	0	50	0	100	100	100	100
Tg5	1	0	16	0	100	100	100	100
Tg6	0	0	6	0	100	NA	NA	100
Tg7	0	0	5	0	100	NA	NA	100

TP, true-positive result defined as evidence of disease progression (increasing Tg level and/or increasing size of metastatic foci), stable disease (stable detectable Tg and stable imaging studies) or inconclusive results of rhTSH-Tg stimulation tests during follow-up period.

FP, false-positive result defined as detectable rhTSH-Tg and no other evidence of disease during the follow-up period.

TN, true-negative result defined as undetectable Tg and no evidence of disease during follow-up period (biochemical and cytological and based on abnormal imaging studies).

FN, false negative defined as undetectable Tg and evidence of disease (biochemical and/or cytological and/or based on abnormal imaging studies).

cancer by the American Thyroid Association indicates that in the absence of structurally evident disease, patients with rhTSH-stimulated Tg levels < 5 ng/mL can be followed on treatment with levothyroxine only, reserving additional therapy for those patients with rising serum Tg levels or other evidence of disease progression during the follow-up period. Based on the data presented in this article, I agree to the recommendations given by the authors saying that a first rhTSH-stimulated Tg at 1 year after initial treatment is an excellent predictor for remission and long-term disease-free survival independent of clinical stage at presentation, and 1 additional negative rhTSH-Tg stimulation test at 3 years together with a negative neck ultrasonography will provide a negative predictive value of 100% and sensitivity of 100% and may be used as a tool selecting the patients who might be followed with baseline Tg measurement and neck ultrasonography every few years. A limitation of this study is its retrospective design, which predicated use of Tg results from different clinical laboratories. On the other hand, this study reflects common clinical practice where Tg measurements occur in various laboratories over time.

M. Schott, MD, PhD

Modified-Release Recombinant Human TSH (MRrhTSH) Augments the Effect of [131]I Therapy in Benign Multinodular Goiter: Results from a Multicenter International, Randomized, Placebo-Controlled Study

Graf H, Fast S, Pacini F, et al (Serviço de Endocrinologia e Metabologia do Hospital de Clínicas da Universidade Federal do Paraná, Curitiba, Brazil; Odense Univ Hosp, Denmark; Univ of Siena, Italy; et al)
J Clin Endocrinol Metab 96:1368-1376, 2011

Background.—Recombinant human TSH (rhTSH) can be used to enhance ^{131}I therapy for shrinkage of multinodular goiter (MG).

Objective, Design, and Setting.—The objective of the study was to compare the efficacy and safety of 0.01 and 0.03 mg modified-release (MR) rhTSH as an adjuvant to ^{131}I therapy, *vs.* ^{131}I alone, in a randomized, placebo-controlled, international, multicenter study.

Patients and Intervention.—Ninety-five patients (57.2 ± 9.6 yr old, 85% females, 83% Caucasians) with MG (median size 96.0, range 31.9–242.2 ml) were randomized to receive placebo (group A, n = 32), MRrhTSH 0.01 mg (group B, n = 30), or MRrhTSH 0.03 mg (group C, n = 33) 24 h before a calculated activity of ^{131}I.

Main Outcome Measures.—The primary end point was a change in thyroid volume (by computerized tomography scan, at 6 months). Secondary end points were the smallest cross-sectional area of the trachea; thyroid function tests; Thyroid Quality of Life Questionnaire; electrocardiogram; and hyperthyroid symptom scale.

Results.—Thyroid volume decreased significantly in all groups. The reduction was comparable in groups A and B (23.1 ± 8.8 and 23.3 ± 16.5%, respectively; $P = 0.95$). In group C, the reduction (32.9 ± 20.7%) was more pronounced than in groups A ($P = 0.03$) and B. The smallest cross-sectional area of the trachea increased in all groups: 3.8 ± 2.9% in A, 4.8 ± 3.3% in B, and 10.2 ± 33.2% in C, with no significant difference among the groups. Goiter-related symptoms were effectively reduced and there were no major safety concerns.

Conclusion.—In this dose-selection study, 0.03 mg MRrhTSH was the most efficacious dose as an adjuvant to ^{131}I therapy of MG. It was well tolerated and significantly augmented the effect of ^{131}I therapy in the short term. Larger studies with long-term follow-up are warranted.

▶ Multinodular goiter (MG) is thought to arise from genetic susceptibility interacting with environmental factors, of which iodine deficiency and cigarette smoking are the most important. The aim of this study was to investigate the new modified-release recombinant human thyrotropin (MRrhTSH) for the treatment of goiter patients. Normally, recombinant human thyrotropin (rhTSH) increases the thyroid radioiodine (^{131}I) uptake (RAIU) by more than 2-fold in patients with MG and in normal subjects. Randomized, placebo-controlled studies have demonstrated that prestimulation with rhTSH (0.3-0.45 mg) increases goiter reduction by 35% to 56% compared with ^{131}I therapy alone.[1-3] The rhTSH doses used in these studies were relatively high, resulting in a marked increase in serum thyroid hormone concentrations, posing a risk in the elderly or patients with cardiovascular disease. Furthermore, studies have demonstrated that rhTSH doses greater than 0.1 mg may result in significant acute thyroid swelling. Although the positive effect of rhTSH on thyroid RAIU appears to be robust in some patients, even with very low doses (ie, 0.01 mg), it is unknown whether the dose of rhTSH is an independent determinant of goiter volume reduction because there are no comparative trials. MRrhTSH is equipotent to rhTSH for increasing thyroid RAIU, but MRrhTSH results in a lower peak plasma TSH concentration. MRrhTSH has altered pharmacokinetics with a delayed time to reach the maximum concentration as compared with aqueous rhTSH. Potentially, this could reduce side effects related to thyroid hyperfunction. In this study, the authors could demonstrate that MRrhTSH with a dose of 0.03 mg together with radioiodine resulted in a significant reduction of the thyroid volume as shown in Fig 1 in the original article (Group C). Considering the high cost for thyroidectomy, including the risk of thyroid hormone replacement (100%), hypoparathyroidism (0.5%-2%), and recurrent laryngeal nerve damage (0.5%-2%) in the hands of an experienced thyroid surgeon, rhTSH-stimulated ablation should be considered a cost-effective viable option because most patients do not become hypothyroid and there is no risk to the parathyroid glands and the recurrent laryngeal nerves. When MRrhTSH becomes available, this therapy should be considered as a first-line alternative treatment for large nontoxic goiters.[4] This international study suggests that the response to rhTSH-stimulated ablation is similar in patients from different genetic backgrounds and with different iodine intake in different countries.

M. Schott, MD, PhD

References

1. Bonnema SJ, Nielsen VE, Boel-Jørgensen H, et al. Improvement of goiter volume reduction after 0.3mg recombinant human thyrotropin-stimulated radioiodine therapy in patients with a very large goiter: a double-blinded, randomized trial. *J Clin Endocrinol Metab*. 2007;92:3424-3428.
2. Nielsen VE, Bonnema SJ, Boel-Jørgensen H, Grupe P, Hegedus L. Stimulation with 0.3-mg recombinant human thyrotropin prior to iodine 131 therapy to improve the size reduction of benign nontoxic nodular goiter: a prospective randomized double-blind trial. *Arch Intern Med*. 2006;166:1476-1482.
3. Silva MN, Rubió IG, Romão R, et al. Administration of a single dose of recombinant human thyrotrophin enhances the efficacy of radioiodine treatment of large compressive multinodular goitres. *Clin Endocrinol (Oxf)*. 2004;60:300-308.
4. Lee SL. Comment on "Modified-release recombinant human TSH (MRrhTSH) augments the effect of 131I therapy in benign multinodular goiter: results from a multicenter international, randomized, placebo-controlled study". *Clinical Thyroidology*. 2011;23:5-7.

Enhanced Survival in Locoregionally Confined Anaplastic Thyroid Carcinoma: A Single-Institution Experience Using Aggressive Multimodal Therapy

Foote RL, Molina JR, Kasperbauer JL, et al (Mayo Clinic Comprehensive Cancer Ctr, Rochester, MN)
Thyroid 21:25-30, 2011

Background.—Historical outcomes in anaplastic thyroid carcinoma (ATC) are poor, with a median survival of only 5 months and <20% of patients surviving 1 year from diagnosis. We hypothesized that survival in newly diagnosed patients with stages IVA and IVB locoregionally confined ATC might be improved by utilizing an aggressive therapeutic approach, prioritizing both the eradication of disease in the neck and preemptive treatment of occult metastatic disease.

Methods.—Between January 1, 2003, and December 31, 2007, 25 new ATC patients were evaluated at our institution. Of these 25 patients, 10 (40%) had metastatic disease at diagnosis and therefore underwent palliative treatment, whereas 5 (20%) had regionally confined disease and desired treatment at their local medical facilities. The remaining 10 consecutive patients (40%) had regionally confined ATC and elected aggressive therapy combining individualized surgery (where feasible), intensity-modulated radiation therapy (IMRT), and radiosensitizing + adjuvant chemotherapy intending four cycles of docetaxel + doxorubicin. Outcomes were assessed on an intention to treat basis.

Results.—There were no deaths from therapy, but hospitalization was required in two patients (20%) because of treatment-related adverse events. Five patients (50%) are alive and cancer-free, all having been followed >32 months (range: 32–89 months; median: 44 months) with a median overall Kaplan–Meier survival of 60 months. Overall survival at 1 and 2 years was 70% and 60%, respectively, compared to <20% historical survival at 1 year in analogous patients previously treated with surgery and conventional postoperative radiation at our and other institutions.

Conclusions.—Although based upon a small series of consecutively treated patients, an aggressive approach combining IMRT and radiosensitizing plus adjuvant chemotherapy appears to improve outcomes, including survival in stages IVA and IVB regionally confined ATC, but remains of uncertain benefit in patients with stage IVC (metastatic) disease. Also uncertain is the optimal chemotherapy regimen to use in conjunction with IMRT. Further multicenter randomized trials are required to define optimal therapy in this rare but deadly cancer.

▶ Anaplastic thyroid carcinoma (ATC) is a malignancy with terrible prognosis. Only about 20% of affected patients survive 1 year from diagnosis, and median survival is only about 5 months. The aim of this study by Foote and coworkers was to investigate the outcome of locally confined tumors of patients with ATC, which were treated by radiation together with a combined chemotherapy with doxorubicin and docetaxel or paclitaxel. The authors could clearly demonstrate a clinical benefit in terms of a prolonged survival in these patients compared with others (Fig 1 in the original article). It has to be mentioned, however, that these patients suffered from a significant toxicity. Nonetheless, these data are somehow encouraging. These data, however, also need to be confirmed in bigger trials.

M. Schott, MD, PhD

Zoledronic Acid in the Treatment of Bone Metastases from Differentiated Thyroid Carcinoma
Orita Y, Sugitani I, Toda K, et al (Okayama Saiseikai General Hosp, Japan; Cancer Inst Hosp, Tokyo, Japan)
Thyroid 21:31-35, 2011

Background.—Currently bisphosphonates are often administered to patients with osteolytic bone metastases from several neoplasms. Based on favorable experience in other cancers with bone metastases and the lack of effective treatment, we started to use zoledronic acid (ZA), a recently developed synthetic bisphosphonate drug, in the treatment of this disease. In the present study, we retrospectively evaluated the efficacy of ZA for bone metastases from differentiated thyroid carcinoma.

Methods.—The study consisted of 50 patients with bone metastases from differentiated thyroid carcinoma treated at the Cancer Institute Hospital of Tokyo between 1976 and 2008. Among them, 28 patients who did not undergo bisphosphonate therapy were defined as group A and 22 patients who received ZA therapy were defined as group B. The primary efficacy endpoint for ZA treatment was the reduction in the percentage of patients who developed skeletal-related events (SREs), including bone fracture, spinal cord compression, and hypercalcemia. A secondary endpoint was the interval between a presentation of bone metastases and appearance of SREs.

Results.—SREs occurred in significantly lower frequency in group B (3 of 22 patients, 14%) than group A (14 of 28 patients, 50%) ($p = 0.007$). The use of ZA significantly retarded the onset of the first SRE ($p = 0.04$). Two group-B patients developed bisphosphonate-related osteonecrosis of the jaw.

Conclusion.—Treatment with ZA was effective in reducing SREs or delaying their appearance in patients with bone metastases from differentiated thyroid carcinoma.

▶ Zoledronic acid (ZA) is a recently developed, highly potent nitrogen-containing bisphosphonate, and it has been shown to have long-term efficacy and safety and thus have the effect in reduction of skeletal-related events in patients with advanced carcinoma. However, trials of ZA in the treatment of skeletal metastases from thyroid carcinomas are very limited. The aim of this study was to retrospectively evaluate the efficacy of ZA for bone metastases from differentiated thyroid carcinoma. As shown in Fig 1 in the original article, patients who received ZA showed a much better (skeletal) event-free survival compared with patients who did not receive this therapy. One limitation of this study might be bias introduced by the fact that the 2 groups of patients were treated at different times. As ZA came to be available worldwide around 2006, group B mainly consisted of relatively new patients, whereas group A mainly consisted of patients who were treated in the year before. However, the therapeutic strategy for patients with thyroid carcinoma has not dramatically changed during these several decades. The other limitation might be the relatively short duration of follow-up after detection of bone metastases, especially in group B (26 months; range, 3-84 months). Therefore, the number of patients who may develop a bisphosphonate-related osteonecrosis of the jaw might be much higher.

M. Schott, MD, PhD

High Expression of the Urokinase Plasminogen Activator and Its Cognate Receptor Associates with Advanced Stages and Reduced Disease-Free Interval in Papillary Thyroid Carcinoma
Ulisse S, Baldini E, Sorrenti S, et al ("Sapienza" Univ of Rome, Italy; et al)
J Clin Endocrinol Metab 96:504-508, 2011

Context.—The urokinase plasminogen activating system is implicated in neoplastic progression, and high tissue levels of urokinase plasminogen activating system components correlate with poor prognosis in various human cancers.

Objective.—The objective of the study was to investigate the prognostic relevance of the urokinase plasminogen activator (uPA), its cognate receptor (uPAR), and the plasminogen activator inhibitor 1 (PAI-1) in human papillary thyroid cancer (PTC).

Design.—The expression of uPA, uPAR, and PAI-1 genes was analyzed in PTC and normal matched tissues by quantitative RT-PCR. The case study consisted of 99 patients (21 males and 78 females) affected by PTC including 77 classical, 15 follicular, four tall cell, and three oncocytic variants. Forty-one patients had lymph node metastases at the time of diagnosis. All the patients underwent thyroidectomy and radioiodine therapy followed by thyroid hormone replacement therapy. Follow-up data were available for 76 patients up to 64 months.

Results.—The uPA, uPAR, and PAI-1 mRNA levels were significantly higher in PTC compared with normal matched tissues by 9.63 ± 1,29-, 4.82 ± 0.45-, and 5.64 ± 0.71-fold, respectively. The increased expression of uPA and uPAR correlated statistically with advanced pT and N status. The uPA was also significantly associated with advanced tumor node metastasis stages. The Kaplan-Meier analysis showed a significant association of uPA and uPAR levels with reduced patient disease-free interval (DFI), and this association was stronger in stage I patients.

Conclusion.—The study demonstrated that in PTC the increased gene expression of uPA and uPAR is associated with tumor invasiveness, advanced stages, and shorter DFI, suggesting their prognostic relevance. These observations warrant further investigation in larger patient populations with longer follow-up.

▶ The urokinase plasminogen activating system (uPAS) consists of the urokinase plasminogen activator (uPA), its cognate receptor (uPAR), and 2 main plasminogen activator inhibitors (PAI), PAI-1 and PAI-2. The uPAS is involved in the extracellular conversion of the inactive plasminogen to the serine protease plasmin, which is implicated in numerous pathophysiological processes including tumor progression. Altogether, patients with papillary thyroid cancer (PTC) have a good prognosis. However, 20% of patients face the morbidity of disease recurrences and PTC-related deaths. As a consequence, the identification of molecular marker(s) to refine the stratification risk of patients with PTC would be of particular interest. The aim of this study was to analyze the potential prognostic values of the expression of uPAS components in patients affected by PTC. The authors could demonstrate that uPA, uPAR, and PAI-1 messenger RNA levels were significantly higher in patients with PTC compared with controls. Importantly, the increased expression of uPA and uPAR correlated statistically with advanced pT and N status (Fig 2 in the original article). These findings may help to establish a more accurate prognosis, make more informed therapeutic decisions, and develop tailored prevention programs, especially for patients with stage I PTC, who are considered at low risk of suffering recurrences. It is also worth drawing attention to the fact that complement DNA samples can be used at the same time to analyze the expression of the uPAS components and to investigate the presence of the V600E BRAF mutation, which is considered a putative prognostic molecular marker in PTC.

M. Schott, MD, PhD

T. Baehring, PhD

Activation of TYRO3/AXL Tyrosine Kinase Receptors in Thyroid Cancer

Avilla E, Guarino V, Visciano C, et al (Dipartimento di Biologia e Patologia Cellulare e Molecolare/Istituto di Endocrinologia ed Oncologia Sperimentale del CNR "G. Salvatore", Naples, Italy; et al)
Cancer Res 71:1792-1804, 2011

Thyroid cancer is the most common endocrine cancer, but its key oncogenic drivers remain undefined. In this study we identified the *TYRO3* and *AXL* receptor tyrosine kinases as transcriptional targets of the chemokine CXCL12/SDF-1 in CXCR4-expressing thyroid cancer cells. Both receptors were constitutively expressed in thyroid cancer cell lines but not normal thyroid cells. AXL displayed high levels of tyrosine phosphorylation in most cancer cell lines due to constitutive expression of its ligand GAS6. In human thyroid carcinoma specimens, but not in normal thyroid tissues, AXL and GAS6 were often coexpressed. In cell lines expressing both receptors and ligand, blocking each receptor or ligand dramatically affected cell viability and decreased resistance to apoptotic stimuli. Stimulation of GAS6-negative cancer cells with GAS6 increased their proliferation and survival. Similarly, siRNA-mediated silencing of AXL inhibited cancer cell viability, invasiveness, and growth of tumor xenografts in nude mice. Our findings suggest that a TYRO3/AXL-GAS6 autocrine circuit sustains the malignant features of thyroid cancer cells and that targeting the circuit could offer a novel therapeutic approach in this cancer.

▶ Thyroid cancer is the most common endocrine malignancy, and its incidence is increasing worldwide. Thyroid cancer histotypes include well-differentiated papillary thyroid carcinoma (PTC) and follicular thyroid carcinoma, poorly differentiated thyroid carcinoma, and anaplastic thyroid carcinoma (ATC). Thyroid cancer features overexpression of specific chemokines and their receptors. CXCR4/SDF-1 axis has an important role in promoting cell growth, invasiveness, and survival in thyroid cancer cells, and its blockade can revert all these phenotypes. In the past, the authors of the present work already analyzed global gene expression profiles of CXCR4-expressing human PTC cells with or without SDF-1a. They identified TYRO3 and AXL, belonging to the TAM family (Tyro3, Axl, and Mer) of tyrosine kinase receptors. TAM-mediated signaling is involved in cell survival, proliferation, migration, and adhesion, as well as vascular smooth muscle homeostasis, platelet function, and erythropoiesis. These receptors are frequently coexpressed in vascular, reproductive, nervous, and immune systems in adults. TAM receptors can be activated by 2 physiological ligands: GAS6 (growth arrest—specific gene 6) and protein S, which are homologous vitamin K—dependent proteins. TAM receptors are involved in cancer development and progression. AXL overexpression is observed in many human cancer types. Gas6 is frequently expressed in cancer, and its level correlates with poor prognosis. The aim of this report is to study TAM receptor involvement in thyroid cancer. The authors show that human PTC/ATC cells and samples, but not normal thyroid, constitutively express AXL, TYRO3, and their ligand GAS6. Moreover, the authors show that AXL, TYRO3, and GAS6 have a critical role in mediating thyroid cancer cell proliferation, invasiveness, and survival (Fig 5 in the original article). Moreover, they also show that silencing of AXL in an ATC cell line strongly affects tumor growth in immunodeficient mice (Fig 7 in the original article). These data strongly suggest that AXL/TYRO3-GAS6 axis can be considered as a novel potential target of thyroid anticancer therapy. Several compounds have already been identified that block AXL signaling by acting at different levels.[1-4] This study suggests that these compounds should be tested in an in vivo setting to establish a new therapy for radioiodine-resistant thyroid cancer, including anaplastic thyroid cancer.

M. Schott, MD, PhD

References

1. Vajkoczy P, Knyazev P, Kunkel A, et al. Dominant-negative inhibition of the Axl receptor tyrosine kinase suppresses brain tumor cell growth and invasion and prolongs survival. *Proc Natl Acad Sci U S A.* 2006;103:5799-5804.
2. Tai KY, Shieh YS, Lee CS, Shiah SG, Wu CW. Axl promotes cell invasion by inducing MMP-9 activity through activation of NF-kappaB and Brg-1. *Oncogene.* 2008;27:4044-4055.

3. Holland SJ, Pan A, Franci C, et al. R428, a selective small molecule inhibitor of Axl kinase, blocks tumor spread and prolongs survival in models of metastatic breast cancer. *Cancer Res.* 2010;70:1544-1554.
4. Rankin EB, Fuh KC, Taylor TE, et al. AXL is an essential factor and therapeutic target for metastatic ovarian cancer. *Cancer Res.* 2010;70:7570-7579.

Primary tumour size is a prognostic parameter in patients suffering from differentiated thyroid carcinoma with extrathyroidal growth: results of the MSDS trial

Krämer JA, on behalf of the MSDS study group (Univ Hosp Münster, Germany; et al)

Eur J Endocrinol 163:637-644, 2010

Objective.—The Multicentre Study Differentiated Thyroid Cancer (MSDS) collective represents a well-defined group of patients with thyroid carcinomas with extrathyroidal extension. The aim of the present study was to evaluate the relationship of the primary tumour size with clinico-pathological features as well as the outcome of patients with minimum and extensive extrathyroidal growth (pT3b- and pT4a-tumours; UICC 2002/2003, 6th ed).

Methods.—The tumour diameter was available in 324 out of 351 MSDS patients (244 females, 80 males). Mean age of patients was 47.7 ± 12.0 years (range, 20.1−69.8 years), and the median follow-up was 6.2 years. The relationship between primary tumour size and the following clinicopathological data was investigated: age, gender, histological tumour type (papillary thyroid carcinomas (PTC) versus follicular thyroid carcinomas (FTC)) and UICC/AJCC TNM classification. In addition, the correlation between primary tumour size and event-free and overall survival was assessed.

Results.—The FTC of our series were significantly larger than PTC (3.46 vs 1.84 cm; $P < 0.001$). Patients suffering from pT3b-tumours presented with significantly smaller tumour size than those with extensive extrathyroidal growth (pT4a-tumours) (1.9 vs 3.0 cm; $P < 0.01$). All patients with distant metastases suffered from tumours >2 cm. Furthermore, event-free and overall survival were significantly correlated with increasing tumour size ($P < 0.05$). Using multivariate analysis, a pT4a-category and a tumour diameter >2 cm remained independent predictors of survival.

Conclusions.—In patients suffering from differentiated thyroid carcinoma with extrathyroidal growth (pT3b and pT4a), the tumour size is an independent predictor of event-free and overall survival (Figs 2 and 3).

▶ The diameter of the primary tumor has been described as a determinant for outcome in differentiated thyroid cancer. It has been suggested that a larger tumor size is related to other phenomena associated with worse prognosis, such as extrathyroidal growth, multifocality, locoregional, and distant metastases.

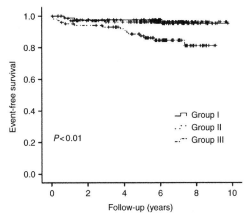

FIGURE 2.—Event-free survival of the MSDS patients according to tumour size in pT3b- and pT4a-carcinomas (6th ed). Group I (≤1.0 cm), group II (>1.0 to ≤2.0 cm) and group III (>2.0 cm) (I versus II: P=NS; I versus III: P<0.05; II versus III: P<0.01, total: P<0.01). (Reprinted from Krämer JA, on behalf of the MSDS study group. Primary tumour size is a prognostic parameter in patients suffering from differentiated thyroid carcinoma with extrathyroidal growth: results of the MSDS trial. *Eur J Endocrinol.* 2010;163:637-644, with permission from European Society of Endocrinology.)

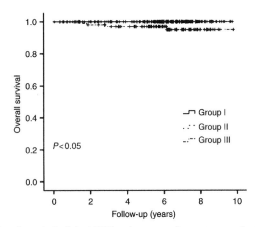

FIGURE 3.—Overall survival of the MSDS patients according to tumour size in pT3b- and pT4a-carcinomas (6th ed). Group I (≤1.0 cm), group II (>1.0 to ≤2.0 cm) and group III (>2.0 cm). (I versus II: P=NS; I versus III: P=NS; II versus III: P<0.05, total: P<0.05). (Reprinted from Krämer JA, on behalf of the MSDS study group. Primary tumour size is a prognostic parameter in patients suffering from differentiated thyroid carcinoma with extrathyroidal growth: results of the MSDS trial. *Eur J Endocrinol.* 2010;163:637-644, with permission from European Society of Endocrinology.)

The aim of this study was to assess the relationship between the primary tumor size and different clinicopathological data using the well-defined prospective Multicentre Study Differentiated Thyroid Cancer collective with thyroid carcinomas with extrathyroidal growth. The large database allowed the scientists to perform a retrospective scientific analysis of a multitude of parameters collected over a follow-up time of up to 9 years. In particular, the correlation between primary tumor size and clinical outcome was assessed. The study was conducted in Germany, Austria, and Switzerland to determine the benefit of adjuvant radiotherapy in patients with differentiated thyroid cancer showing extrathyroidal growth (pT4) with or without lymph node metastases in which patients who agreed to participate were randomly assigned to either external beam radiotherapy (EBRT) or no EBRT. In addition, patients were treated with ^{131}I for remnant ablation. On average, patients with lymph node metastases had significantly larger primary tumors than patients without documented lymph node spread. The study found that patients with tumors > 2 cm (group III) had significantly higher recurrence rates as compared with those with tumors ≤2 cm (Figs 2 and 3). About 5.6% of the patients had locoregional tumor recurrences, and 3.4% presented with distant metastases. The authors point out that > 4 cm has been generally accepted as a significant predictor of a high-risk situation, which, according to the authors, should be applied with caution in view of the poorer prognosis with tumors > 2 cm if extrathyroidal extension is present. Specifically, the lack of division of pT3 tumors into those with and without extrathyroidal extension in the TNM classification should be reconsidered in view of the present finding in this study. The authors opine that using this large prospective multicenter study database allows for retrospective scientific analysis of a multitude of parameters collected during a follow-up period of up to 9 years. The authors did, however, not mention a study by Bilimoria et al[1] of a US database of 52 173 patients with papillary thyroid carcinoma (PTC) in which recurrence rates are shown to be closely related to initial tumor size, beginning with < 1 cm, in which 10-year recurrence rates are approximately 5%, increasing incrementally to recurrence rates of approximately 25% with primary tumors > 8 cm. In addition, 10-year cancer-specific mortality rates ranged from 2% for tumors < 1 cm, which incrementally increased to 19% for tumors > 8 mm. This seems to support the hypothesis that PTC outcome is related to the initial tumor size, increasing progressively with increasingly larger tumors. Limiting the cutoff to 2 cm seems to ignore the well-recognized effect of initial primary tumors ranging to over 8 mm in diameter.[2] These data, including those by Kräemer et al, show that tumor diameter is an independent predictor of overall survival and mortality in patients with thyroid cancer.

M. Schott, MD, PhD

References

1. Bilimoria KY, Bentrem DJ, Ko CY, et al. Extent of surgery affects survival for papillary thyroid cancer. *Ann Surg.* 2007;246:375-381.
2. Mazzaferri EL. Comment on Primary tumour size is a prognostic parameter in patients suffering from differentiated thyroid carcinoma with extrathyroidal growth: results of the MSDS trial. *Clinical Thyroidology.* 2010;10:11-14.

IQGAP1 Plays an Important Role in the Invasiveness of Thyroid Cancer

Liu Z, Liu D, Bojdani E, et al (The Johns Hopkins Univ School of Medicine, Baltimore, MD; et al)
Clin Cancer Res 16:6009-6018, 2010

Purpose.—This study was designed to explore the role of IQGAP1 in the invasiveness of thyroid cancer and its potential as a novel prognostic marker and therapeutic target in this cancer.

Experimental Design.—We examined *IQGAP1* copy gain and its relationship with clinicopathologic outcomes of thyroid cancer and investigated its role in cell invasion and molecules involved in the process.

Results.—We found *IQGAP1* copy number (CN) gain ≥3 in 1 of 30 (3%), 24 of 74 (32%), 44 of 107 (41%), 8 of 16 (50%), and 27 of 41 (66%) of benign thyroid tumor, follicular variant papillary thyroid cancer (FVPTC), follicular thyroid cancer (FTC), tall cell papillary thyroid cancer (PTC), and anaplastic thyroid cancer, respectively, in the increasing order of invasiveness of these tumors. A similar tumor distribution trend of CN ≥4 was also seen. *IQGAP1* copy gain was positively correlated with IQGAP1 protein expression. It was significantly associated with extrathyroidal and vascular invasion of FVPTC and FTC and, remarkably, a 50%–60% rate of multifocality and recurrence of BRAF mutation-positive PTC ($P = 0.01$ and 0.02, respectively). The siRNA knockdown of IQGAP1 dramatically inhibited thyroid cancer cell invasion and colony formation. Coimmunoprecipitation assay showed direct interaction of IQGAP1 with E-cadherin, a known invasion-suppressing molecule, which was upregulated when IQGAP1 was knocked down. This provided a mechanism for the invasive role of IQGAP1 in thyroid cancer. In contrast, IQGAP3 lacked all these functions.

Conclusions.—IQGAP1, through genetic copy gain, plays an important role in the invasiveness of thyroid cancer and may represent a novel prognostic marker and therapeutic target for this cancer.

▶ This study investigated the oncogenic role of IQGAP1 in thyroid cancer and its potential as a novel prognostic marker and therapeutic target in this cancer. The main findings include the genetic copy gain of *IQGAP1* associated with increased IQGAP1 protein expression and increased invasiveness and aggressiveness of thyroid cancer. *IQGAP1* copy gain was preferentially seen in aggressive types of thyroid cancer and highly associated with extrathyroidal and vascular invasion. In *BRAF* mutation–positive papillary thyroid cancer (PTC), *IQGAP1* copy gain was particularly associated with a high tumor recurrence rate of 60%. In vitro knockdown of *IQGAP1* dramatically inhibited thyroid cancer cell invasion (Fig 2 in the original article). The clinical implication of these results is 2-fold: (1) *IQGAP1* copy gain can be used to predict invasiveness and aggressiveness of thyroid cancer and, when coexisting with *BRAF* mutation in PTC, is a particularly powerful predictor for cancer recurrence.

And (2) *IQGAP1* represents a novel potential therapeutic target for thyroid cancer.

M. Schott, MD, PhD

Thyroid Nodules

Shear Wave Elastography: A New Ultrasound Imaging Mode for the Differential Diagnosis of Benign and Malignant Thyroid Nodules
Sebag F, Vaillant-Lombard J, Berbis J, et al (La Timone Univ Hosp, Marseille, France; Laboratory of Clinical Epidemiology, Marseille, France; et al)
J Clin Endocrinol Metab 95:5281-5288, 2010

Context.—Elastography uses ultrasound (US) to assess elasticity. Shear wave elastography (SWE) is anew technique that estimates tissue stiffness in real time and is quantitative and user independent.

Objectives.—The aim of the study was to assess the efficiency of SWE in predicting malignancy and to compare SWE with US.

Design.—Ninety-three patients and 39 control subjects were included in the study. Predictive value of SWE was assessed by correlation between elasticity, US parameters, and histology. Elasticity index (EI) was first analyzed alone. Scores have been constructed with echographic parameters, *i.e.* vascularity, hypoechogenicity, and microcalcifications (Score 1 = US Score), and with the same parameters plus EI (Score 2 = US+SWE Score). For statistical analysis, univariate and multivariate analysis and receiver operating characteristic curves were used.

Results.—A total of 146 nodules from 93 patients were analyzed. Twenty-nine nodules (19.9%) were malignant.Mean($\pm$SD) EI was 150 $\pm$ 95 kPa (range, 30—356) in malignant nodules *vs.* 36 $\pm$ 30 (range, 0—200) kPa in benign nodules ($P < 0.001$, Student's t test). For a positive predictive value of at least 80%, characteristics of tissue elasticity (cutoff, 65 kPa) were: sensitivity = 85.2%, and specificity = 93.9%. Characteristics of the US Score were: sensitivity = 51.9% [95% confidence interval (CI), 33.1; 70.7], and specificity = 97% (95% CI, 93.6; 1). Characteristics of the US+SWE Score were: sensitivity = 81.5% (95% CI, 66.9; 96.1), and specificity = 97.0% (95% CI, 93.6; 1).

Conclusion.—Promising results have been obtained with SWE. This technique may be applied to multinodular goiters. Larger prospective studies are needed to confirm these results and to define the respective places of SWE, US, and FNA (Fig 1, Table 1).

▶ After clinical examination, thyroid ultrasound (US) is used as a first-line procedure to help differentiate benign and malignant nodules. Several US features have been associated with malignancy: microcalcifications, hypoechogenicity, intranodular vascularity, irregular margins, and absent halo sign. All of these features alone are poorly predictive of malignancy. In combination, their specificity increases, but sensitivity decreases. After clinical examination and

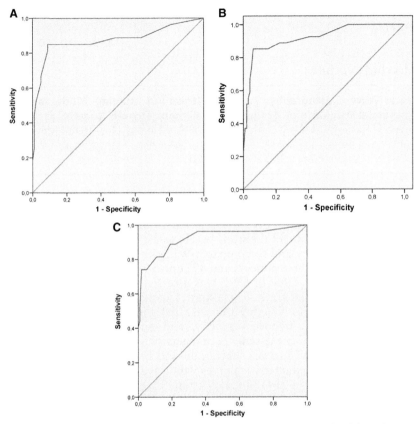

FIGURE 1.—ROC curves (area under the ROC curve) for changes in scores and nodule's malignancy. A, ROC curve for changes in Score 1 (US Score) (AUC = 84.7%). Area under the ROC curve for changes in Score 1 (US Score) and nodule's malignancy. B, ROC curve for the EI of at least 65 kPa (AUC = 93.6%). Area under the ROC curve for changes in index elasticity and nodule's malignancy. C, ROC curve for the Score 2 (US+SWE Score) (AUC = 93.4%). Area under the ROC curve for changes in Score 2 (US+SWE Score) and nodule's malignancy. (Reprinted from Sebag F, Vaillant-Lombard J, Berbis J, et al. Shear wave elastography: a new ultrasound imaging mode for the differential diagnosis of benign and malignant thyroid nodules. *J Clin Endocrinol Metab*. 2010;95:5281-5288, Copyright © 2010, with permission from The Endocrine Society.)

thyroid US, fine-needle aspiration (FNA) biopsy has a central role in differentiating benign from malignant thyroid lesions. In expert centers, FNA provides useful results in 65% to 75% of examined nodules. Approximately 60% to 70% of aspirates prove to be cytologically benign, 5% are positive for papillary carcinoma, and 5% to 15% remain inconclusive. The remaining 15% to 25% of aspirates are indeterminate or suspicious. The latter 2 results offer a challenging dilemma for the clinician. Indeed, FNA is limited by sampling difficulties with inadequately collected specimens and by overlap in morphological signs between benignity and malignancy. When FNA results are indeterminate or suspicious, most clinicians recommend surgical excision. Then, the sensitivity

TABLE 1.—Conventional US Patterns and EI in 126 Patients (Out of 93 Patients) with Complete Data Set for All Those Parameters

	Benign (n = 99)	Cancer (n = 27)	Sensitivity	Specificity
Intranodular vascularity			51.9 (33.1; 70.7)	93.9 (89.2; 98.6)
Present	6	14		
Absent	93	13		
Microcalcifications			66.7 (48.9; 84.5)	84.8 (77.7; 91.9)
Present	15	18		
Absent	84	9		
Macrocalcifications			22.2 (6.5; 37.9)	79.6 (71.7; 87.5)
Present	20	6		
Absent	78	21		
Halo sign			92.6 (82.7; 100)	41.4 (31.7; 51.1)
Absent	58	25		
Present	41	2		
Hypoechogenicity			70.4 (62.4; 78.3)	81.8 (75.1; 88.6)
Present	18	19		
Absent	91	8		
EI			85.2 (71.8; 98.6)	93.9 (89.2; 98.6)
≥65 kPa	6	23		
<65 kPa	93	4		

Data are expressed as number of subjects or percentage (95% CI).

of FNA will increase, whereas its specificity will decrease. The poor quality of FNA specimens may be the source of diagnostic errors with false-negative and false-positive results that reached 25% and 9.9%, respectively, in a recent multi-institutional survey.

Because of the aforementioned problems, there is a need for another way to evaluate thyroid nodules. Over the last few years, a new diagnostic tool has emerged that uses US to assess tissue elasticity and stiffness to differentiate malignant from benign lesions. Stiffness is usually correlated with malignancy because benign lesions are supposed to be softer. Different techniques of elastography have been applied to thyroid nodules, based on real-time elastography and off-line processing of strain images, etc. More recently, a technique has been developed that uses tracking of shear wave propagation through tissue to obtain the elastic modulus.[1] This new shear wave elastography (SWE) is operator independent, reproducible, and quantitative. It gives a local assessment of tissue elasticity at each point of interest of an organ. It has been used with success in the evaluation of breast lesions.[2] One example is shown in Fig 1. The result is not altered by a hard area in the vicinity of the nodule of interest. However, elastography may not be useful in the presence of coarse calcifications because the calcifications are stiff, causing a false-positive rate as high as 25% (Table 1). The technique may be especially valuable in the diagnosis of follicular thyroid cancers because these cancers often lack the US features of papillary thyroid cancer and they usually cannot be diagnosed with precision by FNA. As the authors state, large prospective studies of SWE will be needed to confirm these results and to determine the true utility of this procedure in the evaluation of thyroid nodules.

M. Schott, MD, PhD

References

1. Bercoff J, Tanter M, Fink M. Supersonic shear imaging: a new technique for soft tissue elasticity mapping. *IEEE Trans Ultrason Ferroelectr Freq Control.* 2004;51: 396-409.
2. Tanter M, Bercoff J, Athanasiou A, et al. Quantitative assessment of breast lesion viscoelasticity: initial clinical results using supersonic shear imaging. *Ultrasound Med Biol.* 2008;34:1373-1386.

Real-Time Elastosonography: Useful Tool for Refining the Presurgical Diagnosis in Thyroid Nodules with Indeterminate or Nondiagnostic Cytology

Rago T, Scutari M, Santini F, et al (Univ of Pisa, Italy)
J Clin Endocrinol Metab 95:5274-5280, 2010

Background.—Indeterminate and nondiagnostic patterns represent the main limitation of fine-needle aspiration (FNA) cytology of thyroid nodules, clinical and echographic features being poorly predictive of malignancy. The newly developed real-time ultrasound elastography (USE) has been previously applied to differentiate malignant from benign lesions. The aim of this study was to get further insights into the role of USE in the presurgical diagnosis of nodules with indeterminate or non-diagnostic cytology.

Patients.—The study included 176 patients who had one (n = 138) or multiple (n = 38) nodules with indeterminate or nondiagnostic cytology on FNA, for whom histology was available after thyroidectomy. A total of 195 nodules (142 indeterminate, 53 nondiagnostic) were submitted to USE, and elasticity was scored as 1 (high), 2 (intermediate), or 3 (low).

Results.—In indeterminate lesions, the score 1, describing high elasticity, was strongly predictive of benignity, being found in 102 of 111 benign nodules and in only one of 31 carcinomas ($P < 0.0001$). By combining the scores 2 and 3, USE had a sensitivity of 96.8% and a specificity of 91.8%. In nodules with nondiagnostic cytology, score 1 was found in 39 of 45 benign nodules and in only one of eight carcinomas ($P < 0.0001$). By combining the scores 2 and 3, USE had a sensitivity of 87.5% and a specificity of 86.7%.

Conclusions.—USE may represent an important tool for the diagnosis of thyroid cancer in nodules with indeterminate or nondiagnostic cytology and may prove useful in selecting patients who are candidates for surgery.

▶ This is another study published to investigate the role of real-time ultrasound elastography (USE) in thyroid nodules with indeterminate or nondiagnostic cytology. The authors used a scoring system (1-3) to characterize thyroid nodules (Fig 2 in the original article). Based on that, the authors were able to distinguish benign from malignant nodules with high accuracy (Fig 3 in the original article). Importantly, score 3 was associated with malignancy with high specificity, although the sensitivity was not optimal. Much more rewarding were the negative predictive values of the pattern of high elasticity score 1 to exclude malignancy in both indeterminate and nondiagnostic nodules. Indeed, score 1 was found in 102 of 111 indeterminate lesions with a benign diagnosis at histology and in only 1 of 31 with a final diagnosis of malignancy. Similar findings were observed in the group of nondiagnostic lesions, although sensitivity and specificity were lower. This implies that nodules with high elasticity, which represent the largest proportion of nodules with indeterminate or nondiagnostic cytology, have a minimal probability to bear malignancy. In summary, USE might be an important tool in the presurgical risk stratification in patients with thyroid nodules that will be operated.

M. Schott, MD, PhD

T. Baehring, PhD

Thyroid Ultrasonography

Shear Wave Elastography: A New Ultrasound Imaging Mode for the Differential Diagnosis of Benign and Malignant Thyroid Nodules
Sebag F, Vaillant-Lombard J, Berbis J, et al (Timone Univ Hosp, Marseille, France; Laboratory of Clinical Epidemiology, Marseille, France; et al)
J Clin Endocrinol Metab 95:5281-5288, 2010

Context.—Elastography uses ultrasound (US) to assess elasticity. Shear wave elastography (SWE) is a new technique that estimates tissue stiffness in real time and is quantitative and user independent.

Objectives.—The aim of the study was to assess the efficiency of SWE in predicting malignancy and to compare SWE with US.

Design.—Ninety-three patients and 39 control subjects were included in the study. Predictive value of SWE was assessed by correlation between elasticity, US parameters, and histology. Elasticity index (EI) was first analyzed alone. Scores have been constructed with echographic parameters, *i.e.* vascularity, hypoechogenicity, and microcalcifications (Score 1 = US Score), and with the same parameters plus EI (Score 2 = US+SWE Score). For statistical analysis, univariate and multivariate analysis and receiver operating characteristic curves were used.

Results.—A total of 146 nodules from 93 patients were analyzed. Twenty-nine nodules (19.9%) were malignant. Mean ($\pm$ SD) EI was 150 ± 95 kPa (range, 30—356) in malignant nodules vs. 36 ± 30 (range, 0—200) kPa in benign nodules ($P < 0.001$, Student's t test). For a positive predictive value of at least 80%, characteristics of tissue elasticity (cutoff, 65 kPa) were: sensitivity = 85.2%, and specificity = 93.9%. Characteristics of the US Score were: sensitivity = 51.9% [95% confidence interval (CI), 33.1; 70.7], and specificity = 97% (95% CI, 93.6; 1). Characteristics of the US+SWE Score were: sensitivity = 81.5% (95% CI, 66.9; 96.1), and specificity = 97.0% (95% CI, 93.6; 1).

Conclusion.—Promising results have been obtained with SWE. This technique may be applied to multinodular goiters. Larger prospective

A

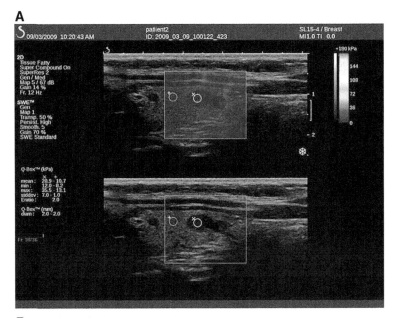

B

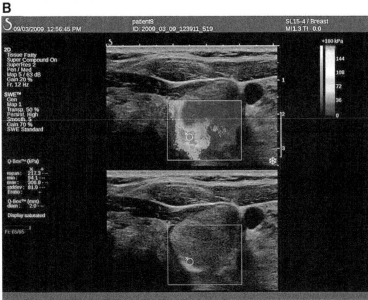

FIGURE 2.—Thyroid nodule images obtained on US elastography of a benign thyroid nodule (A) and a papillary carcinoma (B). (Reprinted from Sebag F, Vaillant-Lombard J, Berbis J, et al. Shear wave elastography: a new ultrasound imaging mode for the differential diagnosis of benign and malignant thyroid nodules. *J Clin Endocrinol Metab*. 2010;95:5281-5288, Copyright © 2010, with permission from The Endocrine Society.)

TABLE 2.—EI of Malignant Thyroid Nodules According to their Histological Subtypes

Characteristics	n	EI, Mean ± sd (kPa)	Range
Solitary nodules (n = 61)			
Papillary carcinoma	9	148 ± 98	40–356
Follicular carcinoma	3	117 ± 72	70–200
Medullary carcinoma	1	263	
Anaplasic carcinoma	1	200	
FTUMP	1	30	
Multiples nodules (n = 83)			
Papillary carcinoma	11	162 ± 109	30–323
Follicular carcinoma	2	250	
FTUMP	1	180	

studies are needed to confirm these results and to define the respective places of SWE, US, and FNA (Fig 2, Table 2).

▶ Over the last few years, a new diagnostic tool has emerged that uses ultrasound (US) to assess tissue elasticity and stiffness to differentiate malignant from benign lesions. Stiffness is usually correlated with malignancy because benign lesions are supposed to be softer. Different techniques of elastography have been applied to thyroid nodules, based on real-time elastography and off-line processing of strain images, external compression, or carotid artery vibrations. However, the widespread applicability of these techniques is limited because they cannot be used in the evaluation of multinodular goiters, which represent about 40% of nodular thyroid glands. There is no consensus about the risk of cancer per patient, regardless of whether 1 or multiple nodules are present. Indeed, the prevalence of carcinoma was found to be lower in patients with a solitary nodule than in those with multinodular thyroid, but the prevalence was equal in another study. More recently, a technique has been developed that uses tracking of shear wave propagation through tissue to obtain the elastic modulus. This new shear wave elastography (SWE) is operator independent, reproducible, and quantitative. It gives a local assessment of tissue elasticity at each point of interest of an organ. It has been used with success in the evaluation of breast lesions. The aim of this study was to investigate the efficiency of SWE in predicting malignancy and to compare SWE with US. The positive predictive value was around 85%, with a specificity of almost 94%. Two examples are shown in Fig 2. A detailed analysis of different carcinoma subtypes are given in Table 2. As indicated, the elasticity index (EI) was significantly higher in papillary carcinoma than in benign nodules. However, follicular and other histological variants of papillary carcinoma are possible. In this study, EI in malignant nodules ranges from 30 to 356 kPa, with 4 of 20 malignant nodules with EI less than 65 kPa, not significantly different from those of benign thyroid nodules. The combination of several conventional US features highly suggestive of papillary carcinoma has been found in 2 of 4 cases. In the 2 other cases, a 9.2-mm papillary carcinoma and a follicular tumor of uncertain malignant potential, none of these conventional US features have been found. In contrast, follicular carcinomas are composed of small microfollicles with variable amounts of colloid. Therefore, their echogenicity and EI may depend on their cellular content. Conventional US is not predictive in follicular lesions, although irregular halo and isoechogenicity or hyperechogenicity have been described in follicular thyroid cancer. In the present study, EI ranges from 70 to 250 kPa, with a possible correlation with stroma content that will need further study. Similar data have been obtained by Rago et al.[1] However, elastography was not efficient for the diagnosis of follicular carcinoma in 2 other studies.[2,3] More studies in correlation with various histological criteria will be helpful in understanding this discrepancy.

M. Schott, MD, PhD

References

1. Rago T, Santini F, Scutari M, Pinchera A, Vitti P. Elastography: new developments in ultrasound for predicting malignancy in thyroid nodules. *J Clin Endocrinol Metab.* 2007;92:2917-2922.
2. Hong Y, Liu X, Li Z, Zhang X, Chen M, Luo Z. Real-time ultrasound elastography in the differential diagnosis of benign and malignant thyroid nodules. *J Ultrasound Med.* 2009;28:861-867.
3. Asteria C, Giovanardi A, Pizzocaro A, et al. US-elastography in the differential diagnosis of benign and malignant thyroid nodules. *Thyroid.* 2008;18:523-531.

Thyroid Disease in Pregnancy

High thyrotrophin levels at end term increase the risk of breech presentation

Kooistra L, Kuppens SMI, Hasaart THM, et al (Univ of Calgary, Canada; Catharina Hosp, Eindhoven, The Netherlands; et al)
Clin Endocrinol 73:661-665, 2010

Objective.—To study the relationship between maternal thyrotrophin (TSH) and breech presentation at term.

Design.—Combined data sets of two prospective studies to obtain adequate epidemiological power.

Patients.—One thousand and fifty-eight healthy pregnant women (58 breech, 1000 cephalic) and 131 women who presented in breech at an obstetrical outpatient clinic.

Measurements.—Maternal thyroid parameters [TSH, free thyroid hormone (FT4), thyroid peroxidase antibody (TPO-Ab)] and foetal presentation were assessed in both groups between 35 and 38 weeks gestation. Power calculations suggested that at least 148 breech cases were required.

Results.—The characteristics of the women in breech in both samples were similar. Women in breech ($n = 58 + 131$) had significantly higher TSH (but not FT4) than those ($n = 1000$) with cephalic presentation (Mann—Whitney U-test, $P = 0 \cdot 003$). Different cut-offs were used to define high TSH in the 916 TPO-Ab-negative women with cephalic presentation: the 90th, 95th and 97·5th percentiles were $2 \cdot 4$ mIU/l ($n = 149$), $2 \cdot 7$ mIU/l

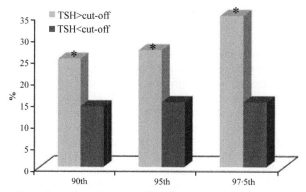

FIGURE 1.—Comparison of prevalence rate of breech presentation at 35—38 weeks between women above and below different percentile cut-offs of thyrotrophin (n total group = 1189, of which 189 breech and 1000 cephalic presentations). (Reprinted from Kooistra L, Kuppens SMI, Hasaart THM, et al. High thyrotrophin levels at end term increase the risk of breech presentation. *Clin Endocrinol.* 2010;73:661-665, with permission from Blackwell Publishing Ltd.)

($n = 77$) and $3 \cdot 2$ mIU/l ($n = 37$). The prevalence rates of breech presentation in these women were all higher compared to the prevalence of breech in women below these cut-offs (df = 1, $P < 0 \cdot 01$). The relative risk of the 149 women with a TSH >90th percentile (>$2 \cdot 4$ mIU/l) to present in breech was $1 \cdot 82$ (95% CI: $1 \cdot 30$—$2 \cdot 56$).

Conclusions.—Women with high TSH at end term are at risk for breech presentation. Substantial evidence for a relation between breech presentation and neurodevelopmental delay exists. As high TSH during gestation has also been linked to poor neurodevelopment, the relation between breech presentation and poor neurodevelopment might be thyroid-related (Fig 1).

▶ Breech presentation occurs in 3% to 5% of term women and is associated with neonatal as well as maternal morbidity and mortality. Breech is often an indication for elective cesarean delivery that, in itself, constitutes a prominent risk factor for decreased reproductive health. According to a recent review, the currently known risk factors associated with breech presentation account for up to only 15% of the variance. The aim of this study was to investigate the correlation between high thyrotropin (TSH) levels and breech presentation. The authors of this study published a previous prospective cohort study of pregnant women aimed at evaluating the relation between breech position at term (> 37 weeks' gestation) and low maternal free thyroid hormone (FT4) levels.[1] The main outcomes of the study were that breech presentation at term delivery was independently related to FT4 levels < 10th percentile at 12 weeks' gestation (odds ratio [OR], 4.7; 95% confidence interval [CI], 1.1-1.9) but was not related to an FT4 level below the 10th percentile at 12 weeks' gestation and was also related to primiparity (OR, 4.7; 95% CI, 1.3-1.5). The study did not find a relationship between serum TSH levels and breech presentation. The conclusion of the study was that women with hypothyroxinemia (FT4 at the lowest 10th percentile) during early gestation without overt thyroid dysfunction are at risk for fetal breech presentation at term (> 37 weeks' gestation).

This study is much larger compared with an initial study of the same group. In this study, the authors found that breech position at birth is related to maternal thyroid hormone status during pregnancy. Indeed, not only was breech delivery almost 2.5-fold more common in women with TSH levels ≥ 2.5 mIU/L, regression analysis confirmed that elevated maternal TSH at 36 weeks' gestation is a key predictor for breech presentation (Fig 1). In addition, high TSH levels were significantly associated with increased thyroid peroxidase antibody levels and a parental history of thyroid disease. In sharp contrast, none of the women with TSH levels below the fifth percentile presented with breech position at term. The study also found no group differences for FT4 levels at 12, 24, and 36 months' gestation. This is a remarkably important study, as breech presentation at term is the most common abnormal fetal presentation and is associated with neonatal and maternal morbidity and mortality. There is considerable evidence of a relationship between subclinical thyroid dysfunction and impaired obstetrical outcome.[2] The authors of this study suggest that research is needed to detect the most appropriate tool for screening of maternal thyroid function during gestation.

M. Schott, MD, PhD

References

1. Pop VJ, Brouwers EP, Wijnen H, Oei G, Essed GG, Vader HL. Low concentrations of maternal thyroxin during early gestation: a risk factor of breech presentation? *BJOG*. 2004;111:925-930.
2. Casey BM, Dashe JS, Wells CE, McIntire DD, Leveno KJ, Cunningham FG. Subclinical hyperthyroidism and pregnancy outcomes. *Obstet Gynecol*. 2006; 107:337-341.

Maternal Thyroid Function during Early Pregnancy and Cognitive Functioning in Early Childhood: The Generation R Study

Henrichs J, Bongers-Schokking JJ, Schenk JJ, et al (Erasmus Med Univ Ctr, Rotterdam, The Netherlands; Erasmus Med Ctr—Sophia Children's Hosp, Rotterdam, The Netherlands; Erasmus Univ, Rotterdam, The Netherlands)
J Clin Endocrinol Metab 95:4227-4234, 2010

Context.—Thyroid hormones are essential for neurodevelopment from early pregnancy onward. Yet population-based data on the association between maternal thyroid function in early pregnancy and children's cognitive development are sparse.

Objective.—Our objective was to study associations of maternal hypothyroxinemia and of early pregnancy maternal TSH and free T_4 (FT_4) levels across the entire range with cognitive functioning in early childhood.

Design and Setting.—We conducted a population-based cohort in The Netherlands.

Participants.—Participants included 3659 children and their mothers.

Main Measures.—In pregnant women with normal TSH levels at 13 wk gestation (SD = 1.7), mild and severe maternal hypothyroxinemia were defined as FT_4 concentrations below the 10th and 5th percentile, respectively. Children's expressive vocabulary at 18 months was reported by mothers using the MacArthur Communicative Development Inventory. At 30 months, mothers completed the Language Development Survey and the Parent Report of Children's Abilities measuring verbal and nonverbal cognitive functioning.

Results.—Maternal TSH was not related to the cognitive outcomes. An increase in maternal FT_4 predicted a lower risk of expressive language delay at 30 months only. However, both mild and severe maternal hypothyroxinemia was associated with a higher risk of expressive language delay across all ages [odds ratio (OR) = 1.44; 95% confidence interval (CI) = 1.09−1.91; P = 0.010 and OR = 1.80; 95% CI = 1.24−2.61; P = 0.002, respectively]. Severe maternal hypothyroxinemia also predicted a higher risk of nonverbal cognitive delay (OR = 2.03; 95% CI = 1.22−3.39; P = 0.007).

Conclusions.—Maternal hypothyroxinemia is a risk factor for cognitive delay in early childhood (Table 3).

▶ Clinical hypothyroidism is associated with subfertility, and in those women who conceive, there is an increased risk of miscarriage, stillbirth, preeclampsia, and preterm delivery. There is also some evidence that subclinical hypothyroidism, defined by an increased serum concentration of thyrotropin (TSH) in the presence of normal levels of free thyroxine (FT_4), may be associated with an increased risk for miscarriage, stillbirth, and preeclampsia. Moreover, there is evidence that subclinical hypothyroidism may affect the brain development of the children. In this article, the authors performed a large population-based cohort study with verbal and nonverbal cognitive measures in early childhood. The aim was to investigate whether low FT_4 concentrations in pregnant women with normal TSH levels negatively affect offspring cognitive development. To

---

TABLE 3.—Maternal Thyroid Function in Early Pregnancy and Nonverbal Cognitive Delay at Age 30 Months

Maternal Thyroid Function Measure	n	Nonverbal Cognitive Delay,[a] OR (95% CI), P
TSH, per SD	2588	0.98 (0.88−1.10), 0.759
FT_4, per SD	2606	0.85 (0.72−1.01), 0.057
Mild hypothyroxinemia[b]	2086[d]	1.37 (0.90 −2.07), 0.139
Severe hypothyroxinemia[c]	2086[d]	2.03 (1.22−3.39), 0.007

Models were adjusted for maternal age, maternal educational level, maternal smoking during pregnancy, maternal prenatal distress, gestational age at blood sampling, birth weight, and child ethnicity. The sample size of the respective analysis is represented by n.
[a]Nonverbal cognitive delay was defined as a score below the 15th age- and gender-specific percentile.
[b]Mild maternal hypothyroxinemia was defined as normal TSH levels and FT_4 concentrations below the 10th percentile.
[c]Severe maternal hypothyroxinemia was defined as normal TSH levels and FT_4 concentrations below the 5th percentile.
[d]Mothers with abnormal TSH levels during early pregnancy were excluded.

this aim, the authors defined mild and severe hypothyroxinemia, representing FT_4 concentrations below the 10th and fifth percentile, respectively, in line with previous research. The authors also examined whether continuous measures of maternal TSH and FT_4 levels in early pregnancy predict verbal cognitive functioning at 18 and 30 months and nonverbal cognitive functioning at 30 months. This study shows that maternal hypothyroxinemia in early pregnancy is a determinant of verbal and nonverbal cognitive functioning in early childhood. The findings of this large population-based study suggest that even in pregnant women with normal TSH levels, low FT_4 concentrations affect fetal brain development and put children at risk for subsequent neurodevelopmental deficits (Table 3). It is tempting to recommend thyroid function screening, including FT_4 measures of women in early pregnancy. Yet, first clinical trials addressing the potentially beneficial effects of iodine treatment or T_4 supplementation in early pregnancy are needed, before the implementation of FT_4 screening programs can be justified.

M. Schott, MD, PhD

Thyroid autoimmunity and miscarriage: a meta-analysis
Chen L, Hu R (Fudan Univ, Shanghai, P. R. China)
Clin Endocrinol (Oxf) 74:513-519, 2011

Objective.—To investigate whether thyroid autoimmunity (TAI) is associated with increased risk of miscarriage in euthyroid women.

Methods.—An electronic search was conducted using the databases Medline, PubMed, EMBASE and the Cochrane library, from inception to October 2010. A systematic review of the studies on the association between TAI and miscarriage was performed. The odd ratios of case–control studies and relative risks of cohort studies were pooled respectively. The software Review Manager (version 4.3.1) was applied for meta-analysis.

Results.—The search strategy identified 53 potentially relevant publications, 22 of which were included in the meta-analysis. A clear association between thyroid autoimmunity and miscarriage was observed with a pooled odds ratio of $2·55$ (95% CI $1·42-4·57$, $P = 0·002$) in eight case-control studies and a pooled relative risk of $2·31$ (95% CI $1·90-2·82$, $P < 0·000\ 01$) in 14 cohort studies. Women with TAI were found to have slightly higher age [age difference, $1·29$ years] (95% CI $0·43-2·16$, $P = 0·003$) and thyroid-stimulating hormone (TSH) levels [TSH difference, $0·61$ mIU/l] (95% CI $0·51-0·71$, $P < 0·000\ 01$) compared with those without TAI.

Conclusion.—Based on the currently available evidence, it appears that the presence of thyroid autoimmunity is associated with an increased risk of spontaneous miscarriage in euthyroid women (Table 3).

▶ The aim of the study by Chen and Hu was to investigate whether thyroid autoimmunity (TAI) is associated with increased risk of miscarriage in euthyroid

TABLE 3.—Meta-Analysis of Studies on Association Between TAI and Miscarriage

	Heterogeneity Test	Model Type	Pooled OR(RR) (95% CI)	OR(RR) *Significance* Test
Case–control studies	$\chi^2 = 36 \cdot 89$, $P < 0 \cdot 00001$	Random effect model	$2 \cdot 55$ $(1 \cdot 42 - 4 \cdot 57)$	$Z = 3 \cdot 13$, $P = 0 \cdot 002$
Cohort studies	$\chi^2 = 16 \cdot 01$, $P = 0 \cdot 25$	Fixed effect model	$2 \cdot 31$ $(1 \cdot 90 - 2 \cdot 82)$	$Z = 8 \cdot 35$, $P < 0 \cdot 00001$

women. To do this, they performed a meta-analysis of formerly published data. As shown in Table 3, the authors found a clear association between TAI and miscarriage with odds ratios of 2.55 (for case-control studies) and 2.31 (for cohort studies). These data, however, do not mean that the relationship is causal. Many factors could affect the outcome of pregnancy, of which TAI is just one aspect. One factor could be autoimmunity. Miscarriage is associated with several autoimmune diseases, especially antiphospholipid syndrome (APS) and systemic lupus erythematous (SLE). The abortion rates of pregnancies complicated with APS and SLE are between 7% and around 20%. Another important point is the thyroid function. Other studies already demonstrated that there is a correlation between thyroid function (especially serum thyrotropin [TSH]) and miscarriage. This meta-analysis revealed that antibody-positive woman had in mean 0.61 mIU/L higher TSH levels compared with antibody-negative subjects. Because of this, levothyroxine replacement during pregnancy, aiming for a TSH at the lower third of the normal range, is strongly recommended. The TSH levels of women planning for pregnancy should also be titrated to this lower target value, if possible.

M. Schott, MD, PhD

High Rate of Persistent Hypothyroidism in a Large-Scale Prospective Study of Postpartum Thyroiditis in Southern Italy

Stagnaro-Green A, Schwartz A, Gismondi R, et al (George Washington Univ School of Medicine and Health Sciences, DC; Univ of Illinois, Chicago; Casa di Cura "Salus", Brindisi, Italy; et al)
J Clin Endocrinol Metab 96:652-657, 2011

Context.—The incidence of postpartum thyroiditis (PPT) varies widely in the literature. Limited data exist concerning the hormonal status of women with PPT at the end of the first postpartum year.

Objective.—Our aim was to conduct a large prospective study of the incidence and clinical course of PPT.

Design.—A total of 4394 women were screened for thyroid function and thyroid autoantibodies at 6 and 12 months postpartum. Women were classified as being at high or low risk of having thyroid disease before any thyroid testing.

Setting.—The study was conducted at two ambulatory clinics in southern Italy, an area of mild iodine deficiency.

Patients.—A total of 4394 pregnant women were studied.

Intervention.—There was no intervention.

Main Outcome Measures.—We measured incidence, clinical presentation, and course of postpartum thyroiditis.

Results.—The incidence of postpartum thyroiditis was 3.9% (169 of 4384). Women classified as being at high risk for thyroid disease had a higher incidence of PPT than women classified as low risk (11.1 *vs.* 1.9%; odds ratio, 6.69; 95% confidence interval, 4.63, 9.68). Eighty-two percent of the 169 women with PPT had a hypothyroid phase during the first postpartum year. At the end of the first postpartum year, 54% of the 169 women had persistent hypothyroidism.

Conclusions.—One of every 25 women in southern Italy developed PPT. Women at high risk for thyroid disease have an increased rate of PPT. The high rate of permanent hypothyroidism at 1 yr should result in a reevaluation of the widely held belief that most women with PPT are euthyroid at the end of the first postpartum year (Table 2).

▶ Postpartum thyroiditis (PPT) is the occurrence of transient thyroid hormonal abnormalities in the first year after delivery in women who were euthyroid before pregnancy. In its classic form, hyperthyroidism occurs within the first 3 to 6 months, followed by hypothyroidism, with a return to the euthyroid state (in the majority of women) before the conclusion of the first postpartum year. The incidence of PPT (in retrospective analyses) varies between 1.1% and 16.7%, with a quantitative review estimating that the incidence of PPT is 1 in every 12 women worldwide. The aim of this (prospective) study was to measure the incidence, clinical presentation, and course of PPT. A total of 4394 pregnant women were studied. The incidence of PPT was 3.9% (169 of 4384). Women classified

TABLE 2.—Clinical Progressions of PPT and Associated Thyroid Function Test Values at 6 and 12 Months

| | Euthyroid at 6 Months | | Hyperthyroid at 6 Months | | Hypothyroid at 6 Months | |
	Hypothyroid at 12 Months	Hyperthyroid at 12 Months	Hypothyroid at 12 Months	Euthyroid at 12 Months	Hypothyroid at 12 Months	Euthyroid at 12 Months
TSH at 6 months (median, IQR)	2.15 (1.58)	1.35 (1.88)	0.02 (0.04)	0.03 (0.05)	6.7 (1.8)[a]	5.2 (0.77)[a]
TSH at 12 months (median, IQR)	7.25 (5.5)[a]	0.04 (0.10)[a]	7.4 (6.0)[a]	2.0 (1.3)[a]	7.9 (3.8)[a]	3.05 (1.2)[a]
FT4 at 6 months	11.5 (2.3)	13.0 (1.8)	27.3 (6.3)	23.7 (4.9)	8.3 (0.69)	9.1 (0.65)
FT4 at 12 months	8.4 (0.85)[a]	17.8 (10.2)[a]	8.0 (0.93)[a]	12.8 (1.4)[a]	8.2 (0.82)[a]	10.9 (1.7)[a]
No. (%) of women with PPT with this progression	38 (22.5%)	4 (2.4%)	23 (13.6%)	27 (16.0%)	31 (18.3%)	46 (27.2%)

Values of thyroid function tests are given as means (SD), except where noted. IQR, Interquartile range.
[a]Values significantly different in paired comparisons between clinical progressions with a common 6-month thyroid status, based on Scheffé tests (for FT4) or Mann-Whitney *U* tests (for TSH).

as being at high risk for thyroid disease had a higher incidence of PPT than women classified as low risk. Eighty-two percent of the 169 women with PPT had a hypothyroid phase during the first postpartum year. At the end of the first postpartum year, 54% of the 169 women had persistent hypothyroidism. Detailed data are given in Table 2.

This study supports the high incidence of a hypothyroid phase in the course of PPT. The most unexpected finding, as stated by the authors, is the high incidence of permanent hypothyroidism in over 50% of their patients. The literature mentioned an incidence of 5% to 20% of permanent hypothyroidism at 12 months postpartum and an incidence of 20% to 60% of permanent hypothyroidism after 5 to 10 years. The authors speculated that the low incidence of PPT in their study represents an underestimation because of limited sampling only at 6 and 12 months postpartum. In addition, the incidence of PPT in this study was lower than that in other reports. This could be attributable to several reasons, as indicated by the authors, including the selection of patients; all their patients were euthyroid in the first trimester of pregnancy, and the thyroid tests were done routinely at 6 and 12 months postpartum. In other studies, thyroid tests were performed every 3 months for 12 months, and this could have yielded a higher incidence of women with PPT.[1]

M. Schott, MD, PhD

Reference

1. Mestman J. Over half of women with postpartum thyroiditis remain hypothyroid one year later. *Clinical Thyroidology.* 2011;23:16-19.

5 Calcium and Bone Metabolism

Introduction

A variety of significant advances in clinical investigation of calcium and bone disorders were made during the last year. Many of the studies presented in this section describe results of the major clinical trials published this past year in the clinically important area of osteoporosis, but the others evaluate various aspects of metabolic bone disease and vitamin D and mineral metabolism. Taken together, these studies highlight many of the major advances in the understanding of the pathophysiology and treatment of calcium and bone disorders. These studies will impact clinical practice significantly in the near future. As with any selected review of the literature, there were many other significant papers published this past year that could not be included in this short chapter. This chapter describes a sample of many of the most important papers in this area over the last year.

The first section focuses on advances in osteoporosis therapy. The first 5 articles discussed summarize findings of major clinical trials with the new osteoporosis agent denosumab. Denosumab is a fully human monoclonal antibody that is a first-in-class receptor activator of nuclear factor κB (RANK) ligand (RANKL) inhibitor. Denosumab acts as an antiresorptive agent by potently suppressing osteoclast activity by blocking the interaction of RANKL with RANK on the surface of osteoclasts and osteoclast precursors. This agent was approved for treatment of postmenopausal osteoporosis in the United States on June 1, 2010.

The first study described the skeletal effects of the clinically approved dose of denosumab 60 mg by subcutaneous injection every 6 months for 2 years in postmenopausal women with low bone density, followed by 2 years off treatment. Denosumab improved bone mineral density (BMD) and decreased markers of bone turnover during treatment as expected during the first two years. The changes seen during the first 2 years almost completely reversed during the 2 years off treatment, emphasizing that even though denosumab is as potent an antiresorptive agent as the bisphosphonates, its effects are short-lived off treatment. This monoclonal antibody is a relatively short-acting biological agent with maximal effects persisting 3-6 months after injection.

The second paper described bone histomorphometry findings in patients treated with denosumab for up to 3 years in the FREEDOM pivotal fracture trial, or denosumab versus alendronate for 1 year in the STAND trial. Denosumab significantly decreased bone resorption and bone formation in both studies, with the effect of denosumab on bone turnover in both trials greater that alendronate in the STAND trial. Further follow-up will be required in order to determine how long decreased bone turnover caused by denosumab is safe.

The third study was a long-term extension of a phase II clinical trial that showed that denosumab was well tolerated and effective over 6 years of continuous treatment in postmenopausal women. The fourth paper demonstrated that denosumab caused a different pattern of changes in markers of bone turnover than other antiresorptive agents in the FREEDOM trial. Serum CTx-telopeptide, a marker of bone resorption, decreased rapidly below the premenopausal reference range and remained there for the duration of the trial in about half of subjects, as did P1NP, a marker of bone formation. This degree of suppression of turnover was greater than typically seen with other antiresorptive agents. The significant reduction in serum CTx-telopeptide correlated with increased bone density, however.

The fifth study compared changes in trabecular and cortical bone microarchitecture as assessed by high-resolution quantitative CT scanning in subjects treated with denosumab or alendronate. Denosumab improved or prevented loss of total, trabecular, and cortical BMD at the radius and tibia, whereas alendronate prevented loss at both sites. A measure of bone strength, known as the polar moment of inertia, increased more in the denosumab group, indicating greater improvement in bone strength with denosumab.

The next article clarified results previously reported in the 10-year Fracture Intervention Trial (FIT) Long-Term Extension (FLEX) Trial. The initial report of this trial indicated that postmenopausal women who continued alendronate for 10 years did not have fewer nonvertebral fractures than those who stopped alendronate at 5 years, but that subjects who continued alendronate for 10 years had fewer clinical vertebral fractures, although not fewer morphometric vertebral fractures. This study clarified that subjects without vertebral fractures at the start of the FLEX trial had reduced nonvertebral fractures over the next 5 years if their baseline FLEX femoral neck BMD T-score was below -2.5, but not if it was above -2.5, or below -2.0.

The seventh study reported the surprising finding that combination therapy with zoledronic acid and teriparatide (recombinant human PTH 1-34) resulted in greater improvement in lumbar spine and hip BMD than either agent alone over 12 months of treatment. Zoledronic acid is a potent long-acting antiresorptive agent, and teriparatide the only currently approved anabolic agent. Previous studies have reported that combination therapy with antiresorptive agents and teriparatide resulted in blunting of the anabolic response to teriparatide.

The eighth study demonstrated that zoledronic acid 5 mg given intravenously once a year and alendronate 70 mg given orally once a week over 2 years were equally effective in improving BMD and suppressing markers of bone turnover in men with osteoporosis. This study is important because very few previous head-to-head comparison studies of therapeutic agents have been published in men with osteoporosis.

The 2 studies that follow evaluated the possibility that long-term alendronate therapy increases the risk of atypical subtrochanteric femoral fractures. The study by Black et al assessed the risk of this type of unusual fracture in 14,195 postmenopausal women treated for up to 10 years with alendronate in the FIT and FLEX clinical trials, and for 18 months with zoledronic acid in the Health Outcomes and Reduced Incidence with Zoledronic Acid Once Yearly (HORIZON) Pivotal Fracture Trial. The study concluded that there was not an increased risk of atypical subtrochanteric fractures in subjects in these clinical trials, but that the studies were not powered to demonstrate conclusive findings. The Abrahamson et al study reported that long-term users of alendronate were at higher risk of typical hip and atypical subtrochanteric/diaphyseal fractures than matched controls, but that higher cumulative doses of alendronate did not increase the risk of this unusual type of fracture more than lower doses. The study concluded that the atypical subtrochanteric/diaphyseal fractures were more likely due to osteoporosis, rather than alendronate therapy of osteoporosis.

The next section of this chapter discusses a variety of studies offering insight into the epidemiology and pathophysiology of osteoporosis. The first study showed that the bone regulatory protein sclerostin is a significant regulator of physiological bone mineralization via upregulation of MEPE, downregulation of PHEX, and increased secretion of MEPE-ASARM peptides in preosteocytes. Mineralization of new bone by osteoblasts was confirmed to be increased significantly by the tri-phosphorylated form of MEPE-ASARM peptides. This study adds significantly to the previous understanding that sclerostin decreases new bone formation by inhibiting the Wnt/β-catenin signaling pathway in osteoblasts.

The next study reported that circulating sclerostin levels in 27 postmenopausal women correlated with their bone marrow plasma levels, and that intermittent PTH therapy with teriparatide reduced their circulating sclerostin levels. These findings imply that decreased sclerostin levels might be one of the mechanisms by which anabolic intermittent PTH therapy improves BMD and reduces fractures. The next study demonstrated that circulating sclerostin levels were decreased by estrogen treatment in 17 postmenopausal women, but not testosterone treatment in 59 elderly men. The study concluded that decreased sclerostin might be one of the mechanisms by which estrogen treatment reduces osteoclast activity in postmenopausal women treated for osteoporosis.

The study that follows reported that circulating serum sclerostin levels are higher in men than women, that serum sclerostin levels increase significantly with aging, and that older subjects have higher serum sclerostin levels for their bone mass than younger subjects in a population-based sample of 362 women and 318 men ages 21 to 97 years. Further studies will be required to assess the reasons for the age-related increase in circulating sclerostin, as well as the potential role of this increase in mediating the age-related decrease in bone formation.

The next study reported that estimation of hip strength by high-resolution quantitative CT scanning (HRQCT) and finite element analysis (FEA) predicted hip fractures in subjects with hip strength of less than 3000 Newtons, as well as overall and osteoporotic fractures elsewhere in the skeleton in an age-stratified random sample of 314 female and 266 male community-based adults aged ≥35 years. These findings imply that estimated hip strength of less than 3000 Newtons may represent a critical level of systemic skeletal fragility in both women and men. The next study provides evidence that grade 1 vertebral deformities should be regarded as osteoporotic fractures. For many years, the consensus has been that minor or low-grade vertebral deformities may be due to congenital anomalies or other causes, but this report showed that this type of deformity is associated with decreased BMD, impaired structure, and reduced strength in 193 women with vertebral fractures compared with 90 controls without such fractures. The results of this study imply that adults with low-grade vertebral fractures should be treated as if they have had osteoporotic fractures.

The next study demonstrated that hip strength may be less than predicted in older adults by areal BMD DXA measurement, and that hip strength decreases more rapidly with age than areal BMD T-score. The study evaluated hip HRQCT and areal BMD by DXA in a randomly sampled age-stratified cohort of 362 women and 317 men ages 21 to 89 years. The findings imply that older adults may be at greater risk of hip fracture because of lower femoral strength than previously assumed using the WHO definition of osteoporosis based on a real BMD T-score measurement.

The next study is a meta-analysis of calcium without vitamin D supplementation in adults older than 40 years. This study concluded that calcium supplements increase the risk of myocardial infarction (MI). The study also showed non-significant increases in risk of stroke, death, and a composite end point including MI, stroke, or sudden death. These findings remain controversial since none of the individual studies included in the meta-analysis demonstrated an increased risk of MI. Nevertheless, the findings suggest that the use of calcium supplements in treatment or prevention of osteoporosis may need to be reassessed.

Two studies that follow provide significant new findings that suggest the skeleton may directly regulate male fertility and reproduction, and glucose homeostasis and energy metabolism. Both fertility and glucose metabolism are mediated via osteoblast production of uncarboxylated osteocalcin in mice. As novel and intriguing as these study findings are, they should be regarded with caution for now, because they have not yet been reproduced in humans. The first study showed that osteoblasts directly regulate testosterone secretion by the testis via osteocalcin in mice, by osteocalcin binding to a G-protein-linked receptor on Leydig cells, and signaling through a cyclic

AMP response element to cause synthesis of enzymes required for testosterone biosynthesis. The second study demonstrated that insulin stimulates osteoblasts to release increased uncarboxylated osteocalcin via osteoclast bone resorption, which then stimulates β-cell insulin secretion, increases β-cell mass, and increases insulin sensitivity. These and other recent similar studies have prompted recognition that the skeleton serves key functions beyond those that have traditionally been recognized.

The next section of this chapter reviews several studies that shed light on issues in metabolic bone disease. The first paper reported that minimally invasive parathyroidectomy is a superior technique compared to traditional full neck exploration in patients with sporadic primary hyperparathyroidism. This study summarizes a case series of 1650 parathyroidectomies performed at a single US academic institution over 19 years.

The next study showed that cinacalcet, an allosteric calcium-sensing receptor (CaSR) calcimimetic agent that increases the sensitivity of the CaSR to calcium, was effective for treatment of hypercalcemia due to primary hyperparathyroidism over a wide range of disease severity for 4.5 years. The study did not demonstrate improvement in BMD in treated subjects, but showed that cinacalcet kept serum calcium within or close to the normal range, and PTH close to the normal range, over this multi-year interval. This and other studies led to the recent FDA approval of cinacalcet for the additional indication of treatment of severe hypercalcemia due to primary hyperparathyroidism, when surgery is not possible.

The next study showed that open-label treatment with human PTH 1-84 100 mcg every other day in 30 adults with hypoparathyroidism for 24 months significantly reduced daily calcium and calcitriol supplement requirements. During this study, serum calcium and 24-hour urinary calcium remained stable, and lumbar spine BMD improved slightly, while hip BMD remained stable and wrist BMD decreased slightly. A 6-month phase III clinical trial with daily PTH 1-84 versus placebo is currently under way to evaluate effectiveness of this agent in treatment of hypoparathyroidism.

The next study showed that frailty in elderly women responds in a biphasic manner to serum 25-hydroxyvitamin D levels. The study showed that frailty was moderately increased in women with baseline serum 25-hydroxyvitamin D <20 ng/mL or ≥30 ng/mL. The study also reported that in nonfrail women at baseline, serum 25-hydroxyvitamin D <20 ng/mL was associated with increased risk of developing frailty or dying over the next 4.5 years of follow-up.

The next section of this chapter discusses several novel therapies for osteoporosis. The first study (5-25) showed that nitroglycerin ointment applied daily for 2 years modestly increased BMD at the lumbar spine, total hip, and femoral neck compared to placebo. Bone specific alkaline phosphatase, a marker of bone formation, increased during the trial, whereas urinary NTx-telopeptide, a marker of bone resorption, decreased. Headaches were the most prominent side effect, but headache frequency decreased after 12 months of treatment. Nitric oxide donors such as nitroglycerin may represent a new form of therapy for osteoporosis.

The study that follows presented 2-year follow-up data from a study of balloon kyphoplasty versus nonsurgical management for vertebral compression fractures. The study showed that kyphoplasty rapidly reduced pain and improved function, disability, and quality of life averaged over 2 years after treatment, compared with medical management, without increasing the risk of subsequent vertebral fractures, and that reduction in back pain was significant at all observation timepoints. The study concluded that balloon kyphoplasty is a useful adjunct for management of painful acute vertebral fractures.

The final study in this chapter showed that odanacatib, a new cathepsin K inhibitor, selectively inhibits osteoclast bone resorption when given at a dose of 50 mg orally each week, and it causes progressive increases in BMD in postmenopausal women over 3 years of follow-up. Bone resorption markers remained suppressed for the duration of treatment, whereas bone formation markers gradually returned toward baseline. Discontinuation of odanacatib resulted in moderately rapid bone loss and transiently increased bone resorption, suggesting that, unlike bisphosphonates, cathepsin K inhibitors do not cause long-term suppression of bone turnover.

In summary, these selected papers give a glimpse of the breadth and depth of clinical research in calcium and bone disorders during the last year. As noted, many other significant papers could not be included due to selection constraints. Some of the studies presented confirm long-held views based on previous observations, whereas others demonstrate previously unsuspected physiological functions of the skeleton. Future clinical investigation will likely clarify recent findings that do not fit within the classical paradigms of skeletal function in health and disease.

Bart L. Clarke, MD

Current Issues in Osteoporosis Therapy

Effects of Denosumab Treatment and Discontinuation on Bone Mineral Density and Bone Turnover Markers in Postmenopausal Women with Low Bone Mass
Bone HG, Bolognese MA, Yuen CK, et al (Michigan Bone and Mineral Clinic, Detroit; Bethesda Health Res Ctr, Maryland; Univ of Manitoba, Winnipeg, Canada; et al)
J Clin Endocrinol Metab 96:972-980, 2011

Context.—Denosumab treatment for 24 months increased bone mineral density (BMD) and reduced bone turnover markers (BTM) in postmenopausal women.

Objective.—The aim was to determine the effects of prior denosumab or placebo injections on BMD, BTM, and safety over 24 months after treatment discontinuation.

Design.—We conducted an off-treatment extension of a phase 3, randomized, double-blind, parallel- group study.

Participants.—A total of 256 postmenopausal women with a mean age of 59 yr and a mean lumbar spine T-score of −1.61 at randomization participated in the study.

Interventions.—Participants received placebo or 60 mg denosumab every 6 months for 24 months, followed by 24 months off treatment.

Main Outcome Measures.—We measured the percentage changes in BMD and BTM, and evaluated safety.

Results.—Of the 256 participants enrolled in the posttreatment phase, 87% completed the study. During 24 months of denosumab treatment, BMD increased (lumbar spine, 6.4%; total hip, 3.6%; 1/3 radius, 1.4%), and BTM decreased (serum C-terminal telopeptide of type 1 collagen, 63%; and N-terminal propeptide of type 1 procollagen, 47%), compared with placebo. After discontinuation, BMD declined, but the previously treated denosumab group maintained higher BMD than the previously treated placebo group at these sites ($P \le 0.05$). Final BMD at month 48 strongly correlated with month 0 BMD. After denosumab discontinuation, BTM increased above baseline within 3 months (serum C-terminal telopeptide of type 1 collagen) or 6 months (N-terminal propeptide of type 1 procollagen) and returned to baseline by month 48. Adverse event rates during the off-treatment phase were similar between groups.

Conclusions.—In postmenopausal women with low BMD, the effects of 60mgdenosumabtreatment for 24 months on BMD and BTM are reversible upon discontinuation, reflecting its biological mechanism of action. Residual BMD measurements remained above those of the group previously treated with placebo.

▶ Denosumab is a fully human monoclonal antibody against receptor activator of nuclear factor-κB (RANK) ligand (RANKL) that was recently approved for treatment of postmenopausal osteoporosis.[1] RANKL is essential for formation, function, and survival of osteoclasts.[2,3] Denosumab binds RANKL secreted by osteoblasts and osteoblast precursors and prevents its interaction with the receptor RANK on osteoclasts and osteoclast precursors.[4] The antibody reversibly inhibits osteoclast-mediated bone resorption and has been shown to prevent bone loss and fractures.[1,5]

This off-treatment extension of a phase 2, randomized, double-blind, parallel-group study of denosumab[6] 60 mg versus placebo by subcutaneous injection every 6 months for 2 years showed that the effects of denosumab were reversible over the next 2 years. Bone mineral density decreased after denosumab was stopped but still remained greater at all sites than that in the placebo group. Serum C-terminal telopeptide of type 1 collagen increased from 63% below baseline after 2 years of therapy to above baseline within 3 months of stopping denosumab. Serum N-terminal propeptide of type 1 procollagen increased from 47% below baseline after 2 years of therapy to above baseline within 6 months of stopping denosumab. Both markers returned to baseline by 48 months after stopping denosumab.

These findings indicate that the monoclonal antibody denosumab potently suppresses bone turnover while preventing bone loss and fractures. However, unlike bisphosphonates, the effect of denosumab wears off quickly after stopping the medication. This allows resumption of normal bone turnover within a short time of stopping denosumab, which may prevent adverse consequences of prolonged suppression of bone turnover.

B. L. Clarke, MD

References

1. Cummings SR, Martin JS, McClung MR, et al. Denosumab for prevention of fractures in postmenopausal women with osteoporosis. *N Engl J Med.* 2009;361: 756-765.
2. Lacey DL, Timms E, Tan HL, et al. Osteoprotegerin ligand is a cytokine that regulates osteoclast differentiation and activation. *Cell.* 1998;93:165-176.
3. Lacey DL, Tan HL, Lu J, et al. Osteoprotegerin ligand modulates murine osteoclast survival in vitro and in vivo. *Am J Pathol.* 2000;157:435-448.
4. Hsu H, Lacey DL, Dunstan CR, et al. Tumor necrosis factor receptor family member RANK mediates osteoclast differentiation and activation induced by osteoprotegerin ligand. *Proc Natl Acad Sci U S A.* 1999;96:3540-3545.
5. McClung MR, Lewiecki EM, Cohen SB, et al. Denosumab in postmenopausal women with low bone mineral density. *N Engl J Med.* 2006;354:821-831.
6. Lewiecki EM, Miller PD, McClung MR, et al. Two-year treatment with denosumab (AMG 162) in a randomized phase 2 study of postmenopausal women with low BMD. *J Bone Miner Res.* 2007;22:1832-1841.

Effects of Denosumab on Bone Histomorphometry: The FREEDOM and STAND Studies

Reid IR, on behalf of the Denosumab Phase 3 Bone Histology Study Group (Univ of Auckland, New Zealand; et al)
J Bone Miner Res 25:2256-2265, 2010

Denosumab, a human monoclonal antibody against RANKL, reversibly inhibits osteoclast-mediated bone resorption and has been developed for use in osteoporosis. Its effects on bone histomorphometry have not been described previously. Iliac crest bone biopsies were collected at 24 and/or 36 months from osteoporotic postmenopausal women in the FREEDOM study (45 women receiving placebo and 47 denosumab) and at 12 months from postmenopausal women previously treated with alendronate in the STAND study (21 continuing alendronate and 15 changed to denosumab at trial entry). Qualitative histologic evaluation of biopsies was unremarkable. In the FREEDOM study, median eroded surface was reduced by more than 80% and osteoclasts were absent from more than 50% of biopsies in the denosumab group. Double labeling in trabecular bone was observed in 94% of placebo bones and in 19% of those treated with denosumab. Median bone-formation rate was reduced by 97%. Among denosumab-treated subjects, those with double labels and those with absent labels had similar levels of biochemical markers of bone turnover. In the STAND trial, indices of bone turnover tended to be lower in the denosumab group than in the alendronate group. Double labeling in trabecular bone was seen in 20% of the denosumab biopsies and in 90% of the alendronate samples. Denosumab markedly reduces bone turnover and also reduces fracture numbers. Longer follow-up is necessary to determine how long such low turnover is safe.

▶ Bone remodeling may be modulated by inhibition of osteoclast bone resorption by blocking receptor activator of nuclear factor kappa B (RANK) ligand (RANKL).[1] RANKL is required for formation, function, and survival of osteoclasts and osteoclast precursors.[2,3] Denosumab is a fully human monoclonal antibody against RANKL that neutralizes this signaling molecule after secretion by osteoblasts and osteoblast precursors before it can interact with RANK on the cell membrane of osteoclasts and osteoclast precursors. Denosumab has been shown to reduce bone turnover, increase bone mineral density,[4] and reduce fractures in postmenopausal women with osteoporosis.[5]

This study presents histomorphometric data from iliac crest bone biopsies taken at 24 and/or 36 months from 45 postmenopausal osteoporotic women receiving denosumab and 47 women receiving placebo in the Fracture REduction Evaluation of Denosumab in Osteoporosis every 6 Months (FREEDOM) study[5] and at 12 months from 21 postmenopausal osteoporotic women continuing alendronate and 15 women switched to denosumab in the Study of Transitioning from AleNdronate to Denosumab (STAND) study.[6] Qualitative evaluation of biopsies was unremarkable. Biopsies from denosumab-treated subjects in the FREEDOM study showed that median eroded surface was reduced by more than 80%, and that osteoclasts were absent from more than 50% of biopsies. Double labeling was present in 94% of placebo subjects and 19% of those treated with denosumab, and median bone formation rate was reduced by 97% in those treated with denosumab. In denosumab-treated subjects, biochemical markers of bone turnover were similar in those with double labels and those with absent labels. In the STAND study, denosumab-treated subjects had lower indices of bone turnover than alendronate-treated subjects. Double labeling of trabecular bone was present in 20% of the denosumab subjects and 90% of the alendronate-treated subjects.

These findings demonstrate that denosumab markedly reduces bone turnover at the same time it reduces fractures. Denosumab suppresses bone turnover more effectively than the bisphosphonate alendronate during treatment. However, bone marker studies show that the effect of denosumab wears off within 6 months of each injection, indicating that this biological agent acts differently from the long-acting bisphosphonate alendronate. Longer-term follow-up will be necessary to determine how long markedly suppressed turnover is safe.

B. L. Clarke, MD

References

1. Lacey DL, Timms E, Tan HL, et al. Osteoprotegerin ligand is a cytokine that regulates osteoclast differentiation and activation. *Cell.* 1998;93:165-176.
2. Hsu H, Lacey DL, Dunstan CR, et al. Tumor necrosis factor receptor family member RANK mediates osteoclast differentiation and activation induced by osteoprotegerin ligand. *Proc Natl Acad Sci USA.* 1999;96:3540-3545.

3. Lacey DL, Tan HL, Lu J, et al. Osteoprotegerin ligand modules murine osteoclast survival in vitro and in vivo. *Am J Pathol.* 2000;157:435-448.
4. McClung MR, Lewiecki EM, Cohen SB, et al. Denosumab in postmenopausal women with low bone mineral density. *N Engl J Med.* 2006;354:821-831.
5. Cummings SR, Martin JS, McClung MR, et al. Denosumab for prevention of fractures in postmenopausal women with osteoporosis. *N Engl J Med.* 2009;361: 756-765.
6. Kendler DL, Roux C, Benhamou CL, et al. Effects of denosumab on bone mineral density and bone turnover in postmenopausal women transitioning from alendronate therapy. *J Bone Miner Res.* 2010;25:72-81.

Effect of Denosumab on Bone Mineral Density and Biochemical Markers of Bone Turnover: Six-Year Results of a Phase 2 Clinical Trial

Miller PD, Wagman RB, Peacock M, et al (Colorado Ctr for Bone Res, Lakewood; Amgen Inc, Thousand Oaks, CA; Indiana Univ School of Medicine, Indianapolis; et al)

J Clin Endocrinol Metab 96:394-402, 2011

Context.—This is a study extension to evaluate the efficacy and safety of long-term treatment with denosumab in postmenopausal women with low bone mass.

Objective.—Our objective was to describe changes in bone mineral density (BMD) and bone turnover markers as well as safety with 6 yr of denosumab treatment.

Design.—We conducted an ongoing 4-yr, open-label, single-arm, extension study of a dose-ranging phase 2 trial. This paper reports a 2-yr interim analysis representing up to 6 yr of continuous denosumab treatment.

Setting.—This multicenter study was conducted at 23 U.S. centers.

Patients.—Of the 262 subjects who completed the parent study, 200 enrolled in the study extension and 178 (89%) completed the first 2 yr.

Intervention.—All subjects received denosumab 60 mg sc every 6 months.

Main Outcome Measures.—We evaluated BMD at the lumbar spine, total hip, femoral neck, and one third radius; biochemical markers of bone turnover; and safety, reported as adverse events.

Results.—Over a period of 6 yr, continuous treatment with denosumab resulted in progressive gains in BMD in postmenopausal women with low bone mass. Reduction in bone resorption was sustained over the course of continuous treatment. Independent of past treatment and discontinuation period, subjects demonstrated responsiveness to denosumab therapy as measured by BMD and bone turnover markers. The safety profile of denosumab did not change over time.

Conclusions.—In this study, denosumab was well tolerated and effective through 6 yr of continuous treatment in postmenopausal women with low bone mass.

▶ Denosumab is a fully human monoclonal antibody directed against the receptor activator of nuclear factor kappa-B (RANK) ligand (RANKL). RANKL is a molecular signal secreted by osteoblasts and osteoblast precursors that stimulates the RANK on osteoclast cell membranes to promote formation, function, and survival of osteoclasts.[1,2] Without RANKL stimulation, osteoclast precursors fail to form fully functional multinucleated osteoclasts or to resorb bone.[3] Denosumab reversibly inhibits osteoclast-mediated bone resorption[4] and prevents bone loss and fractures.[5]

This 2-year interim analysis of a 4-year, open-label, single-arm, extension study of a dose-ranging phase 2 trial[6] showed that prolonged treatment of postmenopausal women with low bone mineral density (BMD) with denosumab over a total of 4 years caused continued increased BMD and sustained decreased markers of bone turnover. Subjects in this extension study were enrolled after completing 2 previous years in a phase 2 study with denosumab at different doses by subcutaneous injection compared with alendronate 70 mg each week or placebo. By the end of 6 years, lumbar spine BMD increased by 13.3%, total hip BMD by 6.1%, and one-third distal radius by 1.9%. This study showed that denosumab remained efficacious and safe over 4 further years of treatment, and that response to denosumab was independent of previous therapy or discontinuation interval.

This study demonstrates that denosumab continues to improve bone density over 6 years of continued therapy. Denosumab potently but reversibly suppresses bone turnover for about 6 months, with gradual recovery of turnover toward the end of each 6-month interval. Changes in bone markers correlate with improvement in BMD. Unlike bisphosphonates, denosumab appears to continue to increase bone density over time without a significant plateauing of effect, possibly because of differences in the way that denosumab transiently decreases bone turnover compared with bisphosphonates, which decrease bone turnover for years.

B. L. Clarke, MD

References

1. Lacey DL, Timms E, Tan HL, et al. Osteoprotegerin ligand is a cytokine that regulates osteoclast differentiation and activation. *Cell.* 1998;93:165-176.
2. Lacey DL, Tan HL, Lu J, et al. Osteoprotegerin ligand modulates murine osteoclast survival in vitro and in vivo. *Am J Pathol.* 2000;157:435-448.
3. Hsu H, Lacey DL, Dunstan CR, et al. Tumor necrosis factor receptor family member RANK mediates osteoclast differentiation and activation induced by osteoprotegerin ligand. *Proc Natl Acad Sci USA.* 1999;96:3540-3545.
4. McClung MR, Lewiecki EM, Cohen SB, et al. Denosumab in postmenopausal women with low bone mineral density. *N Engl J Med.* 2006;354:821-831.
5. Cummings SR, Martin JS, McClung MR, et al. Denosumab for prevention of fractures in postmenopausal women with osteoporosis. *N Engl J Med.* 2009;361: 756-765.
6. Miller PD, Bolognese MA, Lewiecki EM, et al. Effect of denosumab on bone density and turnover in postmenopausal women with low bone mass after long-term continued, discontinued, and restarting of therapy: a randomized blinded phase 2 clinical trial. *Bone.* 2008;43:222-229.

Effects of Denosumab on Bone Turnover Markers in Postmenopausal Osteoporosis

Eastell R, Christiansen C, Grauer A, et al (Univ of Sheffield, UK; Ctr for Clinical and Basic Res, Ballerup, Denmark; Amgen, Inc, Thousand Oaks, CA; et al)
J Bone Miner Res 26:530-537, 2011

Denosumab, a fully human monoclonal antibody to RANKL, decreases bone remodeling, increases bone density, and reduces fracture risk. This study evaluates the time course and determinants of bone turnover marker (BTM) response during denosumab treatment, the percentage of deno-sumab-treated women with BTMs below the premenopausal reference interval, and the correlations between changes in BTMs and bone mineral density (BMD). The BTM substudy of the Fracture REduction Evaulation of Denosumab in Osteoporosis every 6 Months (FREEDOM) Trial included 160 women randomized to subcutaneous denosumab (60 mg) or placebo injections every 6 months for 3 years. Biochemical markers of bone resorption (serum C-telopeptide of type I collagen [CTX] and tartra-teresistant acid phosphatise [TRACP-5b]) and bone formation (serum procollagen type I N-terminal propeptide [PINP] and bone alkaline phos-phatase [BALP]) were measured at baseline and at 1, 6, 12, 24, and 36 months. Decreases in CTX were more rapid and greater than decreases in PINP and BALP. One month after injection, CTX levels in all denosumab-treated subjects decreased to levels below the premenopausal reference interval. CTX values at the end of the dosing period were influenced by baseline CTX values and the dosing interval. The percentage of subjects with CTX below the premenopausal reference interval before each subse-quent injection decreased from 79% to 51% during the study. CTX and PINP remained below the premenopausal reference interval at all time points in 46% and 31% denosumab-treated subjects, respectively. With denosumab, but not placebo, there were significant correlations between CTX reduction and BMD increase ($r= -0.24$ to -0.44). The BTM response pattern with denosumab is unique and should be appreciated by physicians to monitor this treatment effectively.

▶ Denosumab was recently approved for treatment of postmenopausal osteopo-rosis. Denosumab is a fully human monoclonal antibody directed against receptor activator of nuclear factor kappa-B (RANK) ligand (RANKL). RANKL is a glycoprotein secreted by osteoblasts and osteoblast precursors and normally binds to the receptor RANK on the surface of osteoclasts and osteoclast precur-sors, thereby inhibiting the formation, activity, and survival of osteoclasts.[1-3] Denosumab has been shown to reversibly inhibit osteoclast-mediated bone resorption[4] and to prevent bone loss and fractures.[5]

This substudy of the Fracture REduction Evaluation of Denosumab in Osteopo-rosis every 6 Months clinical trial[5] evaluated denosumab effects on markers of bone turnover, proportion of subjects with bone turnover markers below the premenopausal normal range, and correlations between changes in bone turnover markers and bone mineral density. The study evaluated bone turnover markers and bone mineral density in 160 postmenopausal women randomized to receive denosumab 60 mg or placebo by subcutaneous injection every 6 months for 3 years. The serum marker of bone resorption, C-telopeptide of type I collagen (CTx), decreased more rapidly and by a larger amount than the serum markers of bone formation, bone-specific alkaline phosphatase and procollagen type I *N*-terminal propeptide (P1NP). All subjects receiving denosumab had serum CTx levels below the premenopausal normal range 1 month after starting denosumab therapy, but the percentage of subjects with CTx below the premenopausal normal range before each subsequent injection decreased from 79% to 51% during the 3 years of the study. CTx and P1NP remained below the premenopausal normal range for the entire study in 46% and 31% of subjects, respectively. In subjects receiving denosumab, the magnitude of serum CTx reduction correlated with increased bone mineral density.

This study demonstrates that denosumab induces a unique pattern of changes in markers of bone turnover when given as 60 mg by subcutaneous injection every 6 months. This pattern of decreased bone turnover is different from that seen with other antiresorptive agents. This unique pattern indicates that denosumab-induced decreased markers of bone turnover wear off about 6 months after each injection. This pattern of short-term effect on bone turnover may help prevent oversuppression of bone turnover by this potent agent, but also implies that bone turnover will return rapidly toward baseline after denosumab effect wears off.

B. L. Clarke, MD

References

1. Lacey DL, Timms E, Tan HL, et al. Osteoprotegerin ligand is a cytokine that regulates osteoclast differentiation and activation. *Cell.* 1998;93:165-176.
2. Lacey DL, Tan HL, Lu J, et al. Osteoprotegerin ligand modulates murine osteoclast survival in vitro and in vivo. *Am J Pathol.* 2000;157:435-448.
3. Hsu H, Lacey DL, Dunstan CR, et al. Tumor necrosis factor receptor family member RANK mediates osteoclast differentiation and activation induced by osteoprotegerin ligand. *Proc Natl Acad Sci U S A.* 1999;96:3540-3545.
4. McClung MR, Lewiecki EM, Cohen SB, et al. Denosumab in postmenopausal women with low bone mineral density. *N Engl J Med.* 2006;354:821-831.
5. Cummings SR, San Martin J, McClung MR, et al. Denosumab for prevention of fractures in postmenopausal women with osteoporosis. *N Engl J Med.* 2009; 361:756-765.

Microarchitectural Deterioration of Cortical and Trabecular Bone: Differing Effects of Denosumab and Alendronate
Seeman E, Delmas PD, Hanley DA, et al (Univ of Melbourne, Australia; INSERM U831 and Univ of Lyon, France; Univ of Calgary, Alberta, Canada; et al)
J Bone Miner Res 25:1886-1894, 2010

The intensity of bone remodeling is a critical determinant of the decay of cortical and trabecular microstructure after menopause. Denosumab suppresses remodeling more than alendronate, leading to greater gains in areal bone mineral density (aBMD). These greater gains may reflect differing effects of each drug on bone microarchitecture and strength. In a phase 2 double-blind pilot study, 247 postmenopausal women were randomized to denosumab (60 mg subcutaneous 6 monthly), alendronate (70 mg oral weekly), or placebo for 12 months. All received daily calcium and vitamin D. Morphologic changes were assessed using high-resolution peripheral quantitative computed tomography (HR-pQCT) at the distal radius and distal tibia and QCT at the distal radius. Denosumab decreased serum C-telopeptide more rapidly and markedly than alendronate. In the placebo arm, total, cortical, and trabecular BMD and cortical thickness decreased (-2.1% to -0.8%) at the distal radius after 12 months. Alendronate prevented the decline (-0.6% to 2.4%, $p = .051$ to $<.001$ versus placebo), whereas denosumab prevented the decline or improved these variables (0.3% to 3.4%, $p < .001$ versus placebo). Changes in total and cortical BMD were greater with denosumab than with alendronate ($p \leq .024$). Similar changes in these parameters were observed at the tibia. The polar moment of inertia also increased more in the denosumab than alendronate or placebo groups ($p < .001$). Adverse events did not differ by group. These data suggest that structural decay owing to bone remodeling and progression of bone fragility may be prevented more effectively with denosumab.

▶ The fully human monoclonal antibody denosumab is directed against the receptor activator of nuclear factor κB ligand (RANKL), a glycoprotein secreted by osteoblasts and osteoblast precursors. Denosumab was recently approved for treatment of postmenopausal osteoporosis. RANKL normally binds to the receptor activator of nuclear factor κB (RANK) on osteoclasts and osteoclast precursors and is essential for the development and activity of osteoclasts.[1,2] Denosumab prevents RANKL from interacting with RANK on the cell membrane of osteoclasts and osteoclast precursors.[3] Denosumab has been shown to reversibly inhibit osteoclast-mediated bone resorption[4] and to prevent bone loss and fractures.[5] This phase 2 double-blind pilot study showed that denosumab prevented deterioration of microarchitecture and bone strength in the distal radius and tibia of women with postmenopausal osteoporosis more effectively than alendronate, when assessed by high-resolution quantitative CT scanning. The study randomized 247 postmenopausal women to receive denosumab, 60 mg, by subcutaneous injection every 6 months; alendronate, 70 mg, every week; or placebo over 12 months. Total, cortical, and trabecular bone densities and cortical thickness at both the distal radius and tibia decreased in subjects receiving placebo after 12 months. Alendronate prevented the decrease in these parameters, whereas denosumab increased or prevented the decrease in the same parameters. Changes in total and cortical bone densities were greater with denosumab than with alendronate. Polar movement of inertia, an index of bone strength, increased more in denosumab-treated subjects than alendronate-treated subjects or the placebo group.

These findings suggest that denosumab is more effective at preventing deterioration of bone microarchitecture than alendronate or placebo in postmenopausal women. This is important because bone strength depends not only on bone mineral density but also on bone quality, which is partly determined by bone microarchitecture. Different antiresorptive agents decrease bone turnover by different mechanisms and with different potencies. Prevention of bone loss is not the only or most important means by which antiresorptive agents prevent fractures. Any agent that preserves bone microstructural parameters better than other agents will likely prevent more fractures with long-term treatment.

B. L. Clarke, MD

References

1. Lacey DL, Timms E, Tan HL, et al. Osteoprotegerin ligand is a cytokine that regulates osteoclast differentiation and activation. *Cell.* 1998;93:165-176.
2. Lacey DL, Tan HL, Lu J, et al. Osteoprotegerin ligand modulates murine osteoclast survival in vitro and in vivo. *Am J Pathol.* 2000;157:435-448.
3. Hsu H, Lacey DL, Dunstan CR, et al. Tumor necrosis factor receptor family member RANK mediates osteoclast differentiation and activation induced by osteoprotegerin ligand. *Proc Natl Acad Sci U S A.* 1999;96:3540-3545.
4. McClung MR, Lewiecki EM, Cohen SB, et al. Denosumab in postmenopausal women with low bone mineral density. *N Engl J Med.* 2006;354:821-831.
5. Cummings SR, San Martin J, McClung MR, et al. Denosumab for prevention of fractures in postmenopausal women with osteoporosis. *N Engl J Med.* 2009; 361:756-765.

Efficacy of Continued Alendronate for Fractures in Women With and Without Prevalent Vertebral Fracture: The FLEX Trial

Schwartz AV, for the FLEX Research Group (Univ of California—San Francisco; et al)

J Bone Miner Res 25:976-982, 2010

In the Fracture Intervention Trial (FIT) Long Term Extension (FLEX) Trial, 10 years of alendronate (ALN) did not significantly reduce the risk of nonvertebral fractures (NVFs) compared with 5 years of ALN. Continuing ALN reduced the risk of clinical but not morphometric vertebral fractures regardless of baseline vertebral fracture status. In previous studies, ALN efficacy for NVF prevention in women without prevalent vertebral fracture was limited to those with femoral neck (FN) T-scores of −2.5 or less. To determine whether the effect of long-term ALN on fracture differs by vertebral fracture status and femoral neck (FN) T-score, we performed a post hoc analysis using FLEX data, a randomized, double-blind, placebo-controlled trial among 1099 postmenopausal women originally randomized to ALN in the FIT with mean ALN use of 5 years. In the FLEX Trial, women were randomized to placebo (40%) or ALN 5 mg/day (30%) or ALN 10 mg/day (30%) for an additional 5 years. Among women without vertebral fracture at FLEX baseline ($n = 720$), continuation of ALN reduced NVF in women with FLEX baseline FN T-scores of −2.5 or less [relative risk (RR) = 0.50, 95% confidence interval (CI) 0.26−0.96] but not with T-scores of greater than −2.5 and −2 or less (RR 0.79, 95% CI 0.37−1.66) or with T-scores of greater than −2 (RR 1.41, 95% CI 0.75−2.66; p for interaction = .019). Continuing ALN for 10 years instead of stopping after 5 years reduces NVF risk in women without prevalent vertebral fracture whose FN T-scores, achieved after 5 years of ALN, are −2.5 or less but does not reduce risk of NVF in women whose T-scores are greater than −2.

▶ The original Fracture Intervention Trial showed that alendronate prevented vertebral fractures in postmenopausal women with prevalent vertebral fractures or femoral neck T scores below −1.6[1] but did not prevent nonvertebral fractures unless women had prevalent vertebral fractures or femoral neck T score below −2.5 without prevalent vertebral fractures.[2] The Fracture Intervention Trial Long Term Extension (FLEX) trial subsequently showed that subjects who stopped taking alendronate after 5 years of continuous therapy had continued reduced risk of fractures for the next 5 years, except for clinical vertebral fractures, regardless of whether they had baseline vertebral fractures or not.[3] The FLEX trial led to the general clinical recommendation that alendronate therapy should be stopped after 5 years unless fractures have already occurred or bone density is significantly decreased. The FLEX trial did not show reduction of nonvertebral fractures with 5 or 10 years of alendronate therapy when vertebral fractures were present at 5 years of therapy unless femoral neck bone mineral density was less than −2.5.

This study presents a post hoc analysis of the FLEX trial that showed that women without vertebral fractures after 5 years of alendronate therapy also had a reduction in nonvertebral fractures if femoral neck bone mineral density was less than −2.5. These women did not have reduced nonvertebral fractures if femoral neck bone mineral density was above −2.5 or below −2.0. The study concluded that continuing alendronate for 10 years instead of stopping after 5 years reduced nonvertebral fractures in women without prevalent vertebral fractures if they had femoral neck T scores below −2.5.

Because nonvertebral fractures represent a significant percentage of the total fracture burden on society, it is important that osteoporosis therapies reduce nonvertebral fractures in addition to vertebral fractures. Most approved osteoporosis therapies reduce vertebral fractures more effectively than nonvertebral fractures. Alendronate reduces nonvertebral fractures in postmenopausal women with prevalent vertebral fractures if femoral neck bone mineral density is in the osteoporotic range with T scores below −2.5 but not if bone density is better than this. Alendronate also reduces nonvertebral fractures in postmenopausal women without prevalent vertebral fractures if femoral neck bone mineral density is in the osteoporotic range, but not if it is above this threshold. These conclusions do not necessarily apply to other bisphosphonate therapies, so it is not yet clear if other bisphosphonates should be stopped after 5 years of therapy.

B. L. Clarke, MD

References

1. Black DM, Cummings SR, Karpf DB, et al. Randomised trial of effect of alendronate on risk of fracture in women with existing vertebral fractures. Fracture Intervention Trial Group. *Lancet.* 1996;348:1535-1541.
2. Cummings SR, Black DM, Thompson DE, et al. Effect of alendronate on risk of fracture in women with low bone density but without vertebral fractures: results from the Fracture Intervention Trial. *JAMA.* 1998;280:2077-2082.
3. Black DM, Schwartz AV, Ensrud KE, et al. Effects of continuing or stopping alendronate after 5 years of treatment: the Fracture Intervention Trial Long-Term Extension (FLEX): a randomized trial. *JAMA.* 2006;296:2927-2938.

Effects of Intravenous Zoledronic Acid Plus Subcutaneous Teriparatide [rhPTH(1–34)] in Postmenopausal Osteoporosis

Cosman F, Eriksen EF, Recknor C, et al (Helen Hayes Hosp, West Haverstraw, NY; Aker Univ Hosp, Oslo, Norway; United Osteoporosis Ctrs, Gainesville, GA; et al)

J Bone Miner Res 26:503-511, 2011

Clinical data suggest concomitant therapy with bisphosphonates and parathyroid hormone (PTH) may blunt the anabolic effect of PTH; rodent models suggest that infrequently administered bisphosphonates may interact differently. To evaluate the effects of combination therapy with an intravenous infusion of zoledronic acid 5 mg and daily subcutaneous recombinant human (rh) PTH(1−34) (teriparatide) 20 μg versus either agent alone on bone mineral density (BMD) and bone turnover markers, we conducted a 1-year multicenter, multinational, randomized, partial double-blinded, controlled trial. 412 postmenopausal women with osteoporosis (mean age 65 ± 9 years) were randomized to a single infusion of zoledronic acid 5 mg plus daily subcutaneous teriparatide 20 μg ($n = 137$), zoledronic acid alone ($n = 137$), or teriparatide alone ($n = 138$). The primary endpoint was percentage increase in lumbar spine BMD (assessed by dual-energy X-ray absorptiometry [DXA]) at 52 weeks versus baseline. Secondary endpoints included change in BMD at the spine at earlier time points and at the total hip, trochanter, and femoral neck at all time points. At week 52, lumbar spine BMD had increased 7.5%, 7.0%, and 4.4% in the combination, teriparatide, and zoledronic acid groups, respectively ($p < .001$ for combination and teriparatide versus zoledronic acid). In the combination group, spine BMD increased more rapidly than with either agent alone ($p < .001$ versus both teriparatide and zoledronic acid at 13 and 26 weeks). Combination therapy increased total-hip BMD more than teriparatide alone at all times (all $p < .01$) and more than zoledronic acid at 13 weeks ($p < .05$), with final 52-week increments of 2.3%, 1.1%, and 2.2% in the combination, teriparatide, and zoledronic acid groups, respectively. With combination therapy, bone formation (assessed by serum N-terminal propeptide of type I collagen [PINP]) increased from 0 to 4 weeks, declined minimally from 4 to 8 weeks, and then rose throughout the trial, with levels above baseline from 6 to 12 months. Bone resorption (assessed by serum β-C-telopeptide of type I collagen [β-CTX]) was markedly reduced with combination therapy from 0 to 8 weeks (a reduction of similar magnitude to that seen with zoledronic acid alone), followed by a gradual increase after week 8, with levels remaining above baseline for the latter half of the year. Levels for both markers were significantly lower with combination therapy versus teriparatide alone ($p < .002$). Limitations of the study included its short duration, lack of endpoints beyond DXA-based BMD (e.g., quantitative computed tomography and finite-element modeling for bone strength), lack of teriparatide placebo, and insufficient power for fracture outcomes. We conclude that while teriparatide increases spine BMD more than zoledronic acid and zoledronic acid increases hip BMD more than teriparatide, combination therapy provides the largest, most rapid increments when both spine and hip sites are considered.

▶ It has been proposed that the use of combination antiresorptive and anabolic therapies for osteoporosis treatment might stimulate a greater increase in bone density than therapy with either type of therapy alone. Theoretically, simultaneous stimulation of new bone formation and suppression of bone resorption should lead to a marked increase in bone formation and consequent increase in bone mineral density. However, previous studies have reported that simultaneous combination therapy with a potent antiresorptive agent, such as alendronate, and an anabolic agent, such as teriparatide or parathyroid hormone (PTH) 1-84, blunted the anabolic effect of teriparatide.[1-3]

This study evaluated the effect of a single infusion of zoledronic acid, 5 mg, over 15 minutes plus teriparatide, 20 μg, by subcutaneous injection once daily over 1 year versus zoledronic acid alone or teriparatide alone in 412 treatment-naive postmenopausal osteoporotic women. The results showed that the combination therapy led to a more rapid and greater increase in bone mineral density than either therapy alone at the lumbar spine and total hip. Markers of bone formation increased with combination therapy throughout the study, whereas markers of bone resorption decreased rapidly with combination therapy and then increased to above baseline in the latter half of the trial. The authors concluded that while teriparatide increased lumbar spine BMD more than zoledronic acid and zoledronic acid increased total hip BMD more than teriparatide, combination therapy provided the largest and most rapid increases in both.

These findings suggest that combination therapy with teriparatide and zoledronic acid in treatment-naive postmenopausal osteoporotic women improves bone mineral density more rapidly and to a greater degree than either therapy alone. Previous studies of combination therapy with teriparatide or PTH 1-84 and antiresorptive agents have given variable results depending on the antiresorptive agent used,[4-6] whether patients were treatment naive or on previous therapy when combination therapy was started.[2,7] And for patients on previous antiresorptive therapies, whether the antiresorptive therapy was continued or stopped when teriparatide or PTH 1-84 were started.[3] One previous study[2] found that treatment-naive patients randomized to alendronate alone, PTH 1-84 alone, or combination therapy had no evidence of additive benefit from combination therapy at the spine, but that combination therapy increased dual-energy x-ray absorptiometry bone density at the hip to a greater degree than teriparatide. Evaluation of trabecular bone's volumetric bone density by quantitative CT and bone turnover markers in this study suggested that combination therapy with alendronate might reduce the anabolic effect of PTH 1-84. These studies indicate that the response to combination therapies with teriparatide or PTH 1-84 and antiresorptive therapies for osteoporosis depends on the specific clinical situation.

B. L. Clarke, MD

References

1. Keaveny TM, Donley DW, Hoffmann PF, Mitlak BH, Glass EV, San Martin JA. Effects of teriparatide and alendronate on vertebral strength as assessed by finite element modeling of QCT scans in women with osteoporosis. *J Bone Miner Res.* 2007;22:149-157.
2. Black DM, Greenspan SL, Ensrud KE, et al. PaTH Study investigators. The effects of parathyroid hormone and alendronate alone or in combination in postmenopausal osteoporosis. *N Engl J Med.* 2003;349:1207-1215.
3. Cosman F, Wermers RA, Recknor C, et al. Effects of teriparatide in postmenopausal women with osteoporosis on prior alendronate or raloxifene: differences between stopping and continuing the antiresorptive agent. *J Clin Endocrinol Metab.* 2009;94:3772-3780.
4. Lindsay R, Nieves J, Formica C, et al. Randomised controlled study of effect of parathyroid hormone on vertebral-bone mass and fracture incidence among postmenopausal women on oestrogen with osteoporosis. *Lancet.* 1997;350:550-555.
5. Cosman F, Nieves J, Woelfert L, et al. Parathyroid hormone added to established hormone therapy: effects on vertebral fracture and maintenance of bone mass after parathyroid hormone withdrawal. *J Bone Miner Res.* 2001;16:925-931.
6. Ettinger B, San Martin J, Crans G, Pavo I. Differential effects of teriparatide on BMD after treatment with raloxifene or alendronate. *J Bone Miner Res.* 2004; 19:745-751.
7. Finkelstein JS, Hayes A, Hunzelman JL, Wyland JJ, Lee H, Neer RM. The effects of parathyroid hormone, alendronate, or both in men with osteoporosis. *N Engl J Med.* 2003;349:1216-1226.

Efficacy and Safety of a Once-Yearly i.v. Infusion of Zoledronic Acid 5 mg Versus a Once-Weekly 70-mg Oral Alendronate in the Treatment of Male Osteoporosis: A Randomized, Multicenter, Double-Blind, Active-Controlled Study

Orwoll ES, Miller PD, Adachi JD, et al (Oregon Health Sciences Univ, Portland; Colorado Ctr for Bone Res, Lakewood; McMaster Univ, Hamilton, Ontario, Canada; et al)
J Bone Miner Res 25:2239-2250, 2010

Zoledronic acid (ZOL) has shown beneficial effects on bone turnover and bone mineral density (BMD) in postmenopausal osteoporosis. This study compared the efficacy and safety of a once-yearly i.v. infusion of ZOL with weekly oral alendronate (ALN) in men with osteoporosis. In this multicenter, double-blind, active-controlled, parallel-group study, participants

($n = 302$) were randomized to receive either once-yearly ZOL 5 mg i.v. or weekly oral ALN 70 mg for 24 months. Changes in BMD and bone marker levels were assessed. ZOL increased BMD at the lumbar spine, total hip, femoral neck, and trochanter and was not inferior to ALN at 24 months [least squares mean estimates of the percentage increases in lumbar spine BMD of 6.1% and 6.2%; difference approximately 0.13; 95% confidence interval (CI) 1.12−0.85 in the ZOL and ALN groups, respectively]. At month 12, the median change from baseline of markers for bone resorption [serum β-C-terminal telopeptide of type I collagen (β-CTx) and urine N-terminal telopeptide of type I collagen (NTx)] and formation [serum N-terminal propeptide of type I collagen (P1NP) and serum bone-specific alkaline phosphatase (BSAP)] were comparable between ZOL and ALN groups. Most men preferred i.v. ZOL over oral ALN. The incidence of adverse events and serious adverse events was similar in the treatment groups. It is concluded that a once-yearly i.v. infusion of ZOL 5 mg increased bone density and decreased bone turnover markers similarly to once-weekly oral ALN 70 mg in men with low bone density.

▶ Very few head-to-head comparison trials have been performed in postmenopausal women with osteoporosis. The available studies have been done in different populations with different study supplements, making it very difficult to draw comparison between the different drugs. Such studies have not previously been done in men, and none of these studies have been powered to show fracture reduction. Epidemiological studies have shown that 25% to 33% of men will sustain osteoporotic fractures during their lifetime[1] and that morbidity and mortality associated with osteoporotic fractures are greater in men than women.[2,3]

This multicenter randomized study assessed the efficacy and safety of once-yearly intravenous zoledronic acid compared with weekly oral alendronate over 24 months in 302 men with osteoporosis. Intravenous zoledronic acid increased bone mineral density by 6.1% at the lumbar spine, 2.5% at the total hip, 3.2% at the femoral neck, and 3.3% at the greater trochanter, whereas oral alendronate increased bone density by 6.2% at the lumbar spine, 3.0% at the total hip, 3.0% at the femoral neck, and 3.7% at the greater trochanter. The changes in bone density caused by zoledronic acid were noninferior to alendronate. Markers of bone turnover at 12 months were no different between the 2 groups. The incidence of adverse events and serious adverse events was similar with zoledronic acid or alendronate. The study concluded that intravenous zoledronic acid and oral alendronate over 2 years increased bone density and reduced markers of bone turnover similarly in men with osteoporosis.

This is the first head-to-head comparison of 2 bisphosphonates in men with osteoporosis. The study suggests that intravenous zoledronic acid and alendronate are comparable in the way they increase bone mineral density and reduce markers of bone turnover. This study was not powered to show fracture reduction, so no conclusions can be drawn regarding relative effectiveness of these agents in reducing fractures in men. Hopefully, future studies will address the issue of fracture reduction in men.

B. L. Clarke, MD

References

1. Khosla S. Update in male osteoporosis. *J Clin Endocrinol Metab.* 2010;95:3-10.
2. Khosla S, Amin S, Orwoll E. Osteoporosis in men. *Endocr Rev.* 2008;29:441-464.
3. Kamel HK. Male osteoporosis: new trends in diagnosis and therapy. *Drugs Aging.* 2005;22:741-748.

Bisphosphonates and Fractures of the Subtrochanteric or Diaphyseal Femur

Black DM, for the Fracture Intervention Trial and HORIZON Pivotal Fracture Trial Steering Committees (Univ of California at San Francisco; et al)
N Engl J Med 362:1761-1771, 2010

Background.—A number of recent case reports and series have identified a subgroup of atypical fractures of the femoral shaft associated with bisphosphonate use. A populationbased study did not support this association. Such a relationship has not been examined in randomized trials.

Methods.—We performed secondary analyses using the results of three large, randomized bisphosphonate trials: the Fracture Intervention Trial (FIT), the FIT Long-Term Extension (FLEX) trial, and the Health Outcomes and Reduced Incidence with Zoledronic Acid Once Yearly (HORIZON) Pivotal Fracture Trial (PFT). We reviewed fracture records and radiographs (when available) from all hip and femur fractures to identify those below the lesser trochanter and above the distal metaphyseal flare (subtrochanteric and diaphyseal femur fractures) and to assess atypical features. We calculated the relative hazards for subtrochanteric and diaphyseal fractures for each study.

Results.—We reviewed 284 records for hip or femur fractures among 14,195 women in these trials. A total of 12 fractures in 10 patients were classified as occurring in the subtrochanteric or diaphyseal femur, a combined rate of 2.3 per 10,000 patient-years. As compared with placebo, the relative hazard was 1.03 (95% confidence interval [CI], 0.06 to 16.46) for alendronate use in the FIT trial, 1.50 (95% CI, 0.25 to 9.00) for zoledronic acid use in the HORIZON-PFT trial, and 1.33 (95% CI, 0.12 to 14.67) for continued alendronate use in the FLEX trial. Although increases in risk were not significant, confidence intervals were wide.

Conclusions.—The occurrence of fracture of the subtrochanteric or diaphyseal femur was very rare, even among women who had been treated with bisphosphonates for as long as 10 years. There was no significant increase in risk associated with bisphosphonate use, but the study was underpowered for definitive conclusions.

▶ Recent case series and case-control studies have described atypical subtrochanteric or diaphyseal femoral shaft fractures in postmenopausal women who take long-term bisphosphonate therapy.[1-3] Most patients reported with this type of fracture have taken alendronate continuously for at least 5 years, but occasional patients have taken alendronate for less than 5 years, and some have never taken alendronate but have taken other antiresorptive drugs.[4] Some reports indicate that some patients with this type of fracture have never taken a bisphosphonate, raising the possibility that other factors are involved.[5]

This article, as well as one by Abrahamsen et al, are important contributions to the literature in this area.[6] The article by Abrahamsen et al evaluated the risk of subtrochanteric/diaphyseal fractures in long-term alendronate users in Denmark. The authors compared 39 567 alendronate users without prior hip fracture who started therapy between 1996 and 2005 with 158 268 age- and sex-matched nonusers. The hazard ratio for hip fracture in women was 1.37 (95% confidence interval [CI], 1.30-1.46), whereas that for men was 2.47 (95% CI, 2.07-2.95). Risks of subtrochanteric/diaphyseal fracture were not different in patients receiving 9 years of treatment (highest quartile) and those who had stopped therapy after the equivalent of 3 months of treatment (lowest quartile). The study concluded that alendronate-treated patients are at a higher risk of hip and subtrochanteric/diaphyseal fracture than matched control subjects, but that large cumulative doses of alendronate were not associated with a greater absolute risk of subtrochanteric/diaphyseal fractures than small cumulative doses. In the final assessment, the authors stated that these fractures could be because of osteoporosis rather than directly because of alendronate. This article by Black et al performed secondary analyses of 3 large prospective randomized trials of bisphosphonate therapy to assess the relative risk of subtrochanteric fractures in users of alendronate or zoledronic acid. In a review of 284 hip or femur fractures among 14 195 women in these trials, a total of 12 fractures in 10 patients were classified as occurring in the subtrochanteric or diaphyseal femur for a combined rate of 2.3 per 10 000 patient-years. Compared with placebo, the relative hazard ratios were 1.03 (95% CI, 0.06-16.46) for alendronate use in the Fracture Intervention Trial, 1.50 (95% CI, 0.25-9.00) for zoledronic acid use in the Health Outcomes and Reduced Incidence With Zoledronic Acid Once Yearly—Pivotal Fracture Trial, and 1.33 (95% CI, 0.12-14.67) for continued alendronate use in the Fracture Intervention Trial Long-term Extension trial. The authors concluded that the occurrence of subtrochanteric or diaphyseal femoral fractures was very rare, even among women who had been treated with bisphosphonates for as long as 10 years, and that there was no significant increase in risk associated with bisphosphonate use, although the study was underpowered for definitive conclusions.

These articles were unable to show that long-term bisphosphonate use increased the risk of subtrochanteric or diaphyseal femoral fractures. Despite large number of subjects, and long-term follow-up, an obvious increase in risk of fracture was not demonstrated. Larger longer-term studies will be required to demonstrate whether alendronate or other bisphosphonates increase the risk of this rare type of fracture.

B. L. Clarke, MD

References

1. Lenart BA, Neviaser AS, Lyman S, et al. Association of low-energy femoral fractures with prolonged bisphosphonate use: a case control study. *Osteoporos Int.* 2009;20:1353-1362.

2. Neviaser AS, Lane JM, Lenart BA, Edobor-Osula F, Lorich DG. Low-energy femoral shaft fractures associated with alendronate use. *J Orthop Trauma.* 2008; 22:346-350.

3. Park-Wyllie LY, Mamdami MM, Juurlink DM, et al. Bisphosphonate use and the risk of subtrochanteric or femoral shaft fractures in older women. *JAMA.* 2011; 305:783-789.

4. Shane E, Burr D, Ebeling PR, et al. Atypical subtrochanteric and diaphyseal femoral fractures: report of a task force of the American Society for Bone and Mineral Research. *J Bone Miner Res.* 2010;25:2267-2294.

5. Vestergaard P, Schwartz F, Rejnmark L, Mosekilde L. Risk of femoral shaft and sub-trochanteric fractures among users of bisphosphonates and raloxifene. *Osteoporos Int.* 2011;22:993-1001.

6. Abrahamsen B, Eiken P, Eastell R. Cumulative alendronate dose and the long-term absolute risk of subtrochanteric and diaphyseal femur fractures: a register-based national cohort analysis. *J Clin Endocrinol Metab.* 2010;95:5258-5265.

Cumulative Alendronate Dose and the Long-Term Absolute Risk of Subtrochanteric and Diaphyseal Femur Fractures: A Register-Based National Cohort Analysis

Abrahamsen B, Eiken P, Eastell R (Univ of Southern Denmark, Odense, Denmark; Hillerød Hosp, Denmark; Univ of Sheffield, UK)
J Clin Endocrinol Metab 95:5258-5265, 2010

Context.—Bisphosphonates are the mainstay of anti-osteoporotic treatment and are commonly used for a longer duration than in the placebo-controlled trials. A link to development of atypical subtrochanteric or diaphyseal fragility fractures of the femur has been proposed, and these fractures are currently the subject of a U.S. Food and Drug Administration review.

Objective.—Our objective was to examine the risk of subtrochanteric/ diaphyseal femur fractures in long term users of alendronate.

Design.—We conducted an age- and gender-matched cohort study using national healthcare data.

Patients.—Patients were alendronate users, without previous hip fracture, who began treatment between January 1, 1996, and December 31, 2005 (n = 39,567) and untreated controls, (n = 158,268).

Main Outcome Measures.—Subtrochanteric or diaphyseal femur fractures were evaluated.

Results.—Subtrochanteric and diaphyseal fractures occurred at a rate of 13 per 10,000 patient-years in untreated women and 31 per 10,000 patient-years in women receiving alendronate [adjusted hazard ratio (HR) = 1.88; 95% confidence interval (CI) = 1.62−2.17]. Rates for men were six and 31 per 10,000 patient-years, respectively (HR = 3.98; 95% CI = 2.62−6.05). The HR for hip fracture was 1.37 (95% CI = 1.30−1.46) in women and 2.47 (95% CI = 2.07−2.95) in men. Risks of subtrochanteric/diaphyseal fracture were similar in patients who had received 9 yr of treatment (highest quartile) and patients who had stopped therapy after the equivalent of 3 months of treatment (lowest quartile).

Conclusions.—Alendronate-treated patients are at higher risk of hip and subtrochanteric/diaphyseal fracture than matched control subjects. However, large cumulative doses of alendronate were not associated with a greater absolute risk of subtrochanteric/diaphyseal fractures than small cumulative doses, suggesting that these fractures could be due to osteoporosis rather than to alendronate.

▶ Recent case series and case-control studies have described atypical subtrochanteric or diaphyseal femoral shaft fractures in postmenopausal women who take long-term bisphosphonate therapy.[1-3] Most patients reported with this type of fracture have taken alendronate continuously for at least 5 years, but occasional patients have taken alendronate for less than 5 years, and some have never taken alendronate but have taken other antiresorptive drugs.[4] Some reports indicate that some patients with this type of fracture have never taken a bisphosphonate, raising the possibility that other factors are involved.[5]

This article, as well as one by Black et al, are important contributions to the literature in this area.[6] Abrahamsen et al evaluated the risk of subtrochanteric/ diaphyseal fractures in long-term alendronate users in Denmark. The authors compared 39 567 alendronate users without prior hip fracture who started therapy between 1996 and 2005 with 158 268 age- and sex-matched nonusers. The hazard ratio for hip fracture in women was 1.37 (95% confidence interval [CI], 1.30-1.46), whereas that for men was 2.47 (95% CI, 2.07-2.95). Risks of subtrochanteric/diaphyseal fracture were not different in patients receiving 9 years of treatment (highest quartile) and those who had stopped therapy after the equivalent of 3 months of treatment (lowest quartile). The study concluded that alendronate-treated patients are at a higher risk of hip and subtrochanteric/ diaphyseal fracture than matched control subjects, but that large cumulative doses of alendronate were not associated with a greater absolute risk of subtrochanteric/diaphyseal fractures than small cumulative doses. In the final assessment, the authors stated that these fractures could be because of osteoporosis rather than directly because of alendronate. The article by Black et al performed secondary analyses of 3 large prospective randomized trials of bisphosphonate therapy to assess the relative risk of subtrochanteric fractures in users of alendronate or zoledronic acid. In a review of 284 hip or femur fractures among 14 195 women in these trials, a total of 12 fractures in 10 patients were classified as occurring in the subtrochanteric or diaphyseal femur for a combined rate of 2.3 per 10 000 patient-years. Compared with placebo, the relative hazard ratios were 1.03 (95% CI, 0.06-16.46) for alendronate use in the Fracture Intervention Trial, 1.50 (95% CI, 0.25-9.00) for zoledronic acid use in the Health Outcomes and Reduced Incidence With Zoledronic Acid Once Yearly—Pivotal Fracture Trial, and 1.33 (95% CI, 0.12-14.67) for continued alendronate use in the Fracture Intervention Trial Long-term Extension trial. The authors concluded that the occurrence of subtrochanteric or diaphyseal femoral fractures was very rare, even among women who had been treated with bisphosphonates for as long as 10 years, and that there was no significant increase in risk associated with bisphosphonate use, although the study was underpowered for definitive conclusions.

These articles were unable to show that long-term bisphosphonate use increased the risk of subtrochanteric or diaphyseal femoral fractures. Despite large number of subjects, and long-term follow-up, an obvious increase in risk of fracture was not demonstrated. Larger longer-term studies will be required to demonstrate whether alendronate or other bisphosphonates increase the risk of this rare type of fracture.

B. L. Clarke, MD

References

1. Lenart BA, Neviaser AS, Lyman S, et al. Association of low-energy femoral fractures with prolonged bisphosphonate use: a case control study. *Osteoporos Int.* 2009;20:1353-1362.
2. Neviaser AS, Lane JM, Lenart BA, Edobor-Osula F, Lorich DG. Low-energy femoral shaft fractures associated with alendronate use. *J Orthop Trauma.* 2008;22:346-350.
3. Park-Wyllie LY, Mamdani MM, Juurlink DN, et al. Bisphosphonate use and the risk of subtrochanteric or femoral shaft fractures in older women. *JAMA.* 2011; 305:783-789.
4. Shane E, Burr D, Ebeling PR, et al. Atypical subtrochanteric and diaphyseal femoral fractures: report of a task force of the American Society for Bone and Mineral Research. *J Bone Miner Res.* 2010;25:2267-2294.
5. Vestergaard P, Schwartz F, Rejnmark L, Mosekilde L. Risk of femoral shaft and subtrochanteric fractures among users of bisphosphonates and raloxifene. *Osteoporos Int.* 2011;22:993-1001.
6. Black DM, et al. Bisphosphonates and fractures of the subtrochanteric or diaphyseal femur. *N Engl J Med.* 2010;362:1761-1771.

Epidemiology and Pathophysiology of Osteoporosis

Sclerostin is a locally acting regulator of late-osteoblast/pre-osteocyte differentiation and regulates mineralization through a MEPE-ASARM dependent mechanism

Atkins GJ, Rowe PS, Lim HP, et al (Univ of Adelaide, South Australia, Australia; Univ of Kansas Med Ctr, Rainbow Boulevard, Wahl Hall East)
J Bone Miner Res 2011 [Epub ahead of print]

The identity of the cell type responsive to sclerostin, a negative regulator of bone mass, is unknown. Since sclerostin is expressed *in vivo* by mineral-embedded osteocytes, we tested the hypothesis that sclerostin would regulate the behaviour of cells actively involved in mineralization in adult bone, the pre-osteocyte. Differentiating cultures of human primary osteoblasts exposed to recombinant human sclerostin (rhSCL) for 35 days displayed dose- and time-dependent inhibition of *in vitro* mineralization, with late cultures being most responsive in terms of mineralization and gene expression. Treatment of advanced (day 35) cultures with rhSCL markedly increased the expression of the pre-osteocyte marker *E11* and decreased the expression of mature markers, *DMP1* and *SOST*. Concomitantly, MEPE expression was increased by rhSCL at both the mRNA and protein levels, while PHEX was decreased, implying regulation through the MEPE-ASARM axis. We confirmed that mineralization by human osteoblasts is exquisitely sensitive to the tri-phosphorylated ASARM-PO4 peptide. Immunostaining revealed that rhSCL increased the endogenous levels of MEPE-ASARM. Importantly, antibody-mediated neutralization of endogenous MEPE-ASARM antagonized the effect of rhSCL on mineralization, as did the PHEX synthetic peptide, SPR4. Finally, we found elevated *Sost* mRNA expression in long bones of HYP mice, suggesting that sclerostin may drive the increased MEPE-ASARM levels and mineralization defect in this genotype. Our results suggest that sclerostin acts through regulation of the PHEX/MEPE axis at the pre-osteocyte stage and serves as a master regulator of physiological bone mineralization, consistent with its localization *in vivo* and its established role in the inhibition of bone formation.

▶ Sclerostin is a protein produced by the *SOST* gene in osteocytes within the bone matrix that inhibits Wnt signaling in osteoblasts.[1] Inactivating mutations in this gene in humans causes increased osteoblast activity, leading to excess bone formation, which leads to sclerosteosis, a disease characterized by high bone mass phenotype.[2] Deletion of the *SOST* gene in mice leads to a similar high bone mass phenotype.[3] Neutralizing antibodies to sclerostin leads to increased bone formation, increased bone mineral density, and improved bone strength in ovariectomized rats[4] and aged intact male rats.[5] Histomorphometric studies of sclerostin antibody-treated animals have shown that increased bone formation occurs on quiescent bone surfaces, rather than sequentially after bone resorption, in the process known as modeling.[6]

The identity of cells that respond to sclerostin has remained unknown. This study showed that sclerostin inhibited mineralization in differentiating cultures of human primary osteoblasts, with late cultures most responsive in terms of mineralization and gene expression. Treatment of late cultures markedly increased expression of the preosteocyte marker *E11* and decreased expression of the mature osteocyte markers *DMP1* and *SOST*. At the same time, matrix extracellular phosphoglycoprotein (MEPE) levels increased and phosphate-regulating gene with homologies to endopeptidases on the X-chromosome (PHEX) levels decreased, implying that sclerostin regulates the MEPE—acidic serine-aspartate rich MEPE-associated motif (ASARM) axis. The study showed that mineralization by human osteoblasts is inhibited by increased expression of the triphosphorylated ASARM peptide, and immunostaining showed that sclerostin increased endogenous expression of MEPE-ASARM. The antibody to endogenous MEPE-ASARM inhibited this effect of sclerostin on mineralization, as did the PHEX synthetic peptide surface plasmon resonance 4. The long bones of hypophosphatemic mice were shown to have increased *SOST* messenger RNA expression, indicating that sclerostin may increase MEPE-ASARM levels and inhibit mineralization in these mice. These findings indicate that sclerostin regulates the PHEX/MEPE axis at the preosteocyte stage and serves as a major regulator of physiological bone mineralization.

This article clarifies that sclerostin, in addition to inhibiting canonical Wnt signaling and decreasing osteoblast new bone formation by reducing bone morphogenetic protein signaling, acts as a master regulator of bone mineraliza-tion. The cells most sensitive to sclerostin exposure appear to be late osteoblasts and preosteocytes, which are not able to progress to the stage at which they participate in mineralization of newly formed bone matrix. Sclerostin also appears to stimulate the expression of inhibitory MEPE-ASARM levels, which leads to direct inhibition of mineralization of newly formed bone. In summary, sclerostin appears to play several roles in inhibition of new bone formation.

B. L. Clarke, MD

References

1. ten Dijke P, Krause C, de Gorter DJ, Löwik CW, van Bezooijen RL. Osteocyte-derived sclerostin inhibits bone formation: its role in bone morphogenetic protein and Wnt signaling. *J Bone Joint Surg Am.* 2008;90:31-35.
2. Baron R, Rawadi G, Roman-Roman S. Wnt signaling: a key regulator of bone mass. *Curr Top Dev Biol.* 2006;76:103-127.
3. Li X, Ominsky MS, Niu QT, et al. Targeted deletion of the sclerostin gene in mice results in increased bone formation and bone strength. *J Bone Miner Res.* 2008;23: 860-869.
4. Li X, Ominsky MS, Warmington KS, et al. Sclerostin antibody treatment increases bone formation, bone mass, and bone strength in a rat model of postmenopausal osteoporosis. *J Bone Miner Res.* 2009;24:578-588.
5. Li X, Warmington KS, Niu QT, et al. Inhibition of sclerostin by monoclonal anti-body increases bone formation, bone mass, and bone strength in aged male rats. *J Bone Miner Res.* In press.
6. Padhi D, Jang G, Stouch B, Fang L, Posvar E. Single-dose, placebo-controlled, randomized study of AMG 785, a sclerostin monoclonal antibody. *J Bone Miner Res.* In press.

Effects of Parathyroid Hormone Treatment on Circulating Sclerostin Levels in Postmenopausal Women
Drake MT, Srinivasan B, Mödder UI, et al (Mayo Clinic, Rochester, MN; et al)
J Clin Endocrinol Metab 95:5056-5062, 2010

Context.—Intermittent PTH treatment stimulates bone formation, but the mechanism(s) of this effect remain unclear. Sclerostin is an inhibitor of Wnt signaling, and animal studies have demonstrated that PTH suppresses sclerostin production.

Objective.—The objective of the study was to test whether intermittent PTH treatment of postmenopausal women alters circulating sclerostin levels.

Design.—Prospective study.

Setting.—The study was conducted at a clinical research unit.

Participants and Interventions.—Participants included 27 postmeno-pausal women treated with PTH (1-34) for 14 d and 28 control women.

Main Outcome Measures.—Serum sclerostin levels were measured.

Results.—Circulating sclerostin levels decreased significantly in the PTH-treated subjects, from (mean ± SEM) 551 ± 32 to 482 ± 31 pg/ml (-12.7%, $P < 0.0001$) but did not change in the control women (baseline, 559 ± 34 pg/ml; end point, 537 ± 40 pg/ml, $P = 0.207$; $P = 0.017$ for difference in changes between groups). Bone marrow plasma was obtained in a subset of the control and PTH-treated subjects ($n = 19$ each) at the end of the treatment period, and marrow plasma and peripheral serum sclerostin levels were significantly correlated ($R = 0.64$, $P < 0.0001$). Marrow plasma sclerostin levels were 24% lower in PTH-treated compared with control women, but perhaps due to the smaller sample size, this difference was not statistically significant ($P = 0.173$).

Conclusions.—Circulating sclerostin levels correlate with bone marrow plasma levels and are reduced by intermittent PTH therapy in postmenopausal women. Further studies are needed to assess the extent to which decreases in sclerostin production contribute to the anabolic skeletal response to PTH.

▶ Sclerostin is produced by mature osteoblasts and preosteocytes within mineralizing bone matrix, and osteocytes within mature bone, and inhibits Wnt signaling in osteoblasts.[1] Factors that inhibit sclerostin production might therefore be used to improve bone density and bone strength. One recent study showed an inverse correlation between circulating parathyroid hormone (PTH) and sclerostin levels in healthy postmenopausal women,[2] but this study could not prove that increased PTH levels caused the observed decreased sclerostin levels. PTH given intermittently has been shown clinically to stimulate bone formation and reduce fractures,[3] but it has been unclear whether PTH 1-34 (teriparatide), given once daily by subcutaneous injection, acts to suppress sclerostin production.

This study assessed circulating sclerostin levels in a relatively small group of postmenopausal women who were treated with teriparatide. Compared with baseline, teriparatide treatment for 14 days reduced the mean sclerostin level by 12.7%, whereas sclerostin levels did not change in the control group. Because sclerostin acts primarily within the bone microenvironment, bone marrow plasma was obtained from a subset of treated subjects and controls at the end of the treatment interval to demonstrate significant correlation between levels in the circulation and bone marrow. Teriparatide-treated subjects had bone marrow plasma levels 24% lower than controls, although this difference was not statistically different. The study concluded that intermittent PTH 1-34 reduced circulating sclerostin levels after 2 weeks of treatment and that circulating levels correlate with bone marrow plasma levels.

While this study showed that intermittent teriparatide injections reduced circulating sclerostin levels over short-term therapy, it did not demonstrate the amount by which decreased sclerostin production contributed to the anabolic skeletal response to PTH 1-34. Further studies are required to clarify this important issue. The study did not show correlations between teriparatide treatment and serum levels of other potential mediators of PTH 1-34 on bone, including serum Dickkopf-1,[4] receptor activator of nuclear factor κB ligand,[5] and osteoprotegerin,[6] suggesting that the effect on sclerostin may contribute significantly to the anabolic effect of PTH on bone.

B. L. Clarke, MD

References

1. ten Dijke P, Krause C, de Gorter DJ, Löwik CW, van Bezooijen RL. Osteocyte-derived sclerostin inhibits bone formation: its role in bone morphogenetic protein and Wnt signaling. *J Bone Joint Surg Am.* 2008;90:31-35.
2. Mirza FS, Padhi ID, Raisz LG, Lorenzo JA. Serum sclerostin levels negatively correlate with parathyroid hormone levels and free estrogen index in postmenopausal women. *J Clin Endocrinol Metab.* 2010;95:1991-1997.
3. Neer RM, Arnaud CD, Zanchetta JR, et al. Effect of parathyroid hormone (1-34) on fracture and bone mineral density in postmenopausal women with osteoporosis. *N Engl J Med.* 2001;344:1434-1441.
4. Guo J, Liu M, Yang D, et al. Suppression of Wnt signaling by Dkk1 attenuates PTH-mediated stromal cell response and new bone formation. *Cell Metab.* 2010;11:161-171.
5. Huang JC, Sakata T, Pfleger LL, et al. PTH differentially regulates expression of RANKL and OPG. *J Bone Miner Res.* 2004;19:235-244.
6. Onyia JE, Miles RR, Yang X, et al. In vivo demonstration that human parathyroid hormone 1-38 inhibits the expression of osteoprotegerin in bone with the kinetics of an immediate early gene. *J Bone Miner Res.* 2000;15:863-871.

Regulation of Circulating Sclerostin Levels by Sex Steroids in Women and in Men

Mödder UI, Clowes JA, Hoey K, et al (Mayo Clinic, Rochester, MN)
J Bone Miner Res 26:27-34, 2011

Sex steroids are important regulators of bone turnover, but the mechanisms of their effects on bone remain unclear. Sclerostin is an inhibitor of Wnt signaling, and circulating estrogen (E) levels are inversely associated with sclerostin levels in postmenopausal women. To directly test for sex steroid regulation of sclerostin levels, we examined effects of E treatment of postmenopausal women or selective withdrawal of E versus testosterone (T) in elderly men on circulating sclerostin levels. E treatment of postmenopausal women ($n = 17$) for 4 weeks led to a 27% decrease in serum sclerostin levels [versus +1% in controls ($n = 18$), $p < .001$]. Similarly, in 59 elderly men, we eliminated endogenous E and T production and studied them under conditions of physiologic T and E replacement, and then following withdrawal of T or E, we found that E, but not T, prevented increases in sclerostin levels following induction of sex steroid deficiency. In both sexes, changes in sclerostin levels correlated with changes in bone-resorption, but not boneformation, markers ($r = 0.62$, $p < .001$, and $r = 0.33$, $p = .009$, for correlations with changes in serum C-terminal telopeptide of type 1 collagen in the women and men, respectively). Our studies thus establish that in humans, circulating sclerostin levels are reduced by E but not by T. Moreover, consistent with recent data indicating important effects of Wnts on osteoclastic cells, our findings suggest that in humans, changes in sclerostin production may contribute to effects of E on bone resorption.

▶ Sclerostin is produced by mature osteoblasts and preosteocytes within mineralizing bone matrix, and osteocytes within mature bone, and inhibits

Wnt signaling in osteoblasts.[1] Mirza et al demonstrated that postmenopausal women had higher serum sclerostin levels than premenopausal women and that circulating free estradiol index was inversely correlated to circulating sclerostin levels in postmenopausal women.[2] These findings suggested that serum estradiol regulates sclerostin production by osteocytes. However, because correlation does not prove causality, further studies were needed.

This study assessed sex steroid regulation of sclerostin levels in postmenopausal women and older men. Postmenopausal women treated with estrogen for 4 weeks had significantly reduced serum sclerostin levels compared with untreated controls. Older men in whom endogenous production of testosterone and estrogen was eliminated, then physiologically replaced, and then selectively withdrawn had reduced sclerostin levels on estrogen replacement therapy, but not testosterone therapy. Changes in sclerostin levels correlated with changes in markers of bone resorption, but not markers of bone formation. The study concluded that estrogen regulated circulating sclerostin levels in postmenopausal women, and that estrogen, but not testosterone, regulated circulating sclerostin in older men.

The findings of this study imply that changes in sclerostin levels in humans may contribute to the effects of estradiol deficiency on bone resorption. Estradiol deficiency has been shown to play a major role in regulation of bone loss in both postmenopausal women and older men.[3] While this study does not directly show that estradiol regulates sclerostin production at the transcriptional level, the *SOST* promoter has 3 classical estrogen response elements that could allow this to occur.[4] It was somewhat surprising that testosterone in the absence of aromatization to estrogen had no effect on circulating sclerostin levels, although testosterone has been shown to not significantly reduce bone turnover in men.[5,6] Also somewhat surprising, changes in circulating sclerostin did not correlate with markers of bone formation, perhaps because changes in sclerostin may be responsible for only part of the effects of estrogen on maintaining bone formation, or possibly because of longer duration of time required to see changes in markers of bone formation.

B. L. Clarke, MD

References

1. ten Dijke P, Krause C, de Gorter DJ, Löwik CW, van Bezooijen RL, van Bezooijen RL. Osteocyte-derived sclerostin inhibits bone formation: its role in bone morphogenetic protein and Wnt signaling. *J Bone Joint Surg Am.* 2008;90: 31-35.
2. Mirza FS, Padhi ID, Raisz LG, Lorenzo JA. Serum sclerostin levels negatively correlate with parathyroid hormone levels and free estrogen index in postmenopausal women. *J Clin Endocrinol Metab.* 2010;95:1991-1997.
3. Riggs BL, Khosla S, Melton LJ 3rd. Sex steroids and the conservation of the adult skeleton. *Endocr Rev.* 2002;23:279-302.
4. Huang QY, Li GH, Kung AW. The -9247 T/C polymorphism in the SOST upstream regulatory region that potentially affects C/EBP alpha and FOXA1 binding is associated with osteoporosis. *Bone.* 2009;45:289-294.
5. Falahati-Nini A, Riggs BL, Atkinson EJ, O'Fallon WM, Eastell R, Khosla S. Relative contributions of testosterone and estrogen in regulating bone resorption and formation in normal elderly men. *J Clin Invest.* 2000;106:1553-1560.

6. Leder BZ, LeBlanc KM, Schoenfeld DA, Eastell R, Finkelstein JS. Differential effects of androgens and estrogens on bone turnover in normal men. *J Clin Endocrinol Metab.* 2003;88:204-210.

Relation of Age, Gender, and Bone Mass to Circulating Sclerostin Levels in Women and Men

Mödder UI, Hoey KA, Amin S, et al (Mayo Clinic, Rochester, MN)
J Bone Miner Res 26:373-379, 2011

Sclerostin is a potent inhibitor of Wnt signaling and bone formation. However, there is currently no information on the relation of circulating sclerostin levels to age, gender, or bone mass in humans. Thus we measured serum sclerostin levels in a population-based sample of 362 women [123 premenopausal, 152 postmenopausal not on estrogen treatment (ET), and 87 postmenopausal on ET] and 318 men, aged 21 to 97 years. Sclerostin levels (mean ± SEM) were significantly higher in men than women (33.3 ± 1.0 pmol/L versus 23.7 ± 0.6 pmol/L, $p < .001$). In pre- and post-menopausal women not on ET combined ($n = 275$) as well as in men, sclerostin levels were positively associated with age ($r = 0.52$ and $r = 0.64$, respectively, $p < .001$ for both). Over life, serum sclerostin levels increased by 2.4- and 4.6-fold in the women and men, respectively. Moreover, for a given total-body bone mineral content, elderly subjects (age ≥ 60 years) had higher serum sclerostin levels than younger subjects (ages 20 to 39 years). Our data thus demonstrate that (1) men have higher serum sclerostin levels than women, (2) serum sclerostin levels increase markedly with age, and (3) compared with younger subjects, elderly individuals have higher serum sclerostin levels for a given amount of bone mass. Further studies are needed to define the cause of the age-related increase in serum sclerostin levels in humans as well as the potential role of this increase in mediating the known age-related impairment in bone formation.

▶ Sclerostin is a peptide produced by mature osteoblasts and preosteocytes within mineralizing bone matrix, as well as by osteocytes within mature bone, which plays a significant role in regulation of skeletal bone mass. It appears that the majority of sclerostin is produced by osteocytes, with a lesser amount produced by mature osteoblasts and preosteocytes. The main recognized function of sclerostin produced by these different cell types is to inhibit Wnt and canonical β-catenin signaling in osteoblasts.[1] Inhibition of Wnt and canonical β-catenin signaling in osteoblasts by sclerostin results in decreased osteoprogenitor cells and increased apoptosis of mature osteoblasts, which leads to decreased new bone formation and a consequent decrease in bone density.[2,3] Work over the last 10 years has established the Wnt/β-catenin signaling pathway as a major regulator of bone mass.[4,5] However, it has not previously been clear whether circulating sclerostin levels are affected by age, sex, or bone mass.

To answer these questions, this study assessed circulating sclerostin in a population-based sample of 362 women and 318 men aged 21 to 97 years.

The results showed that sclerostin levels were higher in older adults after adjustment for renal function and that men had higher circulating levels than women. In addition, higher sclerostin levels were associated with higher bone mineral content in older adults. The study concluded that circulating sclerostin levels increase with age, sclerostin is higher in men than women, and sclerostin is higher in older adults than younger adults with the same bone density. Further studies will be required to determine the cause of the age-related increase in sclerostin and to assess the role sclerostin may play in the age-related decrease in bone formation.

These findings give important insight into the mechanisms of age-related bone loss. Given that multiple factors play a role in trabecular bone loss beginning in the third decade of life, whereas gonadal sex steroid deficiency plays a major role in cortical bone loss beginning only in the sixth decade,[6] it is possible that sclerostin plays an increasingly important role in bone loss with advancing age. This study showed that women on postmenopausal estrogen therapy had lower circulating sclerostin levels, suggesting that gonadal sex steroids influence or directly regulate circulating sclerostin levels. Additional studies are needed to further clarify the role of sclerostin in regulation of bone mass and age-related bone loss.

B. L. Clarke, MD

References

1. Ten Dijke P, Krause C, de Gorter DJ, Löwik CW, van Bezooijen RL. Osteocyte-derived sclerostin inhibits bone formation: its role in bone morphogenetic protein and Wnt signaling. *J Bone Joint Surg Am.* 2008;90:31-35.
2. van Bezooijen RL, Roelen BAJ, Visser A, et al. Sclerostin is an osteocyte-expressed negative regulator of bone formation, but not a classical BMP antagonist. *J Exp Med.* 2004;199:805-814.
3. Poole KES, van Bezooijen RL, Loveridge N, et al. Sclerostin is a delayed secreted product of osteocytes that inhibits bone formation. *FASEB J.* 2005;19:1842-1844.
4. Krishnan V, Bryant HU, Macdougald OA. Regulation of bone mass by Wnt signaling. *J Clin Invest.* 2006;116:1202-1209.
5. Baron R, Rawadi G. Targeting the Wnt/β-catenin pathway to regulate bone formation in the adult skeleton. *Endocrinology.* 2007;148:2635-2643.
6. Khosla S, Melton LJ 3rd, Riggs BL. The unitary model for estrogen deficiency and the pathogenesis of osteoporosis: is a revision needed? *J Bone Miner Res.* 2011;26: 441-451.

Association of Hip Strength Estimates by Finite Element Analysis with Fractures in Women and Men

Amin S, Kopperdhal DL, Melton LJ III, et al (Mayo Clinic, Rochester, MN; O.N. Diagnostics, Berkeley, CA; et al)
J Bone Miner Res 2011 [Epub ahead of print]

Finite element (FE) analysis of quantitative computed tomography (QCT) scans can estimate site-specific whole bone strength. However, it is uncertain whether the site-specific detail included in FE-estimated proximal femur (hip) strength can determine fracture risk at sites with different biomechanical characteristics. To address this question, we used FE analysis of proximal femur QCT scans to estimate hip strength and load-to-strength ratio during a simulated sideways fall, and measured total hip areal and volumetric bone mineral density (aBMD and vBMD) from QCT images, in an age-stratified, random sample of community adults, age ≥ 35 years. Among 314 women (mean age ± SD: 61 ± 15 years; 235 postmenopausal) and 266 men (62 ± 16 years), 139 women and 104 men had any prevalent fracture, while 55 women and 28 men had a prevalent osteoporotic fracture that had occurred ≥ age 35 years. Odds ratios by age-adjusted logistic regression analysis for prevalent overall and osteoporotic fractures each were similar for FE hip strength and load-to-strength ratio, as well as total hip aBMD and vBMD. C-statistics (estimated areas under ROC curves) were also similar (e.g., 0.84-0.85 [women] and 0.75-0.78 [men] for osteoporotic fractures). In women and men, the association with prevalent osteoporotic fractures increased below an estimated hip strength of ∼3000 N. Despite its site-specific nature, FE-estimated hip strength worked equally well at predicting prevalent overall, and osteoporotic, fractures. Furthermore, an estimated hip strength below 3000 N may represent a critical level of systemic skeletal fragility in both sexes that warrants further investigation.

▶ Prediction of future fractures because of osteoporosis is commonly done in clinical practice by assessment of clinical risk factors, dual-energy X-ray absorptiometry (DXA), bone mineral density (BMD), and/or the Fracture Risk Assessment Tool or other algorithms. However, each of these methods of predicting fracture risk has limitations. Other methods are being investigated to determine if there is a more reliable way to predict fractures. High-resolution peripheral quantitative CT (HRpQCT) scanning is being used to assess skeletal microarchitecture independent of bone density and skeletal geometry in an effort to improve quantitative assessment of fracture risk.[1-4] The information collected with HRpQCT may be analyzed by finite element analysis to predict fracture risk with greater precision than currently available methods.[5,6] However, whether this type of analysis may also be used to predict fracture risk at other skeletal sites, similar to DXA measurement, remains uncertain.

This study evaluated hip strength and load-to-strength ratio during a sideways fall using HRpQCT, as well as total hip areal and volumetric BMD, in a random sample of community-dwelling adults aged 35 years or older. The study included 314 older women and 266 older men, with 139 of the women and 104 of the men having had prevalent fractures that had occurred after the age of 35 years. The odds ratios for prevalent overall and osteoporotic fractures were similar for the finite element analysis hip strength, load-to-strength ratio, total hip areal BMD, and total hip volumetric BMD. In both women and men, the association with prevalent osteoporotic fractures increased below an estimated hip strength of 3000 N. The study concluded that even though finite element analysis of hip strength is specific for the hip, it predicts prevalent overall and osteoporotic fractures equally well and suggests that estimated hip strength of less than 3000 N may be a threshold for significant skeletal fragility.

The limitations of current tools in prediction of future fracture risk may eventually be improved by tools that are able to better assess bone quality. HRpQCT scanning is just one of several tools being developed for eventual clinical application. This technique is able to assess bone microarchitecture as well as hip cross-sectional area and areal and volumetric BMD that adds complementary information to standard DXA bone density testing. This technique, and other tools like it, represents an important advance because many patients with low trauma fractures have either normal or low bone density and do not meet World Health Organization DXA criteria for osteoporosis. The ability to better assess bone strength will eventually lead to better ability to predict fractures.

B. L. Clarke, MD

References

1. Melton LJ 3rd, Riggs BL, Keaveny TM, et al. Structural determinants of vertebral fracture risk. *J Bone Miner Res.* 2007;22:1885-1892.
2. Melton LJ 3rd, Riggs BL, van Lenthe GH, et al. Contribution of in vivo structural measurements and load/strength ratios to the determination of forearm fracture risk in postmenopausal women. *J Bone Miner Res.* 2007;22:1442-1448.
3. Imai K, Ohnishi I, Matsumoto T, Yamamoto S, Nakamura K. Assessment of vertebral fracture risk and therapeutic effects of alendronate in postmenopausal women using a quantitative computed tomography-based nonlinear finite element analysis method. *Osteoporos Int.* 2009;20:801-810.
4. Chevalier Y, Quek E, Borah B, et al. Biomechanical effects of teriparatide in women with osteoporosis treated previously with alendronate and risedronate: results from quantitative computed tomography-based finite element analysis of the vertebral body. *Bone.* 2010;46:41-48.
5. Cody DD, Gross GJ, Hou FJ, Spencer HJ, Goldstein SA, Fyhrie DP. Femoral strength is better predicted by finite element models than QCT or DXA. *J Biomech.* 1999;32:1013-1020.
6. Keyak JH, Rossi SA. Prediction of femoral fracture load using finite element models: an examination of stress- and strain-based failure theories. *J Biomech.* 2000;33:209-214.

Relation of Vertebral Deformities to Bone Density, Structure, and Strength

Melton LJ III, Riggs BL, Keaveny TM, et al (Mayo Clinic, Rochester, MN; Univ of California, Berkeley; et al)
J Bone Miner Res 25:1922-1930, 2010

Because they are not reliably discriminated by areal bone mineral density (aBMD) measurements, it is unclear whether minimal vertebral deformities represent early osteoporotic fractures. To address this, we compared 90 postmenopausal women with no deformity (controls) with 142 women with one or more semiquantitative grade 1 (mild) deformities and 51 women with any grade 2–3 (moderate/severe) deformities. aBMD was measured by dual-energy X-ray absorptiometry (DXA), lumbar spine volumetric bone mineral density (vBMD) and geometry by quantitative computed tomography (QCT), bone microstructure by high-resolution peripheral QCT at the radius (HRpQCT), and vertebral compressive strength and load-to-strength ratio by finite-element analysis (FEA) of lumbar spine QCT images. Compared with controls, women with grade 1 deformities had significantly worse values for many bone density, structure, and strength parameters, although deficits all were much worse for the women with grade 2—3 deformities. Likewise, these skeletal parameters were more strongly associated with moderate to severe than with mild deformities by age-adjusted logistic regression. Nonetheless, grade 1 vertebral deformities were significantly associated with four of the five main variable categories assessed: bone density (lumbar spine vBMD), bone geometry (vertebral apparent cortical thickness), bone strength (overall vertebral compressive strength by FEA), and load-to-strength ratio (45-degree forward bending ÷ vertebral compressive strength). Thus significantly impaired bone density, structure, and strength compared with controls indicate that many grade 1 deformities do represent early osteoporotic fractures, with corresponding implications for clinical decision making.

▶ Prediction of future fractures because of osteoporosis is commonly done in clinical practice by assessment of clinical risk factors, dual-energy X-ray absorptiometry (DXA), bone mineral density (BMD), and/or the Fracture Risk Assessment Tool or other algorithms. However, each of these methods of predicting fracture risk has limitations. Other methods are being investigated to determine if there is a more reliable way to predict fractures. High-resolution peripheral quantitative CT (HRpQCT) scanning is being used to assess skeletal microarchitecture independent of bone density and skeletal geometry in an effort to improve quantitative assessment of fracture risk.[1-4] The information collected with HRpQCT may be analyzed by finite element analysis to predict fracture risk with greater precision than currently available methods.[5,6] However, whether this type of analysis may also be used to predict fracture risk at other skeletal sites, similar to DXA measurement, remains uncertain.

This study evaluated hip strength and load-to-strength ratio during a sideways fall using HRpQCT, as well as total hip areal and volumetric BMD, in a random sample of community-dwelling adults aged 35 years or older. The study included 314 older women and 266 older men, with 139 of the women and 104 of the men having had prevalent fractures that had occurred after the age of 35 years. The odds ratios for prevalent overall and osteoporotic fractures were similar for the finite element analysis hip strength, load-to-strength ratio, total hip areal BMD, and total hip volumetric BMD. In both women and men, the association with prevalent osteoporotic fractures increased below an estimated hip strength of 3000 N. The study concluded that even though finite element analysis of hip strength is specific for the hip, it predicts prevalent overall and osteoporotic fractures equally well and suggests that estimated hip strength of less than 3000 N may be a threshold for significant skeletal fragility.

The limitations of current tools in prediction of future fracture risk may eventually be improved by tools that are able to better assess bone quality. HRpQCT scanning is just one of several tools being developed for eventual clinical application. This technique is able to assess bone microarchitecture as well as hip cross-sectional area and areal and volumetric BMD that adds complementary information to standard DXA bone density testing. This technique, and other tools like it, represents an important advance because many patients with low trauma fractures have either normal or low bone density and do not meet World Health Organization DXA criteria for osteoporosis. The ability to better assess bone strength will eventually lead to better ability to predict fractures.

B. L. Clarke, MD

References

1. Melton LJ 3rd, Riggs BL, Keaveny TM, et al. Structural determinants of vertebral fracture risk. *J Bone Miner Res.* 2007;22:1885-1892.
2. Melton LJ 3rd, Riggs BL, van Lenthe GH, et al. Contribution of in vivo structural measurements and load/strength ratios to the determination of forearm fracture risk in postmenopausal women. *J Bone Miner Res.* 2007;22:1442-1448.
3. Imai K, Ohnishi I, Matsumoto T, Yamamoto S, Nakamura K. Assessment of vertebral fracture risk and therapeutic effects of alendronate in postmenopausal women using a quantitative computed tomography-based nonlinear finite element analysis method. *Osteoporos Int.* 2009;20:801-810.
4. Chevalier Y, Quek E, Borah B, et al. Biomechanical effects of teriparatide in women with osteoporosis treated previously with alendronate and risedronate: results from quantitative computed tomography-based finite element analysis of the vertebral body. *Bone.* 2010;46:41-48.
5. Cody DD, Gross GJ, Hou FJ, Spencer HJ, Goldstein SA, Fyhrie DP. Femoral strength is better predicted by finite element models than QCT or DXA. *J Biomech.* 1999;32:1013-1020.
6. Keyak JH, Rossi SA. Prediction of femoral fracture load using finite element models: an examination of stress- and strain-based failure theories. *J Biomech.* 2000;33:209-214.

Age-Dependence of Femoral Strength in White Women and Men

Keaveny TM, Kopperdahl DL, Melton LJ III, et al (Univ of California—Berkeley; O. N. Diagnostics, Berkeley, CA; Mayo Clinic, Rochester, MN)
J Bone Miner Res 25:994-1001, 2010

Although age-related variations in areal bone mineral density (aBMD) and the prevalence of osteoporosis have been well characterized, there is a paucity of data on femoral strength in the population. Addressing this issue, we used finite-element analysis of quantitative computed tomographic scans to assess femoral strength in an age-stratified cohort of 362 women and 317 men, aged 21 to 89 years, randomly sampled from the population of Rochester, MN, and compared femoral strength with femoral neck aBMD. Percent reductions over adulthood were much greater for femoral strength (55% in women, 39% in men) than for femoral neck aBMD (26% in women, 21% in men), an effect that was accentuated in women. Notable declines in strength started in the mid-40s for women and one decade later for men. At advanced age, most of the strength deficit for women compared with men was a result of this decade-earlier onset of strength loss for women, this factor being more important than sex-related differences in peak bone strength and annual rates of bone loss. For both sexes, the prevalence of "low femoral strength" (<3000 N) was much higher than the prevalence of osteoporosis (femoral neck aBMD *T*-score of −2.5 or less). We conclude that age-related declines in femoral strength are much greater than suggested by age-related declines in femoral neck aBMD. Further, far more of the elderly may be at high risk of hip fracture because of low femoral strength than previously assumed based on the traditional classification of osteoporosis.

▶ Clinical risk factors, decreased bone mineral density (BMD), and FRAX and other models are routinely used to clinically assess the risk of osteoporotic fracture.[1] Low femoral neck BMD measured by dual-energy x-ray absorptiometry (DXA) has been shown to strongly predict the risk of hip fracture.[2] Because most osteoporotic fractures occur in individuals not meeting the criteria for osteoporosis,[3-6] it is possible that risk factors independent of BMD may account for this. It is also possible that the limitations of DXA BMD measurement may be responsible for the inability of this technique to detect all patients at increased risk of fracture. DXA BMD is based on a 2-dimensional assessment of areal bone density and is not able to evaluate specific bone compartments or bone microstructure.

This study evaluated femoral strength by DXA BMD compared with finite element analysis of quantitative CT scan images in a randomly selected population-based sample of 362 women and 317 men aged 21 to 89 years. The results of this cross-sectional study showed that femoral strength decreased faster and by a greater amount than femoral neck DXA BMD with aging. Women were more severely affected than men by femoral strength loss, with marked declines beginning in the mid-40s in women and in the mid-50s in men. Most differences in hip strength between older women and men were because of the earlier age of onset of femoral neck strength loss in women rather than differences in peak bone strength or annual rates of bone loss after menopause. For both women and men, the prevalence of low femoral strength, defined as finite element analysis-estimated strength of less than 3000 N, was much greater than the prevalence of osteoporosis by DXA BMD, defined as BMD T score less than −2.5. The study concluded that decreases in femoral strength because of older age are much greater than that suggested by decreases in femoral neck BMD.

The findings of this study suggest that the risk of hip fracture in older individuals may be much greater than that estimated by femoral neck BMD measurement. Femoral neck BMD strongly correlates with femoral strength but appears to significantly underestimate the full effects of aging on femoral strength. Sex-related differences in peak bone mass and the annual rate of femoral strength appear to have less biomechanical influence on hip strength than the earlier onset of strength loss in women. These findings indicate that the major reason for which women's bones are much weaker than men's bone in old age is the decade-earlier age of onset of bone strength loss in women. If further studies confirm these findings, treatment may need to be started earlier than recommended by current guidelines to prevent significant strength loss and increased fracture risk in aging women.

B. L. Clarke, MD

References

1. Kanis JA, McCloskey EV, Johansson H, Oden A, Melton LJ 3rd, Khaltaev N. A reference standard for the description of osteoporosis. *Bone.* 2008;42:467-475.
2. Cummings SR, Bates D, Black DM. Clinical uses of bone densitometry: scientific review. *JAMA.* 2002;288:1889-1897.
3. Cranney A, Jamal SA, Tsang JF, Josse RG, Leslie WD. Low bone mineral density and fracture burden in postmenopausal women. *CMAJ.* 2007;177:575-580.
4. Pasco JA, Seeman E, Henry MJ, Merriman EN, Nicholson GC, Kotowicz MA. The population burden of fractures originates in women with osteopenia, not osteoporosis. *Osteoporos Int.* 2006;17:1404-1409.
5. Stone KL, Seeley DG, Lui LY, et al. BMD at multiple sites and risk of fracture of multiple types: long term results from the Study of Osteoporotic Fractures. *J Bone Miner Res.* 2003;18:1947-1954.
6. Wainwright SA, Marshall LM, Ensrud KE, et al. Hip fracture in women without osteoporosis. *J Clin Endocrinol Metab.* 2005;90:2787-2793.

Effect of calcium supplements on risk of myocardial infarction and cardiovascular events: meta-analysis

Bolland MJ, Avenell A, Baron JA, et al (Univ of Auckland, New Zealand; Univ of Aberdeen, UK; Dartmouth Med School, NH)

BMJ 341:c3691, 2010

Objective.—To investigate whether calcium supplements increase the risk of cardiovascular events.

Design.—Patient level and trial level meta-analyses.

Data Sources.—Medline, Embase, and Cochrane Central Register of Controlled Trials (1966-March 2010), reference lists of meta-analyses of calcium supplements, and two clinical trial registries. Initial searches were carried out in November 2007, with electronic database searches repeated in March 2010.

Study Selection.—Eligible studies were randomised, placebo controlled trials of calcium supplements (≥ 500 mg/day), with 100 or more participants of mean age more than 40 years and study duration more than one year. The lead authors of eligible trials supplied data. Cardiovascular outcomes were obtained from self reports, hospital admissions, and death certificates.

Results.—15 trials were eligible for inclusion, five with patient level data (8151 participants, median follow-up 3.6 years, interquartile range 2.7-4.3 years) and 11 with trial level data (11 921 participants, mean duration 4.0 years). In the five studies contributing patient level data, 143 people allocated to calcium had a myocardial infarction compared with 111 allocated to placebo (hazard ratio 1.31, 95% confidence interval 1.02 to 1.67, P=0.035). Non-significant increases occurred in the incidence of stroke (1.20, 0.96 to 1.50, P=0.11), the composite end point of myocardial infarction, stroke, or sudden death (1.18, 1.00 to 1.39, P=0.057), and death (1.09, 0.96 to 1.23, P=0.18). The meta-analysis of trial level data showed similar results: 296 people had a myocardial infarction (166 allocated to calcium, 130 to placebo), with an increased incidence of myocardial infarction in those allocated to calcium (pooled relative risk 1.27, 95% confidence interval 1.01 to 1.59, P=0.038).

Conclusions.—Calcium supplements (without coadministered vitamin D) are associated with an increased risk of myocardial infarction. As calcium supplements are widely used these modest increases in risk of cardiovascular disease might translate into a large burden of disease in the population. A reassessment of the role of calcium supplements in the management of osteoporosis is warranted.

▶ Calcium supplementation to maintain adequate calcium intake is recommended for the prevention and treatment of osteoporosis by most clinical guidelines.[1,2] Clinical studies have shown that calcium supplementation alone marginally reduces the risk of fracture.[3,4] Many adults older than 50 years are taking calcium supplements in the belief that these will help reduce their risk of future fracture. Previous observational studies suggested that increased calcium intake may prevent vascular disease,[5-7] consistent with interventional studies that showed calcium supplementation reduced some vascular risk factors.[8-10] Other studies have shown that patients with renal failure, both before and after starting dialysis, have increased vascular calcification and mortality when supplemented with calcium,[11-13] and a recent 5-year randomized trial of calcium supplements in healthy older women showed that calcium supplements increased risk of myocardial infarction (MI) and cardiovascular events.[14,15] The conflicting evidence regarding benefits and risks of calcium supplementation from these studies led to the meta-analysis in this study.

This study evaluated 15 trials of calcium supplementation in around 12 000 adults older than 40 years. Five of the trials included patient-level data, and 11 included trial-level data. The 5 trials with patient-level data contained 143 adults on calcium supplementation with MI and 111 adults on placebo with MI, with a significant difference between the 2 groups. Nonsignificant differences in stroke, composite end point of MI, stroke, or sudden death, and death were seen between the 2 groups. The 11 trials with trial-level data contained 166 adults on calcium supplementation with MI and 130 adults on placebo with MI, again with a significant difference between the 2 groups. The study concluded that calcium supplements without vitamin D are associated with about a 30% increased risk of MI and recommended that the role of calcium supplementation in the management of osteoporosis be reassessed.

The findings of this study are important because they suggest that calcium supplementation in patients with normal renal function may accelerate cardiovascular disease. Closer evaluation of the meta-analysis, however, shows that none of the single studies included showed a significant difference in risk of MI between calcium and placebo. Increased risk of MI was seen mainly with calcium supplementation above the median intake. None of the studies included vitamin D supplementation, which may be protective against cardiovascular disease. None of the trials evaluated cardiovascular events as primary end points, and data on cardiovascular events were not gathered in a standardized manner. Only 2 of the studies had data adjudicated by blinded trial investigators. No cardiovascular outcome data were reported for 7 of the included trials, accounting for about 15% of the total trial participants. Despite these weaknesses, the study conclusions raise concerns regarding calcium supplementation in older adults with osteoporosis. Further studies are needed to evaluate the vascular effects of calcium supplementation without vitamin D.

B. L. Clarke, MD

References

1. American Association of Clinical Endocrinologists medical guidelines for clinical practice for the prevention and treatment of postmenopausal osteoporosis. *Endocrine Pract.* 2003;9:545-564.
2. National Osteoporosis Foundation. *Physician's guide to prevention and treatment of osteoporosis.* National Osteoporosis Foundation; 2008.
3. Bischoff-Ferrari HA, Dawson-Hughes B, Baron JA, et al. Calcium intake and hip fracture risk in men and women: a meta-analysis of prospective cohort studies and randomized controlled trials. *Am J Clin Nutr.* 2007;86:1780-1790.
4. Tang BMP, Eslick GD, Nowson C, Smith C, Bensoussan A. Use of calcium or calcium in combination with vitamin D supplementation to prevent fractures and bone loss in people aged 50 years and older: a meta-analysis. *Lancet.* 2007;370:657-666.
5. Knox EG. Ischaemic-heart-disease mortality and dietary intake of calcium. *Lancet.* 1973;1:1465-1467.
6. Bostick RM, Kushi LH, Wu Y, et al. Relation of calcium, vitamin D, and dairy food intake to ischemic heart disease mortality among postmenopausal women. *Am J Epidemiol.* 1999;149:151-161.
7. Iso H, Stampfer MJ, Manson JE, et al. Prospective study of calcium, potassium, and magnesium intake and risk of stroke in women. *Stroke.* 1999;30:1772-1779.
8. Griffith LE, Guyatt GH, Cook RJ, Bucher HC, Cook DJ. The influence of dietary and nondietary calcium supplementation on blood pressure: an updated meta-analysis of randomized controlled trials. *Am J Hypertens.* 1999;12:84-92.
9. Reid IR, Mason B, Home A, et al. Effects of calcium supplementation on serum lipid concentrations in normal older women: a randomized controlled trial. *Am J Med.* 2002;112:343-347.
10. Reid IR, Home A, Mason B, Ames R, Bava U, Gamble GD. Effects of calcium supplementation on body weight and blood pressure in normal older women: a randomized controlled trial. *J Clin Endocrinol Metab.* 2005;90:3824-3829.
11. Goodman WG, Goldin J, Kuizon BD, et al. Coronary-artery calcification in young adults with end-stage renal disease who are undergoing dialysis. *N Engl J Med.* 2000;342:1478-1483.
12. Block GA, Raggi P, Bellasi A, Kooienga L, Spiegel DM. Mortality effect of coronary calcification and phosphate binder choice in incident hemodialysis patients. *Kidney Int.* 2007;71:438-441.
13. Russo D, Miranda I, Ruocco C, et al. The progression of coronary artery calcification in predialysis patients on calcium carbonate or sevelamer. *Kidney Int.* 2007;72:1255-1261.
14. Reid IR, Mason B, Horne A, et al. Randomized controlled trial of calcium in healthy older women. *Am J Med.* 2006;119:777-785.
15. Bolland MJ, Barber PA, Doughty RN, et al. Vascular events in healthy older women receiving calcium supplementation: randomised controlled trial. *BMJ.* 2008;336:262-266.

Endocrine Regulation of Male Fertility by the Skeleton

Oury F, Sumara G, Sumara O, et al (Columbia Univ, NY; et al)
Cell 144:796-809, 2011

Interactions between bone and the reproductive system have until now been thought to be limited to the regulation of bone remodeling by the gonads. We now show that, in males, bone acts as a regulator of fertility. Using coculture assays, we demonstrate that osteoblasts are able to induce testosterone production by the testes, though they fail to influence estrogen production by the ovaries. Analyses of cells-specific loss- and gain-of-function models reveal that the osteoblast-derived hormone osteocalcin performs this endocrine function. By binding to a G protein-coupled receptor expressed in the Leydig cells of the testes, osteocalcin regulates in a CREB-dependent manner the expression of enzymes that is required for testosterone synthesis, promoting germ cell survival. This study expands the physiological repertoire of osteocalcin and provides the first evidence that the skeleton is an endocrine regulator of reproduction.

▶ This article is important because it establishes for the first time that the skeleton is capable of regulating the reproductive system. The historical perspective has been that the reproductive system regulated the skeleton via gonadal sex steroid secretion,[1,2] particularly during puberty, or via withdrawal of gonadal sex steroid secretion at menopause.[3,4] Recent studies have shown that uncarboxylated osteocalcin produced by osteoblasts acts as a hormone that favors islet β-cell proliferation, insulin secretion and sensitivity, and energy expenditure.[5] The gene *Esp* in osteoblasts inhibits endocrine functions of osteocalcin by favoring its carboxylation through an indirect mechanism.[6,7] Although it was hypothesized 10 years ago that bone mass, energy metabolism, and reproduction might be regulated in a coordinated manner,[8] it has not previously been demonstrated that the skeleton is capable of providing a hormonal stimulus to the reproductive system.

This study shows that osteoblasts in the bone are capable of regulating testosterone production by Leydig cells in the testis via osteocalcin secretion but are not able to regulate estrogen production by the ovary in the same manner. The reason for the gender specificity of this regulatory mechanism is not yet clear. Osteocalcin, long regarded as a marker of bone turnover, is synthesized and secreted into surrounding matrix by osteoblasts during bone formation. Some of this osteocalcin reaches the circulation, where it can be measured as an indirect measure of total skeletal bone formation. Because osteocalcin is incorporated into the matrix, some of the circulating osteocalcin also comes from bone resorption. Osteocalcin is therefore generally regarded as a marker of bone turnover, reflecting both bone formation and bone resorption, because of the dual source of circulating osteocalcin. This study demonstrates that circulating osteocalcin is capable of binding to G protein-coupled receptors in Leydig cells and stimulating expression of enzymes necessary for testosterone production in a cyclic adenosine monophosphate response element-binding dependent manner, thereby resulting in germ cell survival. This study provides the first evidence that the skeleton is an endocrine regulator of reproduction.

These findings indicate that osteocalcin secreted by osteoblasts supports male fertility by stimulating testosterone production by Leydig cells in addition to its endocrine function as a regulator of energy homeostasis. This study expands the biological importance of osteocalcin, begins to explain its molecular mechanism of action, and provides the first evidence that the skeleton is able to regulate fertility, at least in mice.

B. L. Clarke, MD

References

1. Khosla S, Melton LJ III, Atkinson EJ, O'Fallon WM. Relationship of serum sex steroid levels to longitudinal changes in bone density in young versus elderly men. *J Clin Endocrinol Metab.* 2001;86:3555-3561.
2. Riggs BL, O'Fallon WM, Muhs J, O'Connor MK, Kumar R, Melton LJ 3rd. Long-term effects of calcium supplementation on serum parathyroid hormone level, bone turnover, and bone loss in elderly women. *J Bone Miner Res.* 1998;13: 168-174.
3. Manolagas SC, Kousteni S, Jilka RL. Sex steroids and bone. *Recent Prog Horm Res.* 2002;57:386-409.
4. Nakamura T, Imai Y, Matsumoto T, et al. Estrogen prevents bone loss via estrogen receptor alpha and induction of Fas ligand in osteoclasts. *Cell.* 2007;130:811-823.
5. Lee NK, Sowa H, Hinoi E, et al. Endocrine regulation of energy metabolism by the skeleton. *Cell.* 2007;130:456-469.
6. Ferron M, Wei J, Yoshizawa T, et al. Insulin signaling in osteoblasts integrates bone remodeling and energy metabolism. *Cell.* 2010;142:296-308.
7. Fulzele K, Riddle RC, DiGirolamo DJ, et al. Insulin receptor signaling in osteoblasts regulates postnatal bone acquisition and body composition. *Cell.* 2010; 142:309-319.
8. Ducy P, Amling M, Takeda S, et al. Leptin inhibits bone formation through a hypothalamic relay: a central control of bone mass. *Cell.* 2010;100:197-207.

Insulin Signaling in Osteoblasts Integrates Bone Remodeling and Energy Metabolism

Ferron M, Wei J, Yoshizawa T, et al (Columbia Univ, NY; et al)
Cell 142:296-308, 2010

The broad expression of the insulin receptor suggests that the spectrum of insulin function has not been fully described. A cell type expressing this receptor is the osteoblast, a bone-specific cell favoring glucose metabolism through a hormone, osteocalcin, that becomes active once uncarboxylated. We show here that insulin signaling in osteoblasts is necessary for whole-body glucose homeostasis because it increases osteocalcin activity. To achieve this function insulin signaling in osteoblasts takes advantage of the regulation of osteoclastic bone resorption exerted by osteoblasts. Indeed, since bone resorption occurs at a pH acidic enough to decarboxylate proteins, osteoclasts determine the carboxylation status and function of osteocalcin. Accordingly, increasing or decreasing insulin signaling in osteoblasts promotes or hampers glucose metabolism in a bone resorption-dependent manner in mice and humans. Hence, in a feed-forward loop, insulin signals in osteoblasts activate a hormone, osteocalcin, that promotes glucose metabolism.

▶ This article is important because it establishes for the first time that the skeleton is capable of regulating the reproductive system. The historical perspective has been that the reproductive system regulated the skeleton via gonadal sex steroid secretion,[1,2] particularly during puberty, or via withdrawal of gonadal sex steroid secretion at menopause.[3,4] Recent studies have shown that uncarboxylated osteocalcin produced by osteoblasts acts as a hormone that favors islet β-cell proliferation, insulin secretion and sensitivity, and energy expenditure.[5] The gene *Esp* in osteoblasts inhibits endocrine functions of osteocalcin by favoring its carboxylation through an indirect mechanism.[6,7] Although it was hypothesized 10 years ago that bone mass, energy metabolism, and reproduction might be regulated in a coordinated manner,[8] it has not previously been demonstrated that the skeleton is capable of providing a hormonal stimulus to the reproductive system.

This study shows that osteoblasts in the bone are capable of regulating testosterone production by Leydig cells in the testis via osteocalcin secretion but are not able to regulate estrogen production by the ovary in the same manner. The reason for the gender specificity of this regulatory mechanism is not yet clear. Osteocalcin, long regarded as a marker of bone turnover, is synthesized and secreted into surrounding matrix by osteoblasts during bone formation. Some of this osteocalcin reaches the circulation, where it can be measured as an indirect measure of total skeletal bone formation. Because osteocalcin is incorporated into the matrix, some of the circulating osteocalcin also comes from bone resorption. Osteocalcin is therefore generally regarded as a marker of bone turnover, reflecting both bone formation and bone resorption, because of the dual source of circulating osteocalcin. This study demonstrates that circulating osteocalcin is capable of binding to G protein-coupled receptors in Leydig cells and stimulating expression of enzymes necessary for testosterone production in a cyclic adenosine monophosphate response element-binding dependent manner, thereby resulting in germ cell survival. This study provides the first evidence that the skeleton is an endocrine regulator of reproduction.

These findings indicate that osteocalcin secreted by osteoblasts supports male fertility by stimulating testosterone production by Leydig cells in addition to its endocrine function as a regulator of energy homeostasis. This study expands the biological importance of osteocalcin, begins to explain its molecular mechanism of action, and provides the first evidence that the skeleton is able to regulate fertility, at least in mice.

B. L. Clarke, MD

References

1. Khosla S, Melton LJ III, Atkinson EJ, O'Fallon WM. Relationship of serum sex steroid levels to longitudinal changes in bone density in young versus elderly men. *J Clin Endocrinol Metab.* 2001;86:3555-3561.

2. Riggs BL, O'Fallon WM, Muhs J, O'Connor MK, Kumar R, Melton LJ 3rd. Long-term effects of calcium supplementation on serum parathyroid hormone level, bone turnover, and bone loss in elderly women. *J Bone Miner Res.* 1998;13: 168-174.
3. Manolagas SC, Kousteni S, Jilka RL. Sex steroids and bone. *Recent Prog Horm Res.* 2002;57:386-409.
4. Nakamura T, Imai Y, Matsumoto T, et al. Estrogen prevents bone loss via estrogen receptor alpha and induction of Fas ligand. *Cell.* 2007;130:811-823.
5. Lee NK, Sowa H, Hinoi E, et al. Endocrine regulation of energy metabolism by the skeleton. *Cell.* 2007;130:456-469.
6. Ferron M, Wei J, Yoshizawa T, et al. Insulin signaling in osteoblasts integrates bone remodeling and energy metabolism. *Cell.* 2010;142:296-308.
7. Fulzele K, Riddle RC, DiGirolamo DJ, et al. Insulin receptor signaling in osteoblasts regulates postnatal bone acquisition and body composition. *Cell.* 2010; 142:309-319.
8. Ducy P, Amling M, Takeda S, et al. Leptin inhibits bone formation through a hypothalamic relay: a central control of bone mass. *Cell.* 2000;100:197-207.

Metabolic Bone Disease

The Superiority of Minimally Invasive Parathyroidectomy Based on 1650 Consecutive Patients With Primary Hyperparathyroidism

Udelsman R, Lin Z, Donovan P (Yale Univ School of Medicine, New Haven, CT; Yale-New Haven Hosp, CT)
Ann Surg 253:585-591, 2011

Objective.—To compare the results of minimally invasive parathyroidectomy (MIP) and conventional parathyroid surgery.

Background.—Primary hyperparathyroidism is a common endocrine disorder often treated by surgical intervention. Outpatient MIP, employing image-directed focused exploration under cervical block anesthesia, has replaced traditional surgical approaches for many patients with primary hyperparathyroidism. This retrospective review of a prospective database compared MIP with conventional parathyroid surgery.

Methods.—One thousand six hundred fifty consecutive patients underwent surgery for primary hyperparathyroidism by a single surgeon between 1990 and 2009 at 2 tertiary care academic hospitals. Conventional bilateral cervical exploration under general anesthesia was performed in 613 patients and MIP was performed in 1037 cases. Cure rates, complication rates, pathologic findings, length of hospital stay, and total hospital costs were compared.

Results.—Minimally invasive parathyroidectomy is associated with improvements in the cure rate (99.4%) and the complication rate (1.45%) compared to conventional exploration with a cure rate of 97.1% and a complication rate of 3.10%. In addition, the hospital length of stay and total hospital charges were also improved compared to conventional surgery.

Conclusions.—Minimally invasive parathyroidectomy is a superior technique and should be adopted for the majority of patients with sporadic primary hyperparathyroidism.

▶ This article suggests that minimally invasive parathyroidectomy is a better approach than full neck exploration in patients with sporadic primary hyperparathyroidism. The first successful parathyroidectomy was done in Vienna by Dr Felix Mandl in 1925 in a patient with severe osteitis fibrosa cystica using full neck exploration.[1] Three normal glands were identified without preoperative imaging, and a fourth enlarged parathyroid gland was removed, with dramatic cure of the patient's hypercalcemia. The patient unfortunately developed recurrent disease 6 years later and eventually died of the disease.[2] Since that time, full neck exploration was the standard recommendation for most patients with primary hyperparathyroidism because all 4 parathyroid glands could be visualized at surgery, it was less likely that an abnormal gland or glands would be missed, and all visually abnormal glands could be removed. With advances in sestamibi and ultrasound preoperative parathyroid gland imaging,[3] however, minimally invasive approaches became popular because single adenomas could be localized reliably before surgery. In addition, advances in local and regional anesthesia allowed limited exploration on an outpatient basis,[4] and rapid and accurate intraoperative parathyroid hormone assays allowed surgeons to determine the adequacy of parathyroid gland removal during surgery.[5] The minimally invasive approach to parathyroidectomy became very popular with patients and surgeons over the last 20 years.

This study reports the large experience of a single academic surgeon with full neck exploration and minimally invasive parathyroidectomy over almost 20 years. About two-thirds of cases were done using a minimally invasive approach and the rest with traditional full neck exploration surgery. Both the cure and complication rates were better using the minimally invasive approach, and length of hospital stay and total hospital charges were reduced compared with full neck surgery. The study concluded that minimally invasive surgery is a better approach for sporadic primary hyperparathyroidism than full neck exploration and advocates using the minimally invasive approach in most patients with this disorder.

The minimally invasive approach offers obvious advantages compared with full neck exploration. However, occasional abnormal glands can be missed without full neck exploration. Preoperative imaging with sestamibi—single-photon emission computed tomography scanning, sestamibi-^{123}I subtraction scanning, neck ultrasound, 4D-CT scanning, or other techniques is very helpful in localizing abnormal parathyroid glands, but these imaging studies occasionally do not localize an abnormal gland or detect multiglandular disease, and false-positive scans occasionally complicate surgical decisions. This study was not a randomized clinical trial, but the experience reported nevertheless mirrors the current experience at other major surgical centers in the United States.

B. L. Clarke, MD

References

1. Mandl F. Therapeutischer versuch bein falls von osteitis fibrosa generalisata mittles. Extirpation eines epithelkorperchen tumors. *Wien Klin Wochenschr Zentral.* 1926; 143:245-284.
2. Carney JA. The glandulae parathyroideae of Ivar Sandström. Contributions from two continents. *Am J Surg Pathol.* 1996;20:1123-1144.
3. Irvin GL III, Sfakianakis G, Yeung L, et al. Ambulatory parathyroidectomy for primary hyperparathyroidism. *Arch Surg.* 1996;31:1074-1078.
4. Chen H, Sokoll LJ, Udelsman R. Outpatient minimally invasive parathyroidectomy: a combination of sestamibi-SPECT localization, cervical block anesthesia, and intraoperative parathyroid hormone assay. *Surgery.* 1999;126:1016-1022.
5. Udelsman R. Six hundred fifty-six consecutive explorations for primary hyperparathyroidism. *Ann Surg.* 2002;235:665-670.

Cinacalcet HCl Reduces Hypercalcemia in Primary Hyperparathyroidism across a Wide Spectrum of Disease Severity

Peacock M, Bilezikian JP, Bolognese MA, et al (Indiana Univ School of Medicine, Indianapolis; Columbia Univ, NY; Bethesda Health Res, MD; et al)
J Clin Endocrinol Metab 96:E9-E18, 2011

Context.—Primary hyperparathyroidism (PHPT) is characterized by elevated serum calcium (Ca) and increased PTH concentrations.

Objective.—The objective of the investigation was to establish the efficacy of cinacalcet in reducing serum Ca in patients with PHPT across a wide spectrum of disease severity.

Design and Setting.—The study was a pooled analysis of data from three multicenter clinical trials of cinacalcet in PHPT.

Patients.—Patients were grouped into three disease categories for analysis based on the following: 1) history of failed parathyroidectomy (n = 29); 2) meeting one or more criteria for parathyroid-ectomy but without prior surgery (n = 37); and 3) mild asymptomatic PHPT without meeting criteria for either above category (n = 15).

Intervention.—The intervention in this study was treatment with cinacalcet for up to 4.5 yr.

Outcomes.—Measurements in the study included serum Ca, PTH, phosphate, and bone-specific alkaline phosphatase, and areal bone mineral density (aBMD). Vital signs, safety biochemical and hematological indices, and adverse events were monitored throughout the study period.

Results.—The extent of cinacalcet-induced serum Ca reduction, proportion of patients achieving normal serum Ca (≤ 10.3 mg/dl), reduction in serum PTH, and increase in serum phosphate were similar across all three categories. Except for decreased aBMD at the total femur indicated for parathyroidectomy group at 1 yr, no significant changes in aBMD occurred. The efficacy of cinacalcet was maintained for up to 4.5 yr of follow-up. AEs were mild and similar across the three categories.

Conclusions.—Cinacalcet is equally effective in the medical management of PHPT patients across a broad spectrum of disease severity, and overall cinacalcet is well tolerated.

▶ This study demonstrates for the first time that cinacalcet is effective in normalizing serum calcium and reducing plasma parathyroid hormone (PTH) in a heterogeneous sample of patients with primary hyperparathyroidism, including patients with and without indication for parathyroidectomy and patients with a history of failed parathyroidectomy. No previous studies have addressed the comparative efficacy of cinacalcet across a range of disease severity. Cinacalcet is an allosteric calcimimetic compound targeted to the calcium-sensing receptor (CaSR), which increases the sensitivity of the CaSR on parathyroid cells to extracellular calcium concentration, thereby decreasing PTH secretion.[1-3] Cinacalcet has been shown to be effective in treatment of intractable primary hyperparathyroidism,[4] long-term treatment of primary hyperparathyroidism,[5] inoperable parathyroid carcinoma,[6] and secondary hyperparathyroidism because of renal failure.[7] Cinacalcet is approved in the United States for treatment of secondary hyperparathyroidism in patients with chronic kidney disease on dialysis or hypercalcemia because of parathyroid carcinoma. Cinacalcet is approved in Europe for treatment of intractable hypercalcemia in patients with primary hyperparathyroidism for whom parathyroidectomy is indicated, but surgery is clinically inappropriate or is contraindicated.

This article summarizes the results of 3 separate small multicenter clinical trials of cinacalcet in patients with primary hyperparathyroidism. The study cohort included patients who had failed parathyroidectomy and had more severe primary hyperparathyroidism, patients who had indications for parathyroidectomy but not had surgery and had less severe hyperparathyroidism, and patients with mild asymptomatic primary hyperparathyroidism. The findings indicate that cinacalcet was similarly efficacious in all 3 groups in terms of normalizing serum calcium, increasing serum phosphorus, and reducing plasma PTH. Plasma PTH decreased more slowly than serum calcium but never normalized. Bone mineral density (BMD) by dual-energy x-ray absorptiometry did not improve but remained stable, except for decreased hip BMD in the parathyroidectomy group at 1 year. Cinacalcet appeared to be effective over long-term follow-up of up to 4 years.

These findings suggest that cinacalcet may be useful in the medical management of patients with a wide range of severity of primary hyperparathyroidism. Because surgery is highly effective at curing primary hyperparathyroidism, cinacalcet will likely be useful mainly in patients with more severe forms of the disease who are not able to be cured by surgery. This includes patients who have failed surgery, patients not eligible for surgery because of comorbidities, or patients who refuse surgery for personal reasons. This study showed that cinacalcet has a favorable safety and efficacy profile for long-term use.

B. L. Clarke, MD

References

1. Brown EM, Gamba G, Riccardi D, et al. Cloning and characterization of an extracellular Ca(2+)-sensing receptor from bovine parathyroid. *Nature*. 1993;366: 575-580.
2. Nemeth EF, Fox J. Calcimimetic Compounds: a Direct Approach to Controlling Plasma Levels of Parathyroid Hormone in Hyperparathyroidism. *Trends Endocrinol Metab*. 1999;10:66-71.
3. Chang W, Tu C, Chen TH, et al. Expression and signal transduction of calcium-sensing receptors in cartilage and bone. *Endocrinology*. 1999;140:5883-5893.
4. Marcocci C, Chanson P, Shoback D, et al. Cinacalcet reduces serum calcium concentration in patients with intractable primary hyperparathyroidism. *J Clin Endocrinol Metab*. 2009;94:2766-2772.
5. Peacock M, Bolognese MA, Borofsky M, et al. Cinacalcet treatment of primary hyperparathyroidism: biochemical and bone densitometric outcomes in a five-year study. *J Clin Endocrinol Metab*. 2009;94:4860-4867.
6. Silverberg SJ, Rubin MR, Faiman C, et al. Cinacalcet hydrochloride reduces the serum calcium concentrations in inoperable parathyroid carcinoma. *J Clin Endocrinol Metab*. 2007;92:3803-3808.
7. Harris RZ, Padhi D, Marbury TC, Noveck RJ, Salfi M, Sullivan JT. Pharmacokinetics, pharmacodynamics, and safety of cinacalcet hydrochloride in hemodialysis patients at doses of up to 200 mg once daily. *Am J Kid Dis*. 2004;44:1070-1076.

Therapy of hypoparathyroidism with intact parathyroid hormone
Rubin MR, Sliney J Jr, McMahon DJ, et al (Columbia Univ, NY)
Osteoporos Int 21:1927-1934, 2010

Summary.—Hypoparathyroidism, a disorder characterized by low parathyroid hormone (PTH), is generally treated with oral calcium and vitamin D supplementation. We investigated the effects of PTH(1−84) treatment in 30 hypoparathyroid subjects for 24 months. PTH(1−84) treatment in hypoparathyroidism significantly reduced supplemental calcium and 1,25-dihydroxyvitamin D requirements without generally altering serum and urinary calcium levels.

Introduction.—Hypoparathyroidism, a disorder characterized by low PTH, is associated with hypocalcemia, hypercalciuria, and increased bone mineral density (BMD). Conventional therapy with calcium and 1,25-dihydroxyvitamin D can maintain the serum calcium concentration, but doses are high, and control is variable. We investigated the effects of human PTH(1−84) treatment in hypoparathyroidism.

Methods.—Thirty subjects with hypoparathyroidism were treated in an open-label study of PTH(1−84) 100 µg every other day by subcutaneous injection for 24 months, with monitoring of calcium and vitamin D supplementation requirements, serum and 24 h urinary calcium excretion, and BMD by dual energy X-ray absorptiometry.

Results.—Requirements for supplemental calcium decreased significantly ($3,030 \pm 2,325$ to $1,661 \pm 1,267$ mg/day (mean ± SD); $p<0.05$), as did requirements for supplemental 1,25- dihydroxyvitamin D (0.68 ± 0.5 to 0.40 ± 0.5 µg/day; $p<0.05$). Serum calcium levels and 24 h urinary calcium excretion were mostly unchanged at 24 months. BMD increased at the lumbar spine by $2.9 \pm 4\%$ from baseline ($p<0.05$), while femoral neck BMD remained unchanged and distal one third radial BMD decreased by $2.4 \pm 4\%$ ($p<0.05$).

Conclusion.—PTH(1—84) treatment in hypoparathyroidism significantly reduces supplemental calcium and 1,25-dihydroxyvitamin D requirements without generally altering serum and urinary calcium levels.

▶ This is the first study to demonstrate that full-length parathyroid hormone (PTH)(1-84) is effective in treating hypoparathyroidism. Hypoparathyroidism is the last recognized hormone deficiency disorder that does not have the missing hormone available and approved for therapeutic use.[1] Most patients have postsurgical hypoparathyroidism, but acquired hypoparathyroidism may be because of autoimmune destruction of the parathyroid glands, genetic disorders, other comorbid conditions such as hemochromatosis, or other unrecognized causes.[2,3] Patients with hypoparathyroidism have low serum calcium, relatively increased serum phosphorus, decreased or absent serum PTH, decreased serum 1,25-dihydroxyvitamin D, and relatively increased urinary calcium excretion.[4]

Current management of hypoparathyroidism includes relatively high doses of oral calcium and 1,25-dihydroxyvitamin D supplementation. However, this approach may lead to worsening hypercalciuria that causes some patients to develop nephrocalcinosis, calcium-containing kidney stones, or renal dysfunction.[5-7] Patients treated with calcium and 1,25-dihydroxyvitamin D often have better control of their serum calcium, but they may develop rapid swings in their serum calcium, with rapid development of significant hypercalcemia or life-threatening hypocalcemia. Treatment with PTH(1-84) may keep serum calcium closer to goal range most of the time, minimize swings in serum calcium, and/or reduce hypercalciuria.

This study evaluated treatment of 30 patients with hypoparathyroidism with PTH(1-84) 100 µg by subcutaneous injection every other day for 24 months. Treatment with native PTH(1-84) resulted in supplemental calcium requirements decreasing from 3.0 to 1.6 g each day and supplemental 1,25-dihydroxyvitamin D decreasing from 0.68 to 0.40 µg each day. Serum and 24-hour urinary calcium levels were unchanged at 24 months. Subjects had a mild increase in bone mineral density at the lumbar spine, no change at the femoral neck, and a mild decrease at the one-third distal radius. The study concluded that PTH(1-84) treatment of hypoparathyroidism reduced calcium and 1,25-dihydroxyvitamin D supplement requirements while stabilizing serum and urinary calcium levels.

This study showed that treatment of patients with hypoparathyroidism from multiple causes significantly reduced calcium and 1,25-dihydroxyvitamin D supplemental requirements while keeping serum and urinary calcium stable. These findings have prompted a 6-month phase III randomized placebo-controlled clinical trial with PTH(1-84) in a larger number of adult patients with hypoparathyroidism. This study is currently nearing completion and will be used to seek Food and Drug Administration approval of PTH(1-84) to treat hypoparathyroidism.

B. L. Clarke, MD

References

1. Marx SJ. Hyperparathyroid and hypoparathyroid disorders. *N Engl J Med.* 2000; 343:1863-1875.
2. Shoback D. Clinical practice. Hypoparathyroidism. *N Engl J Med.* 2008;359: 391-403.
3. Thakker R. Genetics of endocrine and metabolic disorders: parathyroid. *Rev Endocr Metab Disord.* 2004;5:37-51.
4. Rubin MR, Levine MA. Hypoparathyroidism and pseudohypoparathyroidism. In: *Primer on the Metabolic Bone Diseases and Disorders of Mineral Metabolism.* 7th ed. Washington, DC: American Society for Bone and Mineral Research; 354-361.
5. Christiansen C, Rødbro P, Christensen MS, Hartnack B, Transbøl I. Deterioration of renal function during treatment of chronic renal failure with 1,25-dihydroxy-cholecalciferol. *Lancet.* 1978;2:700-703.
6. Kurokawa K. Calcium-regulating hormones and the kidney. *Kidney Int.* 1987;32: 760-771.
7. Litvak J, Moldawer MP, Forbes AP, Henneman PH. Hypocalcemic hypercalciuria during vitamin D and dihydrotachysterol therapy of hypoparathyroidism. *J Clin Endocrinol Metab.* 1958;18:246-252.

Mineral and Vitamin D Metabolism

Circulating 25-Hydroxyvitamin D Levels and Frailty Status in Older Women

Ensrud KE, for the Study of Osteoporotic Fractures Research Group (Univ of Minnesota, Minneapolis; et al)

J Clin Endocrinol Metab 95:5266-5273, 2010

Context.—Vitamin D deficiency and frailty are common with aging, but the association between these conditions is uncertain.

Objective.—To determine the association between 25-hydroxyvitamin D (25(OH)D) levels and prevalent and incident frailty status among older women.

Design.—Cross-sectional and longitudinal analyses of a prospective cohort study.

Setting.—Four U.S. centers.

Participants.—6307 women aged ≥69 years.

Main Outcome Measures.—Frailty status classified as robust, intermediate stage, or frail at baseline; and robust, intermediate stage, frail, or dead (all-cause mortality) at follow-up an average of 4.5 years later.

Results.—At baseline, there was a U-shaped association between 25(OH) D level and odds of frailty with the lowest risk among women with levels 20.0–29.9 ng/ml (referent group). Compared with this group, the odds of frailty were higher among those with levels <15.0 ng/ml [multivariable odds ratio (MOR) 1.47, 95% confidence interval (CI), 1.19–1.82], those with levels 15.0–19.9 ng/ml (MOR 1.24, 95% CI 0.99–1.54), and those with levels ≥30 ng/ml (MOR 1.32, 95% CI 1.06–1.63). Among 4551 non-frail women at baseline, the odds of frailty/death (vs. robust/intermediate) at follow-up appeared higher among those with levels 15.0–19.9 ng/ml (MOR 1.21, 95% CI 0.99–1.49), but the CI overlapped 1.0. The odds of death (vs. robust/intermediate/frail at follow-up) was higher among those with levels <15.0 ng/ml (MOR 1.40, 95% CI 1.04—1.88) and those with levels 15.0—19.9 ng/ml (MOR 1.30, 95% CI 0.97—1.75), although the latter association did not quite reach significance.

Conclusion.—Lower (<20 ng/ml) and higher (≥30 ng/ml) levels of 25(OH)D among older women were moderately associated with a higher odds of frailty at baseline. Among nonfrail women at baseline, lower levels (<20 ng/ml) were modestly associated with an increased risk of incident frailty or death at follow-up.

▶ This study demonstrates that frailty in older women is moderately associated with serum 25-hydroxyvitamin D levels < 20 or ≥30 ng/mL at baseline, and that among nonfrail older women at baseline serum 25-hydroxyvitamin D level < 20 ng/mL was associated with increased risk of incident frailty or death over 4.5 years of follow-up. Lower serum 25-hydroxyvitamin D level and frailty are both increasingly common with aging. Several studies have shown that frailty predicts adverse health outcomes, including incident disability, falls, fractures, and mortality.[1-4] Weakness and slowness are potential outcomes of vitamin D deficiency, and are components of frailty. Low serum 25-hydroxyvitamin D levels have been variably associated with poorer physical performance and increased risk of falls, fractures, and death in postmenopausal women and older men.

This study evaluated the correlation between serum 25-hydroxyvitamin D level and baseline and incident frailty in older women. Surprisingly, baseline frailty was lowest with serum 25-hydroxyvitamin D levels in the range of 20 to 29 ng/mL and greater with serum 25-hydroxyvitamin D levels < 20 or ≥30 ng/mL. No obvious reason was found for greater frailty with serum 25-hydroxyvitamin D levels of 30 ng/mL or higher, where it might have been expected that frailty would be lower. In the two-thirds of women who were nonfrail at baseline, the odds of frailty or death 4.5 years later were nonsignificantly higher with baseline serum 25-hydroxyvitamin D levels of 15.0 to 19.9 ng/mL, and the odds of death were higher in those with baseline serum 25-hydroxyvitamin D levels < 15 ng/mL and nonsignificantly higher in those with levels in the 15.0 to 19.9 ng/mL range. The study concluded that baseline serum 25-hydroxyvitamin D levels < 20 or ≥30 ng/mL predicted frailty in older women and that nonfrail women at baseline have a greater risk of frailty or death if serum 25-hydroxyvitamin D levels are < 20 ng/mL.

This study is important because only 1 previous study has reported an association between the continuum of frailty and serum 25-hydroxyvitamin D levels, and this study showed an association in men but not in women.[5] Three other studies have assessed the association between baseline serum 25-hydroxyvitamin D level and incident frailty and have reported conflicting results.[6,7] This study indicates that the association between serum 25-hydroxyvitamin D level and frailty is nonlinear and that serum 25-hydroxyvitamin D levels ≥30 ng/mL are associated with increased frailty. Further studies will be required to clarify why what are widely regarded as optimal vitamin D levels are associated with increased frailty.

B. L. Clarke, MD

References

1. Fried LP, Tangen CM, Walston J, et al. Frailty in older adults: evidence for a phenotype. *J Gerontol A Biol Sci Med Sci.* 2001;56:M146-M156.
2. Ensrud KE, Ewing SK, Taylor BC, et al. Frailty and risk of falls, fracture, and mortality in older women: the study of osteoporotic fractures. *J Gerontol A Biol Sci Med Sci.* 2007;62:744-751.
3. Cawthon PM, Marshall LM, Michael Y, et al. Frailty in older men: prevalence, progression, and relationship with mortality. *J Am Geriatr Soc.* 2007;55:1216-1223.
4. Rockwood K, Howlett SE, MacNight C, et al. Prevalence, attributes, and outcomes of fitness and frailty in community-dwelling older adults: report from the Canadian study of health and aging. *J Gerontol A Biol Sci Med Sci.* 2004;59:1310-1317.
5. Shardell M, Hicks GE, Miller RR, et al. Association of low vitamin D levels with the frailty syndrome in men and women. *J Gerontol A Biol Sci Med Sci.* 2009;64:69-75.
6. Puts MT, Visser M, Twisk JW, Deeg DJ, Lips P. Endocrine and inflammatory markers as predictors of frailty. *Clin Endocrinol (Oxf).* 2005;63:403-411.
7. Semba RD, Bartali B, Zhou J, Blaum C, Ko CW, Fried LP. Low serum micronutrient concentrations predict frailty among older women living in the community. *J Gerontol A Biol Sci Med Sci.* 2006;61:594-599.

Novel Osteoporosis Therapies

Effect of Nitroglycerin Ointment on Bone Density and Strength in Postmenopausal Women: A Randomized Trial

Jamal SA, Hamilton CJ, Eastell R, et al (Univ of Toronto, Ontario, Canada; Univ of Sheffield, England; et al)

JAMA 305:800-807, 2011

Context.—Nitroglycerin stimulates bone formation and inhibits bone resorption, is in-expensive, and is widely available. Its effects on bone density, bone structure, and bone strength are unknown.

Objectives.—To determine if nitroglycerin increases lumbar spine bone mineral density (BMD) and to evaluate changes in hip BMD, bone geometry, and density at the radius and tibia, and markers of bone turnover.

Design, Setting, and Participants.—A single-center, double-blind, placebo-controlled randomized trial conducted in Toronto, Ontario, Canada, for 24 months starting in November 2005 and completed in March 2010, of 243 postmenopausal women with lumbar spine T scores of between 0 and −2.0 who completed a 1-week run-in period taking nitroglycerin ointment.

Intervention.—Nitroglycerin ointment (15 mg/d) or placebo applied at bedtime for 24 months.

Main Outcome Measures.—Areal BMD at the lumbar spine, femoral neck, and total hip. Secondary outcomes included indices of bone geometry and strength at the distal radius and tibia, and biomarkers of bone formation (bone-specific alkaline phosphatase) and bone resorption (urine N-telopeptide).

Results.—At 2 years, women randomized to the nitroglycerin group had significant increases in areal BMD at the lumbar spine (from 1.05 to 1.14 g/cm^2 vs placebo from 1.06 to 1.08 g/cm^2; percentage change, 6.7%; 95% confidence interval [CI], 5.2%-8.2%; *P* < .001); total hip (from 0.92 to 0.97 g/cm ^{2} vs placebo from 0.93 to 0.92 g/cm^2; 6.2%; 95% CI, 5.6%-7.0%; *P* < .001); and femoral neck (from 0.88 to 0.93 g/cm^2 vs placebo from 0.87 to 0.86 g/cm^2; 7.0%; 95% CI, 5.5%-8.5%; *P* < .001). At 2 years, nitroglycerin also increased volumetric trabecular BMD (11.9% and 8.5%), cortical thickness (13.9% and 24.6%), periosteal circumference (7.4% and 2.9%), polar section modulus (10.7% and 9.8%), and polar moment of inertia (7.3% and 14.5%) at the radius and tibia, respectively (all *P* < .001); and increased bone-specific alkaline phosphatase by 34.8% and decreased urine N-telopeptide by 54.0% (*P* < .001). Incidence of serious adverse events did not differ between nitroglycerin (5 [4.2%]) and placebo (5 [4.3%]) groups. Among those women who continued treatment for 24 months, headaches were reported by 40 (35%) in nitroglycerin and 6 (5.4%) in placebo groups during the first month, decreasing substantially after 12 months.

Conclusion.—Among postmenopausal women, nitroglycerin ointment modestly increased BMD and decreased bone resorption.

Trial Registration.—isrctn.org Identifier: ISRCTN94484747.

▶ New agents from nontraditional categories may help to prevent or treat osteoporosis. Nitroglycerin is widely used as a coronary vasodilator to treat angina. Nitric oxide is a related compound that inhibits osteoclast activity and serves as a signaling molecule in osteoblasts and osteocytes.[1,2] Nitric oxide donors, such as nitroglycerin, isosorbide mononitrate, and isosorbide dinitrate, have been shown to prevent bone loss because of estrogen deficiency and glucocorticoids in rats and mice.[3,4] Continuous administration of nitrates causes tachyphylaxis to their effects, but intermittent treatment of angina in older women with nitrates is associated with higher hip bone mineral density (BMD) compared with nonusers or women using it continuously.[5] One observational study showed that women taking nitrates have a lower risk of all fractures, including hip fractures.[6] A short-term randomized controlled trial with isosorbide mononitrate once a day at bedtime decreased a marker of bone resorption and increased a marker of bone formation.[7] A randomized controlled trial of nitroglycerin ointment did not demonstrate increased BMD at the lumbar spine, femoral neck, or total hip, but compliance with treatment was poor because of side effects.[8]

This is the first study to report efficacy of once daily nitroglycerin ointment on changes in lumbar spine and hip BMD, bone geometry and strength at the distal radius and tibia, and markers of bone turnover over 2 years. The study randomized 243 postmenopausal women with normal or moderately osteopenic lumbar spine BMD T-scores ranging between 0 and −2.0 to nitroglycerin ointment 15 mg each day or placebo at bedtime. After 2 years of treatment, women receiving nitroglycerin ointment had significant increases in lumbar spine, total hip, and femoral neck BMD ranging from 6.2% to 7.0% compared with placebo. Bone geometry also improved with increased trabecular volumetric BMD, cortical thickness, periosteal circumference, polar section modulus (reflecting increased bone bending strength), and polar moment of inertia (reflecting increased bone twisting strength), all of which improve bone strength. Bone-specific alkaline phosphatase increased by 34%, and urine N-terminal telopeptide of type I collagen decreased by 54%. Adverse events did not differ between the treatment group and placebo, except for headaches, which were more common in those receiving nitroglycerin. The study concluded that nitroglycerin ointment improved BMD, decreased bone resorption, and increased bone formation in postmenopausal women with normal or low BMD.

This study demonstrated that nitroglycerin ointment improved BMD and had favorable effects on bone turnover. The findings suggest that nitroglycerin uncouples bone turnover, leading to increased bone formation and decreased bone resorption. Nitric oxide donor preparations, including nitroglycerin ointment, have not yet been shown to reduce fractures. Thirty-eight subjects discontinued participation in the nitroglycerin ointment group, versus 21 subjects in the placebo group, mostly because of headaches or other health complications. Headaches were responsible for more than half of the dropouts during the run-in phase and about 25% of the dropouts in women randomized to nitroglycerin. It is possible that different preparations, doses, or administration schedules would reduce headache frequency without altering beneficial effects on bone.

B. L. Clarke, MD

References

1. Brandi ML, Hukkanen M, Umeda T, et al. Bidirectional regulation of osteoclast function by nitric oxide synthase isoforms. *Proc Natl Acad Sci USA*. 1995;92: 2954-2958.
2. Collin-Osdoby P, Nickols GA, Osdoby P. Bone cell function, regulation, and communication: a role for nitric oxide. *J Cell Biochem*. 1995;57:399-408.
3. Wimalawansa SJ, De Marco G, Gangula P, Yallampalli C. Nitric oxide donor alleviates ovariectomy-induced bone loss. *Bone*. 1996;18:301-304.
4. Wimalawansa SJ, Chapa MT, Yallampalli C, Zhang R, Simmons DJ. Prevention of corticosteroid-induced bone loss with nitric oxide donor nitroglycerin in male rats. *Bone*. 1997;21:275-280.
5. Jamal SA, Browner WS, Bauer DC, Cummings SR. Intermittent use of nitrates increases bone mineral density: the study of osteoporotic fractures. *J Bone Miner Res*. 1998;13:1755-1759.
6. Rejnmark L, Vestergaard P, Mosekilde L. Decreased fracture risk in users of organic nitrates: a national case-control study. *J Bone Miner Res*. 2006;21: 1811-1817.
7. Jamal SA, Cummings SR, Hawker GA. Isosorbide mononitrate increases bone formation and decreases bone resorption in postmenopausal women: a randomized trial. *J Bone Miner Res*. 2004;19:1512-1517.
8. Wimalawansa SJ, Grimes JP, Wilson AC, Hoover DR. Transdermal nitroglycerin therapy may not prevent early postmenopausal bone loss. *J Clin Endocrinol Metab*. 2009;94:3356-3364.

Balloon kyphoplasty for the treatment of acute vertebral compression fractures: 2-year results from a randomized trial

Boonen S, Van Meirhaeghe J, Bastian L, et al (Katholieke Universiteit Leuven, Belgium; Algemeen Ziekenhuis Sint-Jan Brugge-Oostende AV, Belgium; Klinikum Leverkusen, Germany; et al)

J Bone Miner Res 2011 [Epub ahead of print]

Vertebral fractures are often painful and lead to reduced quality of life and disability. We compared the efficacy and safety of balloon kyphoplasty to non-surgical therapy over 24 months in patients with acute painful fractures. Adults with one to three vertebral fractures were randomized within 3 months from onset of pain to undergo kyphoplasty (n=149) or non-surgical therapy (n=151). Quality of life, function, disability, and pain were assessed over 24 months. Kyphoplasty was associated with greater improvements in SF-36 PCS scores when averaged across the 24-month follow-up period, compared with non-surgical therapy (overall treatment effect 3.24 points, 95% confidence interval [CI] 1.47−5.01; p=0.0004); the treatment difference remained statistically significant at 6 months (3.39 points, 95% CI 1.13−5.64; p=0.003) but not at 12 (1.70 points, 95% CI −0.59 to 3.98; p=0.15) or 24 months (1.68 points, 95% CI −0.63 to 3.99; p=0.15). Greater improvement in back pain was observed over 24 months for kyphoplasty (overall treatment effect -1.49 points, 95% CI −1.88 to −1.10; p<0.0001); the difference between groups remained statistically significant at 24 months (−0.80 points, 95% CI −1.39 to −0.20; p=0.009). There were two device-related serious adverse events in the second year that occurred at index vertebrae (a spondylitis and an anterior cement migration). There was no statistically significant difference between groups in the number of patients (47.5% for kyphoplasty, 44.1% for control) with new radiographic vertebral fractures; fewer fractures occurred (∼18%) within the second year. Compared with non-surgical management, kyphoplasty rapidly reduces pain and improves function, disability, and QOL without increasing the risk of additional vertebral fractures. The differences from non-surgical management are statistically significant when averaged across 24 months. Most outcomes are not statistically different at 24 months, but the reduction in back pain remains statistically significant at all time points.

▶ This study is important because it provides 2-year follow-up of outcomes of balloon kyphoplasty in a large cohort performed for acute painful vertebral fractures.[1] Current therapies for painful vertebral fractures include nonsurgical treatment with pain medication, bed rest, physical therapy, and back bracing or surgical therapy with vertebroplasty or kyphoplasty.[2] Back pain from vertebral fractures may resolve slowly or incompletely, and physical deformities resulting from vertebral fracture may affect function, mobility, and psychosocial outcomes.[3,4] Patients with vertebral fractures have reduced quality of life measured by physical, activities of daily living, emotional, and leisure parameters, in addition to increased back pain, deterioration of physical function, and worse general health perception.[5-8]

This study was performed to assess the success of balloon kyphoplasty compared with standard nonsurgical treatment in treatment of acute osteoporotic vertebral fractures. The trial randomized 300 subjects with 1 to 3 vertebral fractures within 3 months of onset of pain to receive kyphoplasty or standard therapy. Subjects were not blinded to treatment, and nonsurgical treatment was not standardized across study sites. Roughly 25% of subjects dropped out of the study by 2 years. Subjects receiving kyphoplasty reported greater improvements in Short-Form (SF)-36 Physical Component Summary quality-of-life assessment scores when averaged across 2 years compared with the standard therapy group. Kyphoplasty treatment was statistically better for the first 6 months only, however. Back pain was reduced in the kyphoplasty group at 24 months. One episode each of vertebral infectious spondylitis and anterior cement migration and vertebral recollapse occurred in the kyphoplasty group during the second year of follow-up, but there was not an increase in new radiographic vertebral fractures. The study concluded that kyphoplasty rapidly reduces pain and improves function, disability, and quality of life without increasing the risk of new vertebral fractures, compared with nonsurgical management, when averaged over 2 years. Unlike most outcomes measured, back pain remained significantly less in the kyphoplasty group at 2 years.

This study indicates that maximum improvement in disability and pain after kyphoplasty for painful acute vertebral fractures occurs during the first year after treatment. Subjects receiving nonsurgical treatment gradually improve over time and catch up to the group receiving kyphoplasty by 2 years in most parameters followed, except for back pain, which remains less in the kyphoplasty group at 2 years. One limitation of this study is that it did not compare kyphoplasty to sham injections, as done in 2 vertebroplasty trials that did not show improvement because of vertebroplasty. Nevertheless, the improvement in back pain, SF-36 bodily pain, and quality-of-life ratings over 24 months suggests that kyphoplasty provided effects beyond short-term effects of a nonspecific intervention.

B. L. Clarke, MD

References

1. Wardlaw D, Cummings SR, Van Meirhaeghe J, et al. Efficacy and safety of balloon kyphoplasty compared with non-surgical care for vertebral compression fracture (FREE): a randomised controlled trial. *Lancet.* 2009;373:1016-1024.
2. Lyritis GP, Mayasis B, Tsakalakos N, et al. The natural history of the osteoporotic vertebral fracture. *Clin Rheumatol.* 1989;8:66-69.
3. Silverman SL. The clinical consequences of vertebral compression fracture. *Bone.* 1992;13:S27-S31.
4. Lyles KW, Gold DT, Shipp KM, Pieper CF, Martinez S, Mulhausen PL. Association of osteoporotic vertebral compression fractures with impaired functional status. *Am J Med.* 1993;94:595-601.
5. Silverman SL, Minshall ME, Shen W, et al. The relationship of health-related quality of life to prevalent and incident vertebral fractures in postmenopausal women with osteoporosis: results from the Multiple Outcomes of Raloxifene Evaluation Study. *Arthritis Rheum.* 2001;44:2611-2619.

6. Borgström F, Zethraeus N, Johnell O, et al. Costs and quality of life associated with osteoporosis-related fractures in Sweden. *Osteoporos Int.* 2006;17:637-650.
7. Cook DJ, Guyatt GH, Adachi JD, et al. Quality of life issues in women with vertebral fractures due to osteoporosis. *Arthritis Rheum.* 1993;36:750-756.
8. Oleksik AM, Ewing S, Shen W, van Schoor NM, Lips P. Impact of incident vertebral fractures on health related quality of life (HRQOL) in postmenopausal women with prevalent vertebral fractures. *Osteoporos Int.* 2005;16:861-870.

Odanacatib in the Treatment of Postmenopausal Women With Low Bone Mineral Density: Three-Year Continued Therapy and Resolution of Effect

Eisman JA, Bone HG, Hosking DJ, et al (Univ of New South Wales, Sydney, Australia; Michigan Bone and Mineral Clinic, Detroit; Nottingham City Hosp, UK; et al)
J Bone Miner Res 26:242-251, 2011

The selective cathepsin K inhibitor odanacatib (ODN) progressively increased bone mineral density (BMD) and decreased bone-resorption markers during 2 years of treatment in postmenopausal women with low BMD. A 1-year extension study further assessed ODN efficacy and safety and the effects of discontinuing therapy. In the base study, postmenopausal women with BMD *T*-scores between −2.0 and −3.5 at the lumbar spine or femur received placebo or ODN 3, 10, 25, or 50 mg weekly. After 2 years, patients ($n = 189$) were rerandomized to ODN 50 mg weekly or placebo for an additional year. Endpoints included BMD at the lumbar spine (primary), total hip, and hip subregions; levels of bone turnover markers; and safety assessments. Continued treatment with 50 mg of ODN for 3 years produced significant increases from baseline and from year 2 in BMD at the spine (7.9% and 2.3%) and total hip (5.8% and 2.4%). Urine cross-linked N-telopeptide of type I collagen (NTx) remained suppressed at year 3 (−50.5%), but bone-specific alkaline phosphatase (BSAP) was relatively unchanged from baseline. Treatment discontinuation resulted in bone loss at all sites, but BMD remained at or above baseline. After ODN discontinuation at month 24, bone turnover markers increased transiently above baseline, but this increase largely resolved by month 36. There were similar overall adverse-event rates in both treatment groups. It is concluded that 3 years of ODN treatment resulted in progressive increases in BMD and was generally well tolerated. Bone-resorption markers remained suppressed, whereas bone-formation markers returned to near baseline. ODN effects were reversible: bone resorption increased transiently and BMD decreased following treatment discontinuation.

▶ This study summarizes important data on a new category of agent for the treatment of postmenopausal osteoporosis. Currently available categories of therapeutic agents for osteoporosis include bisphosphonates, estrogens, selective estrogen receptor modulators, calcitonin, denosumab, and teriparatide. All these categories except teriparatide primarily suppress bone resorption and secondarily decrease bone formation. The coupled decrease in bone formation limits the increase in bone mineral density (BMD) with these medications, and there is some concern that these agents may oversuppress bone remodeling in postmenopausal women. Odanacatib is a new, potent, orally active cathepsin K inhibitor that selectively inhibits cathepsin K, the main enzyme secreted by bone-resorbing osteoclasts into resorption lacunae, thereby impairing but not completely shutting down osteoclast activity.[1-4] Proton pumps in the osteoclast membrane over the resorption lacunae secrete acid into the resorption lacunae to help solubilize minerals at about pH 4.5, while cathepsin K degrades organic matrix with collagenolytic activity at acidic pH.[5,6] This study is a 1-year extension of the previous 2-year dose-ranging study of odanacatib,[7] with subjects randomized to odanacatib 50 mg or placebo each week in postmenopausal women. The previous 2-year dose-ranging study showed that odanacatib treatment increased BMD and decreased bone resorption and formation with less effect on bone formation markers, did not suppress the osteoclast resorption marker TRAP5b, and was generally well tolerated. This study showed that odanacatib caused further increases in lumbar spine and total hip BMD, with urinary cross-linked N-telopeptide of type I collagen remaining decreased at year 3 and serum bone alkaline phosphatase remaining unchanged from baseline. Treatment discontinuation resulted in rapid bone loss at all skeletal sites, with a temporary increase in bone turnover markers above baseline shortly thereafter. The markers returned to baseline within 12 months of discontinuation of odanacatib. Adverse events were similar between the treatment and placebo groups, with the exception that urinary tract infections were more common in the treatment group.

These findings indicate that selective inhibition of cathepsin K secreted by osteoclasts during bone resorption results in improvement in BMD without a plateauing of response, moderate reduction in bone resorption, and transient less marked reduction in bone formation. To determine whether odanacatib effect on BMD eventually plateaus, a further extension to 5 years is underway. Because odanacatib does not accumulate in bone, it is not surprising that its effect wanes rapidly after discontinuation and that the increase in BMD seen during 2 years of therapy is lost rapidly over 1 year after discontinuation of therapy. These findings are similar to those seen with discontinuation of hormone therapy, denosumab, and teriparatide. Odanacatib appears to be a promising new therapeutic agent for postmenopausal osteoporosis.

B. L. Clarke, MD

References

1. Stoch SA, Wagner JA. Cathepsin K inhibitors: a novel target for osteoporosis therapy. *Clin Pharmacol Ther.* 2008;83:172-176.
2. Adami S, Supronik J, Hala T, et al. Effect of one year treatment with the cathepsin-K inhibitor, balicatib, on bone mineral density (BMD) in postmenopausal women with osteopenia/osteoporosis. *J Bone Miner Res.* 2006;21:S24.
3. Papanastasiou P, Ortmann CE, Olson M, et al. Effect of three month treatment with the cathepsin-K inhibitor, balicatib, on biochemical markers of bone turnover in postmenopausal women: evidence for uncoupling of bone resorption and bone formation. *J Bone Miner Res.* 2006;21:S59.

4. Kumar S, Dare L, Vasko-Moser JA, et al. A highly potent inhibitor of cathepsin K (relacatib) reduces biomarkers of bone resorption both in vitro and in an acute model of elevated bone turnover in vivo in monkeys. *Bone.* 2007;40:122-131.
5. Gauthier JY, Chauret N, Cromlish W, et al. The discovery of odanacatib (MK-0822), a selective inhibitor of cathepsin K. *Bioorg Med Chem Lett.* 2008;18: 923-928.
6. Stoch S, Zajic S, Stone J, et al. Effect of the cathepsin K inhibitor odanacatib on bone resorption biomarkers in healthy postmenopausal women: two double-blind, randomized, placebo-controlled phase I studies. *Clin Pharmacol Ther.* 2009;86: 175-182.
7. Bone HG, McClung MR, Roux C, et al. Odanacatib, a cathepsin-k inhibitor for osteoporosis: a two-year study in postmenopausal women with low bone mineral density. *J Bone Miner Res.* 2010;25:937-947.

6 Adrenal Cortex

Introduction

This year's selections emphasize recurrent themes in adrenal diseases, and the articles highlight novel investigative studies with potential application to the diagnosis and treatment of these diseases. Several articles focus on malignant adrenocortical tumors. There is controversy about the best surgical approach to the resection of primary adrenocortical carcinomas (ACC). A report by Brix et al from Germany suggests there is no difference in clinical outcome between laparoscopic and open adrenalectomies, but other reports suggest patients who have undergone laparoscopic surgery have early development of local recurrence and peritoneal carcinomatosis. The outcome may hinge on the experience of the surgeon performing the surgery, the success in achieving completeness of the initial resection, and if patients have been treated in specialized centers as an article by Fassnacht et al seems to suggest. As indicated by Turbendian et al, extension of tumor into large vessels at the time of the initial resection carries worse prognosis. The management of hepatic metastases from ACC is challenging and could involve partial hepatectomy or radiation therapy. Cazejust et al from France report on the possible use of transcatheter arterial embolization as another option. There is an ongoing search for biomarkers of tumorigenesis that could predict tumor behavior and become targets for therapy. Positive results have been reported in articles by Sbiera et al on steroidogenic factor-1 (SF-1), Adam et al on epidermal growth factor (EGF) receptor, Kanczkowski et al on Toll-like receptor 4 (TLR4) and cluster of differentiation 14 (CD14), and Ragazzon et al on p53 and β-catenin. The differential diagnosis of adrenal masses has been greatly facilitated by imaging techniques using CT and MRI. For indeterminate adrenal tumors, Nunes et al propose using 18F-FDG PET.

Several interesting articles focus on the diagnosis and treatment of primary aldosteronism (PA). Selective adrenal venous sampling to distinguish between adrenal adenomas and hyperplasia is being further refined as highlighted by articles by Solar et al and Mathur et al. Renin assays are evolving as reported by Morganti et al, and a possible new way of treating PA with an aldosterone synthase inhibitor is reported by Amar et al. The hypertension of primary aldosteronism is not only a consequence of the mineralocorticoid effect of aldosterone but, as described by Kontak et al, there may be a sympathetic component involved. An article by Boulkroun et al provides interesting observation on the molecular pathology of the

237

peritumoral zona glomerulosa in patients with PA and suggests the adenoma is a manifestation of diffuse adrenocortical pathology. In more than a third of patients with aldosterone-secreting adenomas, hypertension persists after adrenalectomy. Genetic studies by Wang et al attempt to identify susceptibility for persistent hypertension in these patients.

Patients with spontaneous or iatrogenic Cushing's syndrome exhibit memory and mood impairment, which appears to relate to hippocampal damage by glucocorticoids. Brown et al suggest that glutamate may be involved in this effect. Extending the effect of glucocorticoids to the medial prefrontal cortex, Barsegyan et al provide evidence that the dual effect of glucocorticoids of enhancing consolidation but impairing working memory occur through a common neural mechanism. Patients with ACTH-independent macronodular adrenocortical hyperplasia have expression of various types of G protein-coupled receptors. Assie et al report on increased expression of a $\alpha 2A$ adrenergic receptor in such patients that could be a potential target for pharmacological treatment. Osteoporosis is a common complication of chronic corticosteroid therapy. Xia et al showed in an elegant study that glucocorticoids lead to cell death and loss of bone mass through autophagy.

Patients with hereditary pheochromocytoma, such as von Hippel-Lindau syndrome often present with bilateral adrenal medullary disease, and the surgical treatment involves bilateral adrenalectomy. Benhammou et al from the NIH report on successful partial adrenalectomy in these patients. Taking advantage of a comprehensive register in Sweden, Bjornsdottir et al examined the obstetrical outcome of patients with autoimmune Addison's disease. Given the size of the series, the observations are of interest. Finally, the possible metabolic consequence of apparently nonfunctioning adrenal masses is once again emphasized in a study from Greece by Peppa et al.

David E. Schteingart, MD

Adrenal Hormone Secretion and Pathology

Laparoscopic Versus Open Adrenalectomy for Adrenocortical Carcinoma: Surgical and Oncologic Outcome in 152 Patients
Brix D, German Adrenocortical Carcinoma Registry Group (Univ of Würzburg, Germany; et al)
Eur Urol 58:609-615, 2010

Background.—The role of laparoscopic adrenalectomy in the treatment of patients with adrenocortical carcinoma (ACC) is controversial.

Objective.—Our aim was to compare oncologic outcome in patients with ACC who underwent either open adrenalectomy (OA) or laparoscopic adrenalectomy (LA) for localised disease.

Design, Setting, and Participants.—We conducted a retrospective analysis of 152 patients with stage I-III ACC with a tumour ≤10 cm registered with the German ACC Registry.

Intervention.—Patients were stratified into two groups according to the surgical procedure (LA or OA). For comparison, we used both a matched pairs approach by selecting for each patient from the LA group ($n = 35$) one corresponding patient from the OA group ($n = 117$) and multivariate analysis in all 152 patients.

Measurements.—Disease-specific survival was chosen as the predefined primary end point. Secondary end points were recurrence-free survival, frequency of tumour capsule violation and postoperative peritoneal carcinomatosis, and incidence and reasons for conversion from LA to OA.

Results and Limitations.—LA and OA did not differ with regard to the primary end point using either the matched pairs approach (hazard ratio [HR] for death: 0.79; 95% confidence interval [CI], 0.36—1.72; $p = 0.55$) or multivariate analysis (HR for death: 0.98; 95% CI, 0.51—1.92; $p = 0.92$). Similarly, adjusted recurrence-free survival was not different between LA and OA (HR: 0.91; 95% CI, 0.56—1.47; $p = 0.69$). Frequency of tumour capsule violation and peritoneal carcinomatosis were comparable between groups. In 12 of 35 patients of the LA group, surgery was converted to open surgery with no impact on the clinical outcome.

Conclusions.—For localised ACC with a diameter of ≤10 cm, LA by an experienced surgeon is not inferior to OA with regard to oncologic outcome (Fig 1).

▶ The optimal treatment of stages I, II, and III adrenocortical carcinoma (ACC) is surgical resection of the primary tumor. Complete curative resection has the best chance for cure or long-term remission. This first attempt at surgical resection needs to be optimal. Ideally, the resection should be carried out by an experienced and technically skilled surgeon, with the objective of complete tumor extraction and exploration for local extension and lymph node involvement. A real concern is breaching the tumor capsule and spreading tumor into the

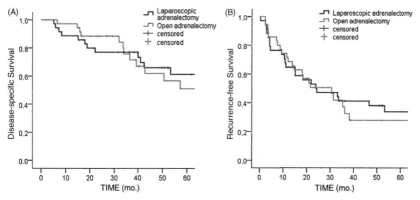

FIGURE 1.—Kaplan-Meier estimates of (A) disease-specific survival and (B) recurrence-free survival of 35 patients with laparoscopic adrenalectomy versus 35 matched patients with open adrenalectomy (OA). In 12 of 35 patients, minimally invasive adrenalectomy was converted to OA (see Fig. 2). (Reprinted from Brix D, German Adrenocortical Carcinoma Registry Group. Laparoscopic Versus Open Adrenalectomy for Adrenocortical Carcinoma: Surgical and Oncologic outcome in 152 Patients. *Eur Urol.* 2010;58:609-615. Copyright 2010, with permission from European Association of Urology.)

peritoneal cavity during the procedure. For these reasons, we at the University of Michigan advocate open adrenalectomy with wide en bloc tumor resection in all cases. Laparoscopic surgery is currently popular, and it offers the advantage of smaller incisions and shorter postoperative recovery. Many surgeons choose this approach to remove adrenal masses even if malignant, as long as the tumor is not too large. The choice of approach, open adrenalectomy versus laparoscopic resection, remains controversial. Brix et al in Germany compared in a retrospective study the surgical and oncological outcome of 152 patients with stages I to III ACC with tumors < 10 cm. The primary end point was disease-specific survival, while secondary end points were recurrence-free survival, frequency of tumor capsule violation, and postoperative peritoneal carcinomatosis. As shown in Fig 1, their finding was that laparoscopic surgery was not inferior to the open adrenalectomy in terms of these potential complications. Our experience differs from these findings. We often see patients operated laparoscopically in smaller surgical centers by less experienced surgeons who present months later with local recurrence and peritoneal dissemination out of proportion of those who undergo open procedures. We therefore strongly advocate open procedures for all patients with ACC.[1]

D. E. Schteingart, MD

Reference

1. Miller BS, Ammori JB, Gauger PG, Broome JT, Hammer GD, Doherty GM. Laparoscopic resection is inappropriate in patients with known or suspected adrenocortical carcinoma. *World J Surg.* 2010;34:1380-1385.

Improved Survival in Patients with Stage II Adrenocortical Carcinoma Followed Up Prospectively by Specialized Centers

Fassnacht M, on behalf of the German ACC Registry Group (Univ of Würzburg, Germany; et al)
J Clin Endocrinol Metab 95:4925-4932, 2010

Context.—Median survival in stage II adrenocortical carcinoma (ACC) differs widely in published series ranging between 23 and more than 60 months. We hypothesized that these results may have been affected by a referral bias because many patients may contact specialized centers only after recurrence.

Objective.—The objective of the study was a comparison of outcome in patients with stage II ACC who were followed up prospectively early after surgery and were counseled by a specialized center (prospective group) with patients who registered with the German ACC registry later than 4 months after diagnosis (retrospective group).

Patients/Methods.—The study was a cohort analysis in 149 adult patients with stage II ACC.

Results.—Patients who were followed up prospectively (n = 30) had a lower recurrence rate and a superior 5-yr survival compared with the

119 patients in the retrospective group (30 *vs.* 74%, *P* < 0.01 and 96 *vs.* 55%, *P* < 0.05, respectively). In the retrospective group, 67% of the patients had registered only after disease recurrence. In the remaining patients, the recurrence rate was low (21%), and the 5-yr survival was greater than 95%. More patients in the prospective group received adjuvant mitotane (53 *vs.* 16%, *P* < 0.001), and adjuvant mitotane was associated with improved survival [hazard risk 0.35 (95% confidence interval 0.13–0.97); *P* = 0.04]. However, the survival advantage was maintained when only patients without mitotane therapy were analyzed.

Conclusions.—Patients who are followed up prospectively after surgery for stage II ACC and receive early specialized care have a much better prognosis than previously reported due to a major referral bias in previous series and use of adjuvant mitotane. These findings will impact on the perception of prognosis in newly diagnosed stage II ACC.

▶ Outcome of patients with adrenocortical carcinoma (ACC) varies with the treatment approach and the experience of the treatment team. Patients with a presumptive diagnosis of ACC should be treated ideally in specialized centers and followed closely from the time of their initial diagnosis. Decisions regarding the type of surgery, adjuvant radiation therapy or chemotherapy, use of mitotane, reoperation, systemic cytotoxic chemotherapy, or newer targeted therapy protocols can only be made in centers experienced in the management of ACC. Being that ACC is rare, only few centers are qualified to optimally follow these patients. Fassnacht et al confirm this concept in a study of a cohort of 149 patients in stage II ACC. As shown in Fig 1 in the original article, 30 were followed prospectively from the time of their diagnosis and had lower recurrence rates than 119 patients in a retrospective group, more than half of whom registered only after disease recurrence. Adjuvant therapy with mitotane was more prevalent among the prospective group, and it is not clear if this treatment, as shown in Fig 4 in the original article, influenced outcome.

D. E. Schteingart, MD

Adrenocortical carcinoma: The influence of large vessel extension
Turbendian HK, Strong VE, Hsu M, et al (New York Presbyterian Hosp—Weill Cornell; Memorial Sloan Kettering Cancer Ctr, NY)
Surgery 148:1057-1064, 2010

Background.—The impact of large vessel extension (LVE) as a prognostic factor for adrenocortical carcinoma (ACC) is not fully understood. This study aimed to assess outcome of ACC in the presence and absence of LVE.

Methods.—A retrospective review of 57 patients undergoing curative intent resection for ACC over 10 years is presented comparing those with and without LVE. LVE was defined as vascular wall invasion or intraluminal extension of the neoplasm into the inferior vena cava or renal vein.

Preoperative diagnostics, operative details, pathology, overall survival (OS), and recurrence-free survival (RFS) were analyzed.

Results.—Multivariable regression analysis showed a significant association for decreased survival with Stage III and IV disease and LVE. Patients with LVE had more functional neoplasms, greater preoperative serum hormone levels, and more positive margins than those without LVE. Median OS was 6 years and RFS 3 years. Kaplan-Meier analysis demonstrated a significant decrease in OS and RFS with LVE. Median OS with and without LVE was 18 vs 111 months and median RFS was 11 vs 64 months. Three-year OS with and without LVE were 29% vs 93% and 3 year RFS was 15% vs 67%.

Conclusion.—In addition to systemic and lymph node metastases, LVE is associated with poorer OS and RFS (Fig 1).

▶ Many factors determine the clinical course of patients diagnosed with adrenocortical carcinoma (ACC). Limited disease, smaller tumors, and histological patterns of low-grade malignancy seem to have a better prognosis. Larger tumors with local invasion, lymph node involvement, high mitotic index, and

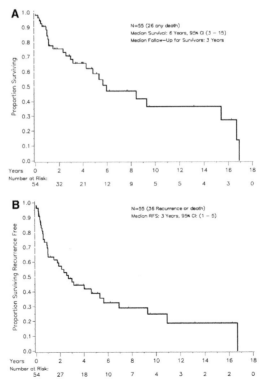

FIGURE 1.—Kaplan-Meier survivals: *A,* Overall Survival for all patients; *B,* Kaplan-Meier recurrence-free survival. (Reprinted from Turbendian HK, Strong VE, Hsu M, et al. Adrenocortical carcinoma: The influence of large vessel extension. *Surgery.* 2010;148:1057-1064, Copyright 2010, with permission from Mosby, Inc.)

high immunohistochemical biomarkers such as Ki67 are associated with worse outcome. Occasionally, large primary tumors are complicated by large vessel invasion, including the inferior vena cava wall and lumen and the right atrium. Surgical resection of this tumor extension is technically feasible, including partial resection of the affected vascular wall and placement of a patch. However, the prognosis of patients with large vessel extension is worse than without extension. Turbendian et al performed a retrospective review of 57 patients undergoing curative intent resection of ACC and compared patients with large vessel extension with those without. As illustrated in Fig 1, overall survival was only 18 months for patients with large vessel extension as compared with 111 months in those without and recurrence-free survival was 11 versus 64 months. As suggested by the authors, these patients should be considered for adjuvant or neoadjuvant chemotherapy or radiation therapy and possibly early cytotoxic chemotherapy.

D. E. Schteingart, MD

Transcatheter Arterial Chemoembolization for Liver Metastases in Patients with Adrenocortical Carcinoma
Cazejust J, De Baère T, Auperin A, et al (Institut Gustave Roussy, Villejuif, France)
J Vasc Interv Radiol 21:1527-1532, 2010

Purpose.—To retrospectively evaluate the effectiveness, tolerance, and predictors of response to transcatheter arterial chemoembolization for treatment of liver metastases from adrenocortical carcinoma.

Materials and Methods.—Twenty-nine patients with progressive liver metastases from adrenocortical carcinoma were treated with transcatheter arterial chemoembolization. Rate and duration of tumor response were defined according to Response Evaluation Criteria In Solid Tumors. The size of liver metastases, percentage of liver involvement, and Lipiodol uptake were studied as potential predictive factors of response. Time to liver and metastatic lesion progression were considered as endpoints.

Results.—Three months after transcatheter arterial chemoembolization, a liver morphologic response was observed in six of 29 patients (21%), stabilization in 18 (62%), and progression in five (17%). According to per-lesion analysis ($n = 103$), a morphologic response was observed in 23 lesions (22%), stabilization in 67 (65%), and progression in 13 (13%). Higher response rates were observed in cases in which the diameter of the target metastasis was 3 cm or smaller ($P = .002$) and in cases of high Lipiodol uptake (> 50%; $P < .0001$). On per-patient and per-lesion bases, progression rates were 32% and 55% at 6 months and 23% and 38% at 12 months. The median time to progression was 9 months and median survival was 11 months after the first procedure.

Conclusions.—Transcatheter arterial chemoembolization should be considered as part of the therapeutic arsenal to treat liver metastases from adrenocortical carcinoma. The size of liver metastases and the percentage of Lipiodol uptake may help identify patients likely to benefit most from transcatheter arterial chemoembolization.

▶ Stage IV adrenocortical carcinoma (ACC) usually involves hepatic metastases. With single small lesions, there is a possibility of ablating them surgically, by radiation therapy, or by radiofrequency ablation. Most of these approaches have limited responses but may improve the clinical manifestations of the disease in cases of hormone-secreting tumors and, by decreasing the tumor burden, improve the response to systemic chemotherapy. Cazejust et al in France used transcatheter arterial embolization of liver metastases in 29 patients with progressive liver metastases from ACC. They observed morphological responses in 21%, stable disease in 62%, and progression in 17%. Best responses were observed with lesions < 3 cm in diameter and higher lipiodol uptake. Some postprocedure complications were recorded, requiring hospitalization for 3 to 6 days, but most patients recovered well. The chemoembolization involved cisplatin mixed with iodized oil and gelatin sponge pledgets and administered intra-arterially through the hepatic artery. This study offers another tool for the management of ACC patients with single hepatic metastases. Some of the patients included in the study had metastatic disease in the lungs and bone. The benefit of treatment with hepatic chemoembolization in such patients is questionable. The rationale for the use of this technique is the assumption that hepatic metastases shorten overall survival, while chemoembolization elicits responses in 83% of patients, lasting 6 to 12 months. However, we do not have a comparison with patients with similar clinical presentation treated with or without chemoembolization to determine if this procedure is better able to extend time to progression or overall survival.

D. E. Schteingart, MD

High Diagnostic and Prognostic Value of Steroidogenic Factor-1 Expression in Adrenal Tumors

Sbiera S, Schmull S, Assie G, et al (Univ of Würzburg, Germany; Université Paris Descartes, France; et al)
J Clin Endocrinol Metab 95:E161-E171, 2010

Context.—No immunohistochemical marker has been established to reliably differentiate adrenocortical tumors from other adrenal masses. A panel of markers like melan-A and inhibin-α is currently used for this purpose but suffers from limited diagnostic accuracy. We hypothesized that expression of steroidogenic factor-1 (SF-1), a transcription factor involved in adrenal development, is of value for the differential diagnosis of adrenal masses and predicts prognosis in adrenocortical carcinoma (ACC).

Patients and Methods.—SF-1 protein expression was assessed by immunohistochemistry on tissue samples from 167 ACC, 52 adrenocortical adenomas (ACA), six normal adrenal glands, six normal ovaries and 73 neoplastic nonsteroidogenic tissues. In an independent cohort of 33 ACC and 58 ACA, SF-1 mRNA expression was analyzed. SF-1 expression was correlated with clinical outcome in patients with ACC.

Results.—SF-1 protein staining was detectable in 158 of 161 (98%) evaluable ACC samples including 49 (30%) with strong SF-1 staining and in all normal and benign steroidogenic tissues. In addition, SF-1 mRNA expression was present in all 91 analyzed adrenocortical tumors. In contrast, SF-1 expression was absent in all nonsteroidogenic tumors. Strong SF-1 protein expression significantly correlated with poor clinical outcome: tumor stage-adjusted hazard ratio for death 2.46 [95% confidence interval (CI) = 1.30−4.64] and for recurrence 3.91 (95% CI = 1.71−8.94). Similar results were obtained in the independent cohort using RNA analysis [tumor stage-adjusted hazard ratio for death 4.69 (95% CI = 1.44−15.30)].

Conclusion.—SF-1 is a highly valuable immunohistochemical marker to determine the adrenocortical origin of an adrenal mass with high sensitivity and specificity. In addition, SF-1 expression is of stage-independent prognostic value in patients with ACC.

▶ Steroidogenic factor 1 (SF-1) is postulated as another possible marker of adrenal tumorigenesis with potential prognostic and therapeutic value. Sbiera et al analyzed tissue samples from 167 adrenocortical carcinoma (ACC), 52 adrenocortical adenomas, 6 normal adrenal glands, and 73 neoplastic nonsteroidogenic tissues for SF-1 by immunohistochemistry, and in an independent cohort, by messenger RNA expression. They correlated SF-1 expression (low vs high) with clinical outcome. SF-1 was detectable in all malignant and benign adrenocortical tumors and in normal steroidogenic tissues, but, as expected, it was not present in nonsteroidogenic tissues. As shown in Fig 2 in the original article, strong SF-1 expression in ACC correlated with poor prognosis for recurrence and death. Although SF-1 is involved in steroidogenesis, it appears to be also involved in fetal adrenal development and could function as an adrenocortical growth factor. It has been observed that patients with cortisol-secreting ACC and Cushing syndrome have worse prognosis and exhibit a more rapidly progressive disease. This study, however, did not find a correlation between high SF-1 expression and hormonal status. The authors conclude that SF-1 expression can be used to distinguish adrenocortical from other neoplastic lesions and that they may be able to predict a more aggressive tumor progression. If SF-1 plays a role in adrenal tumorigenesis, it could be another potential target for antitumor therapy.

D. E. Schteingart, MD

Epidermal growth factor receptor in adrenocortical tumors: analysis of gene sequence, protein expression and correlation with clinical outcome

Adam P, Hahner S, Hartmann M, et al (Univ of Tübingen, Germany; Univ of Würzburg, Germany; et al)

Mod Pathol 23:1596-1604, 2010

Adrenocortical carcinoma is a rare but highly malignant neoplasm with still limited treatment options. Epidermal growth factor receptor (EGFR) has been shown to be overexpressed in many solid tumors, but its expression in adrenocortical carcinoma has been studied only in a limited number of cases. Therefore, we analyzed the expression of EGFR in 169 adrenocortical carcinoma samples and compared it with 31 adrenocortical adenomas. Additionally, in 30 cases of adrenocortical carcinoma, exons 18–21 of the *EGFR* gene were cloned and sequenced. EGFR expression was found in 128 of 169 adrenocortical carcinoma samples (76%), and in 60 of these samples (=36%) strong membrane staining was detected. However, there was no significant correlation with clinical outcome. In addition, all 30 sequenced cases revealed unmutated *EGFR* genes. In contrast, only 1 out of 31 adrenocortical adenomas weakly expressed the EGFR (3%). In summary, EGFR was overexpressed in more than three-quarters of adrenocortical carcinoma cases of this series. However, no mutations of the *EGFR* gene were found and EGFR expression was not of prognostic relevance. As EGFR is hardly expressed in adrenocortical adenomas, our results suggest that its expression in adrenocortical tumors indicates a malignant phenotype, which may be used in the differential diagnosis between adrenocortical adenomas and carcinomas (Fig 2).

▶ Ideal management of adrenocortical carcinoma (ACC) requires a better understanding of its pathogenesis and molecular pathology. Therapies directed at specific molecular defects hope to block tumor progression and improve life expectancy. With support of gene array studies of benign and malignant adrenocortical tumors, unique patterns of gene expression have been encountered in ACC. For example, overexpression of insulin-like growth factor (IGF) has been demonstrated in most ACCs, and clinical trials with IGF receptor antagonists are currently underway with modest results. There have also been attempts to correlate specific molecular defects with malignancy grade and prognosis. The study by Adam et al from Germany analyzed the expression of epidermal growth factor receptor (EGFR) in 169 ACC samples and compared it with 31 adrenocortical adenomas. EGFR expression was found in 76% of ACC and in only 3% of adenomas. No mutations were found in EGFR in malignant tumors, and their expression was not of prognostic significance. As shown in Fig 2, a correlation with morphologic features, according to the Weiss score (higher score, more malignant features) and immunohistochemical markers such as Ki67, no significant Kaplan-Meier survival differences with different EGFR staining intensity. The conclusion of this study is that expression of EGFR could be used as a feature of malignancy in the differential diagnosis of adrenal

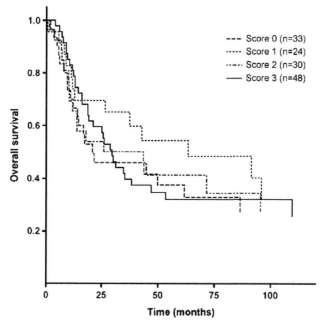

Time (months)

FIGURE 2.—Kaplan—Meier survival analysis comparing adrenocortical carcinoma patients with different epidermal growth factor receptor (EGFR) staining intensity of their primary tumor. Only patients with detailed follow-up information are included in this analysis. (Reprinted from Adam P, Hahner S, Hartmann M, et al. Epidermal growth factor receptor in adrenocortical tumors: analysis of gene sequence, protein expression and correlation with clinical outcome. *Mod Pathol.* 2010;23:1596-1604, Copyright 2010, with permission from Macmillan Publishers Ltd: Modern Pathology.)

masses with borderline histologic profile, but EGFR expression does not have prognostic value.

D. E. Schteingart, MD

Abrogation of TLR4 and CD14 Expression and Signaling in Human Adrenocortical Tumors

Kanczkowski W, Tymoszuk P, Ehrhart-Bornstein M, et al (Technical Univ of Dresden, Germany; et al)
J Clin Endocrinol Metab 95:E421-E429, 2010

Context.—Adrenocortical carcinoma (ACC) is a rare tumor with poor prognosis. The expression of innate immunity receptor Toll-like receptor 4 (TLR4) was recently reported in various human tumors, and TLR4 was shown to regulate tumor immune escape processes, proliferation, and resistance to chemotherapeutical agents.

Objective.—The aim of this study was to investigate TLR4 expression, signaling, and function in the process of tumorigenesis in the human adrenal cortex.

Measurements and Main Results.—Real-time PCR analysis of human ACC (n = 8), adenoma (n = 8), and ACC cell lines (SW13, NCI-H295R, and HAC15) revealed a significant down-regulation of TLR4, MD2 (myeloid differentiation protein-2), and cluster of differentiation 14 (CD14) mRNA compared with normal human adrenal cortex and adreno-cortical cells in primary culture. Furthermore, immunohistochemistry revealed an abrogation of TLR4 and CD14 expression in ACC but not adenoma tissues. Western blot analysis of MAPK, AKT, activator protein-1, and nuclear factor-κB signaling revealed that the ACC cell lines are unresponsive to lipopolysaccharide action. Restoration of TLR4 signaling by stable transfection of TLR4-CD14 plasmid into NCI-H295R cells sensitized them to lipopolysaccharide incubation as shown by nuclear factor-κB activation and decreased cell viability and induced apoptosis in these cells.

Conclusion.—Our results demonstrate a significant reduction in the expression of TLR4 and CD14 and an inactivation of TLR4 signaling in ACCs. Furthermore, our data show that reintroduction of TLR4 expression in ACCs may provide a novel therapeutic strategy for adrenal cancer.

▶ Therapies directed at specific molecular defects hope to block tumor progression and improve life expectancy. With the support of gene array studies of benign and malignant adrenocortical tumors, unique patterns of gene expression have been encountered in adrenocortical carcinoma (ACC). Similar to other studies reviewed here, Kanczkowski et al, in Dresden, investigated innate immunity receptor toll-like receptor 4 (TLR4) expression, signaling, and function in the process of tumorigenesis in the human adrenal cortex. Using real-time polymerase chain reaction, analysis of human ACC and adenoma tissue and ACC cell lines showed significant downregulation of TLR4, myeloid differentiation protein 2, and cluster of differentiation 14 (CD14) mRNA compared with normal human adrenal cortex and adrenocortical cells in primary cultures. Immunohistochemistry showed abrogation of TLR4 and CD14 in ACC, but not in adenoma tissues. Western blot analysis of MAPK, AKT, activator protein 1, and nuclear factor κB showed that ACC lines were unresponsive to lipopolysaccharide action, but restoration of TLR4 by stable transfection sensitized NCI-H295R ACC cells to this activator, decreasing cell viability and inducing apoptosis in these cells. The study suggests another possible molecular mechanism of tumorigenesis and potential target for therapy, but there is a long way to go before these concepts find clinical application. These type of studies provide proof of concept for possible targeted therapy, but the next step will have to be preclinical animal studies, which, even if successful, do not guarantee clinical efficacy.

D. E. Schteingart, MD

Transcriptome Analysis Reveals that p53 and β-Catenin Alterations Occur in a Group of Aggressive Adrenocortical Cancers
Ragazzon B, Libé R, Gaujoux S, et al (Université Paris Descartes, France; et al)
Cancer Res 70:8276-8281, 2010

Adrenocortical carcinoma (ACC) is a rare disease with an overall poor but heterogeneous prognosis. This heterogeneity could reflect different mechanisms of tumor development. Gene expression profiling by transcriptome analysis led to ACC being divided into two groups of tumors with very different outcomes. Somatic inactivating mutations of the tumor suppressor gene *TP53* and activating mutations of the proto-oncogene *β-catenin (CTNNB1)* are the most frequent mutations identified in ACC. This study investigates the correlation between p53 and β-catenin alterations and the molecular classification of ACC by transcriptome analysis of 51 adult sporadic ACCs. All *TP53* and *CTNNB1* mutations seemed to be mutually exclusive and were observed only in the poor-outcome ACC group. Most of the abnormal p53 and β-catenin immunostaining was also found in this group. Fifty-two percent of the poor-outcome ACC group had *TP53* or *CTNNB1* mutations and 60% had abnormal p53 or β-catenin immunostaining. Unsupervised clustering transcriptome analysis of this poor-outcome group revealed three different subgroups, two of them being associated with p53 or β-catenin alterations, respectively. Analysis of p53 and β-catenin target gene expressions in each cluster confirmed a profound and anticipated effect on tumor biology, with distinct profiles logically associated with the respective pathway alterations. The third group had no p53 or β-catenin alteration, suggesting other unidentified molecular defects. This study shows the important respective roles of p53 and β-catenin in ACC development, delineating subgroups of ACC with different tumorigenesis and outcomes.

► Heterogeneity of clinical presentation in adrenocortical carcinoma (ACC) may be related to stage of the disease at diagnosis and the malignancy grade of the tumor judged by histological criteria, according to the Weiss score. Molecular differences among tumors may be another important factor in their phenotypic presentation. Several groups have carried out transcriptome analysis of ACC in search of specific mutations associated with aggressive phenotypes. Ragazzon et al analyzed 51 tumors for inactivating mutations of the tumor suppressor gene *TP53* and activating mutations of the protooncogene *CTNNB1*, involved in the β-catenin pathway. Their cluster of clinically aggressive phenotypes showed alteration of 1 of these 2 genes, although not concurrently. The authors were able to identify subgroups of poor outcome ACC that are associated with frequent genetic alterations, specifically, *TP53* inactivating mutations and *CTNNB1* activating mutations that would promote the development of aggressive tumors. Molecular profiling of ACC could help determine more accurately their prognosis and selection of appropriate therapy.

D. E. Schteingart, MD

18F-FDG PET for the Identification of Adrenocortical Carcinomas among Indeterminate Adrenal Tumors at Computed Tomography Scanning

Nunes ML, Rault A, Teynie J, et al (Centre Hospitalier Universitaire de Bordeaux, Pessac, France)
World J Surg 34:1506-1510, 2010

Background.—18F-fluorodeoxyglucose positron emission tomography (18F-FDG PET) has been proposed for the evaluation of adrenal tumors. However, only scarce data are available to evaluate its usefulness for the identification of primary adrenal carcinomas in patients with no previous history of cancer and equivocal tumors on computed tomography (CT) scan. The objective of the present study was to evaluate the diagnostic performance of 18F-FDG-PET to predict malignancy in such patients.

Methods and Patients.—This was a retrospective study carried out from 2006 to 2009 in a single university hospital center. Twenty-three consecutive patients without previous history of cancer investigated for adrenal tumors without features of benign adrenocortical adenoma on CT scan but no obvious ACC underwent 18F-FDG PET. All patients underwent adrenalectomy because of CT scan characteristics regardless of the results of 18F-FDG PET. The ratio of maxSUV adrenal tumor on maxSUV liver (adrenal/liver maxSUV ratio) during 18F-FDG PET was compared to Weiss pathological criteria.

Results.—Seventeen patients had an adrenal adenoma, 2 had small size adrenal carcinomas (<5 cm), 1 had an angiosarcoma, and 3 had noncortical benign lesions. An adrenal/liver maxSUV ratio above 1.6 provided 100% sensitivity, 90% specificity, and 100% negative predictive value for the diagnosis of malignant tumor.

Conclusions.—Because of its excellent negative predictive value, 18F-FDG-PET may be of help in avoiding unnecessary surgery in patients with non-secreting equivocal tumors at CT scanning and low 18F-FGD uptake.

▶ Imaging criteria for identifying benign adrenal masses are a measurement of < 10 unenhanced density on unenhanced CT and contrast washout of > 60% at 15 minutes after contrast injection. Sensitivity of unenhanced CT is 98%, specificity 92%, and washout sensitivity and specificity almost 100%. Lipid-rich benign lesions can also be detected by their drop in signal with chemical shift MRI with comparable sensitivity and specificity. The problem is with indeterminate adrenal masses that do not reach the cutoff criteria. Nunes et al propose the use of 18F-fluorodeoxyglucose positron emission tomography (18F-FDG PET) as helpful in determining which of these lesions are likely to be malignant. An adrenal/liver max standardized uptake value ratio above 1.6 provided 100% sensitivity, 90% specificity, and 100% negative predictive value for diagnosing malignancy. The PET would also be helpful in detecting metastases and helping to stage the tumor. In a series of 23 patients, they discovered 2 adrenocortical carcinoma (ACC) and 1 angiosarcoma, while the rest were benign adrenocortical adenomas. They conclude that 18F-FDG PET can be useful in patients with indeterminate adrenal masses. Of interest in this series is that the 2 patients with small ACC were treated by laparoscopic surgery and developed local recurrence and peritoneal carcinomatosis. We have observed these complications frequently with laparoscopic resections and have strongly recommended open adrenalectomies in all cases of ACC regardless of tumor size or surgical skill.

D. E. Schteingart, MD

Primary Aldosteronism

Adrenal Venous Sampling: Where Is the Aldosterone Disappearing to?
Solar M, Ceral J, Krajina A, et al (Univ Hosp Hradec Kralove, Sokolska, Czech Republic)
Cardiovasc Intervent Radiol 33:760-765, 2010

Adrenal venous sampling (AVS) is generally considered to be the gold standard in distinguishing unilateral and bilateral aldosterone hypersecretion in primary hyperaldosteronism. However, during AVS, we noticed a considerable variability in aldosterone concentrations among samples thought to have come from the right adrenal glands. Some aldosterone concentrations in these samples were even lower than in samples from the inferior vena cava. We hypothesized that the samples with low aldosterone levels were unintentionally taken not from the right adrenal gland, but from hepatic veins. Therefore, we sought to analyze the impact of unintentional cannulation of hepatic veins on AVS. Thirty consecutive patients referred for AVS were enrolled. Hepatic vein sampling was implemented in our standardized AVS protocol. The data were collected and analyzed prospectively. AVS was successful in 27 patients (90%), and hepatic vein cannulation was successful in all procedures performed. Cortisol concentrations were not significantly different between the hepatic vein and inferior vena cava samples, but aldosterone concentrations from hepatic venous blood (median, 17 pmol/l; range, 40–860 pmol/l) were markedly lower than in samples from the inferior vena cava (median, 860 pmol/l; range, 460–4510 pmol/l). The observed difference was statistically significant ($P < 0.001$). Aldosterone concentrations in the hepatic veins are significantly lower than in venous blood taken from the inferior vena cava. This finding is important for AVS because hepatic veins can easily be mistaken for adrenal veins as a result of their close anatomic proximity.

▶ This is another study trying to improve on adrenal venous sampling, the gold standard in the differential diagnosis of primary aldosteronism. The question being examined is the error in calculating an aldosterone:cortisol ratio in the right adrenal vein, the one most difficult to catheterize. Errors in determining lateralization occur when the hepatic vein rather than the right adrenal vein is cannulated. Under those circumstances, both the aldosterone and cortisol levels are low, indicating that the catheter is not in the adrenal vein. To make things confusing, there is occasionally a discrepancy between aldosterone and cortisol levels (aldosterone low, cortisol similar to that in the inferior vena cava [IVC]), suggesting that there is a predominance of the contralateral side. Solar et al studied 30 patients referred to them for adrenal venous sampling. They catheterized not only the adrenal veins but also the hepatic vein, a frequent source of erroneous sampling. The interesting finding is that although cortisol levels matched that in the IVC, hepatic vein aldosterone level was lower than that in the IVC. They suggest greater hepatic extraction of aldosterone than cortisol, leading to an apparent low aldosterone:renin ratio and misdiagnosis of the dominant side.

D. E. Schteingart, MD

Consequences of Adrenal Venous Sampling in Primary Hyperaldosteronism and Predictors of Unilateral Adrenal Disease

Mathur A, Kemp CD, Dutta U, et al (Natl Cancer Inst, BD; Eunice Kennedy Shriver Natl Insts of Child Health and Human Development (NICHD), MD; et al)

J Am Coll Surg 211:384-390, 2010

Background.—In patients with primary hyperaldosteronism, distinguishing between unilateral and bilateral adrenal hypersecretion is critical in assessing treatment options. Adrenal venous sampling (AVS) has been advocated by some to be the gold standard for localization of the responsible lesion, but there remains a lack of consensus for the criteria and the standardization of technique.

Study Design.—We performed a retrospective study of 114 patients with a biochemical diagnosis of primary hyperaldosteronism who all underwent CT scan and AVS before and after corticotropin (ACTH) stimulation. Univariate and multivariate analyses were performed to determine what factors were associated with AVS lateralization, and which AVS values were the most accurate criteria for lateralization.

Results.—Eighty-five patients underwent surgery at our institution for unilateral hyperaldosteronism. Of the 57 patients who demonstrated unilateral abnormalities on CT, AVS localized to the contralateral side in 5 patients and revealed bilateral hyperplasia in 6 patients. Of the 52 patients who showed bilateral disease on CT scan, 43 lateralized with AVS. The most accurate criterion on AVS for lateralization was the post-ACTH stimulation value. Factors associated with AVS lateralization included a low renin value, high plasma aldosterone-to plasma-renin ratio, and adrenal mass ≥3 cm on CT scan.

Conclusions.—Because 50% of patients would have been inappropriately managed based on CT scan findings, patients with biochemical evidence of primary hyperaldosteronism and considering adrenalectomy should have AVS. The most accurate measurement for AVS lateralization was the post-ACTH stimulation value. Although several factors predict successful AVS lateralization, none are accurate enough to perform AVS selectively.

▶ A presumptive biochemical diagnosis of primary aldosteronism is made when serum aldosterone level is higher than 15 ng/dL and plasma renin is suppressed with an aldosterone:renin ratio > 20. The 2 major types of primary aldosteronism are an aldosterone-secreting adenoma and idiopathic bilateral adrenocortical hyperplasia. Successful surgical treatment depends on the distinction between the 2 and proper lateralization of the lesion. MRI and CT yield mislateralization in about one-third of the patients, and selective venous sampling has become the gold standard for determining the actively secreting side. The test involves simultaneous catheterization of the right and left adrenal veins, sampling before and after an adrenocorticotropic hormone (ACTH) infusion, and measurement of the aldosterone:cortisol (A:C) ratio to ensure proper placement of the catheter. The manner the procedure is performed varies among centers, and several articles over the past few years have stressed potential technical difficulty, especially when attempting to catheterize the right adrenal vein. Mathur et al attempt to standardize the procedure and establish criteria for interpreting the results. In a retrospective study of 114 patients evaluated at the National Institutes of Health, they conclude that the most accurate measurement for adrenal venous sampling lateralization is the post-ACTH stimulation A:C ratio. Unfortunately, the article does not give clear criteria for right:left and central:peripheral A:C ratios. Young et al propose using a 4:1 ratio between right and left A:C ratios in unilateral disease and a 10:1 ratio after ACTH stimulation between adrenal vein and inferior vena cava.[1]

D. E. Schteingart, MD

Reference

1. Young WF, Stanson AW, Thompson GB, Grant CS, Farley DR, VanHeerden JA. Role for adrenal venous sampling in Primary Aldosteronism. *Surgery.* 2004; 136(6):1227-1235.

A comparative study on inter and intralaboratory reproducibility of renin measurement with a conventional enzymatic method and a new chemiluminescent assay of immunoreactive renin
Morganti A, on behalf of the European study group for the validation of DiaSorin liaison direct renin assay (Univ of Milan, Italy)
J Hypertens 28:1307-1312, 2010

Background.—The activity of the renin—angiotensin system is usually evaluated as plasma renin activity (PRA, ngAI/ml per h) but the reproducibility of this enzymatic assay is notoriously scarce. We compared the inter and intralaboratory reproducibilities of PRA with those of a new automated chemiluminescent assay, which allows the direct quantification of immunoreactive renin [chemiluminescent immunoreactive renin (CLIR), µU/ml].

Methods.—Aliquots from six pool plasmas of patients with very low to very high PRA levels were measured in 12 centres with both the enzymatic and the direct assays. The same methods were applied to three control plasma preparations with known renin content.

Results.—In pool plasmas, mean PRA values ranged from 0.14 ± 0.08 to 18.9 ± 4.1 ngAI/ml per h, whereas those of CLIR ranged from 4.2 ± 1.7 to 436 ± 47 µU/ml. In control plasmas, mean values of PRA and of CLIR were always within the expected range. Overall, there was a significant correlation between the two methods ($r = 0.73$, $P < 0.01$). Similar correlations were found in plasmas subdivided in those with low, intermediate and high PRA. However, the coefficients of variation among laboratories found for PRA were always higher than those of CLIR, ranging from 59.4 to 17.1% for PRA, and from 41.0 to 10.7% for CLIR ($P < 0.01$). Also, the mean intralaboratory variability was higher for PRA than for CLIR, being respectively, 8.5 and 4.5% ($P < 0.01$).

Conclusion.—The measurement of renin with the chemiluminescent method is a reliable alternative to PRA, having the advantage of a superior inter and intralaboratory reproducibility.

▶ Sensitive and reproducible renin assays are essential for accurate diagnosis of low-renin states, including primary aldosteronism. The earliest renin assay developed in the 1960s and still used today was an enzymatic assay based on the generation of angiotensin I when incubating the enzyme renin with renin substrate. Results were expressed as plasma renin activity (PRA) in ngAI/ml/h and served well through the years for research and clinical use. Because results depend on the duration of incubation, there may be problems with reproducibility. Later on, attempts were made to measure renin directly by radioimmunoassay, but the most recent attempt is a chemiluminescent assay of immunoreactive renin, expressed as µU/ml. Morganti, on behalf of a European group, reported on a multicenter comparative study of sensitivity and reproducibility of the enzymatic and the chemiluminescent assays. They compared samples in the low, medium, and high range of renin concentration and found a good correlation between the 2 methods ($r = 0.73$; $P < .01$). They conclude that the chemiluminescent direct assay is a reliable alternative to PRA with superior interlaboratory and intralaboratory reproducibility.

D. E. Schteingart, MD

Reversible Sympathetic Overactivity in Hypertensive Patients with Primary Aldosteronism

Kontak AC, Wang Z, Arbique D, et al (Univ of Texas Southwestern Med Ctr, Dallas; et al)
J Clin Endocrinol Metab 95:4756-4761, 2010

Context.—Aldosterone has been shown to exert a central sympathoexcitatory action in multiple animal models, but evidence in humans is still lacking.

Objectives.—Our objective was to determine whether hyperaldosteronism causes reversible sympathetic activation in humans.

Methods.—We performed a cross-sectional comparison of muscle sympathetic nerve activity (SNA, intraneural microelectrodes) in 14 hypertensive patients with biochemically proven primary aldosteronism (PA) with 20 patients with essential hypertension (EH) and 18 age-matched normotensive (NT) controls. Seven patients with aldosterone-producing adenoma (APA) were restudied 1 month after unilateral adrenalectomy.

Results.—Mean blood pressure values in patients with PA and EH and NT controls was $145 \pm 4/88 \pm 2$, $150 \pm 4/90 \pm 2$, and $119 \pm 2/76 \pm 2$ mm Hg, respectively. The major new findings are 2-fold: 1) baseline SNA was significantly higher in the PA than the NT group (40 ± 3 *vs.* 30 ± 2 bursts/min, $P = 0.014$) but similar to the EH group (41 ± 3 bursts/min) and 2) after unilateral adrenalectomy for APA, SNA decreased significantly from 38 ± 5 to 27 ± 4 bursts/min ($P = 0.01$), plasma aldosterone levels fell from 72.4 ± 20.3 to 11.4 ± 2.3 ng/dl ($P < 0.01$), and blood pressure decreased from $155 \pm 8/94 \pm 3$ to $117 \pm 4/77 \pm 2$ mm Hg ($P < 0.01$).

Conclusion.—These data provide the first evidence in humans that APA is accompanied by reversible sympathetic overactivity, which may contribute to the accelerated hypertensive target organ disease in this condition.

▶ It is generally agreed that the mechanism of hypertension in patients with primary aldosteronism is mineralocorticoid-mediated sodium retention and volume expansion. Aldosterone also has direct effects on the heart and kidneys, inducing fibrosis. There may be other contributing factors in the pathogenesis of hypertension in primary aldosteronism, including a central sympathoexcitatory action of aldosterone. This putative effect had been shown in animal models but not in humans. Kontak et al compared muscle sympathetic nerve activity (SNA) in 14 patients with primary aldosteronism, 20 patients with essential hypertension, and 18 age-matched normotensive controls. Studies were repeated in some patients with primary aldosteronism after adrenalectomy. As shown in Fig 4 in the original article, SNA was significantly increased in primary aldosteronism and essential hypertension and was consistently reversed after adrenalectomy. These studies suggest a possible benefit of sympathetic blockers in treating patients with primary aldosteronism.

D. E. Schteingart, MD

Adrenal Cortex Remodeling and Functional Zona Glomerulosa Hyperplasia in Primary Aldosteronism

Boulkroun S, Samson-Couterie B, Dzib J-FG, et al (Paris Cardiovascular Res Ctr, France; Institut des Hautes Études Scientifiques, Bures sur Yvette, France; et al)
Hypertension 56:885-892, 2010

Primary aldosteronism is the most common form of secondary hypertension with hypokalemia and suppressed renin-angiotensin system caused by autonomous aldosterone production. Our aim was to compare zona glomerulosa (ZG) structure and function between control adrenals and the peritumoral tissue from patients operated on for aldosterone-producing adenoma. ZG morphology and CYP11B1, CYP11B2, and disabled 2 expression were studied in 15 control adrenals and 25 adrenals with aldosterone-producing adenoma. A transcriptome analysis was done using publicly available data sets. In control adrenals, ZG was discontinuous, and CYP11B2 expression was focal or partly continuous and localized to 3 structures, foci, megafoci, and aldosterone-producing cell clusters. CYP11B2 expression was restricted to a limited number of ZG cells expressing Dab2 but not CYP11B1; aldosterone-producing cell clusters were composed of cells with an intermediate phenotype expressing CYP11B2 but not disabled 2 or CYP11B1. In peritumoral tissue, large remodeling of the adrenal cortex was observed with increased nodulation and decreased vascularization that were not correlated with CYP11B2 expression. In 17 out of 25 adrenals, hyperplasia of adjacent ZG was observed with persistent expression of CYP11B2 that was extended to the entire ZG. In all of the adrenals from patients with aldosterone-producing adenoma, CYP11B2 expression was present in foci, megafoci, and aldosterone-producing cell clusters. Transcriptome profiling indicates a close relationship between peritumoral and control adrenal cortex. In conclusion, adrenal cortex remodeling, reduced vascularization, and ZG hyperplasia are major features of adrenals with aldosterone-producing adenoma. Transcriptional phenotyping is not in favor of this being an intermediate step toward the formation of aldosterone-producing adenoma.

▶ The 2 major types of primary aldosteronism are aldosterone-secreting adrenocortical adenoma and bilateral adrenocortical hyperplasia. It has been assumed that the adenomas are monoclonal and arise in an otherwise normal or suppressed adrenal cortex. In contrast, hyperplasia involves both glands. The mechanism by which these 2 types develop is unknown. In this interesting article, Boulkroun et al studied the uninvolved adrenal cortex surrounding adenomas and found significant pathology. They compared 25 adrenals with aldosterone-secreting adenomas with 15 control adrenals from patients undergoing enlarged nephrectomies. They studied the morphology of the zona glomerulosa, expression of CYP11B1, CYP11B2, and disabled 2 (a specific marker of zona glomerulosa) and performed a transcriptome analysis of the cortex. They observed large remodeling of the adrenal cortex in the peritumoral tissue, with evidence of hyperplasia of the adjacent zona glomerulosa and persistent expression of CYPB2. These observations do not clarify if the peritumoral changes are a result of paracrine effects of aldosterone by the adenoma or a manifestation of an overall cortical pathology from which the adenoma emerges. It also speaks against adenomectomies with preservation of the non-adenomatous gland in the surgical approach to these patients.

D. E. Schteingart, MD

Association of DNA Polymorphisms Within the CYP11B2/CYP11B1 Locus and Postoperative Hypertension Risk in the Patients With Aldosterone-producing Adenomas

Wang B, Zhang G, Ouyang J, et al (China PLA General Hosp, Beijing, People's Republic of China; First Affiliated Hosp of Gannan Med Univ, Ganzhou, People's Republic of China; et al)

Urology 76:1018.e1-1018.e7, 2010

Objectives.—Hypertension often persists after adrenalectomy for primary aldosteronism. Traditional factors associated with postoperative hypertension were evaluated, but whether genetic determinants were involved remains poorly understood. The aim of this study was to investigate the association of DNA polymorphisms within steroid synthesis genes (CYP11B2, CYP11B1) and the postoperative resolution of hypertension in Chinese patients undergoing adrenalectomy for aldosterone-producing adenomas (APA).

Methods.—Ninety-three patients with APA were assessed for postoperative resolution of hypertension. All patients were genotyped for rs1799998 (C-344 T), intron 2 conversion, rs4539 (A2718G) within CYP11B2 and rs6410 (G22 5A), rs6387 (A2803G) within CYP11B1. The associations between CYPB11B2/CYP11B1 polymorphisms and persistent postoperative hypertension were assessed by multivariate analysis.

Results.—CYP11B2-CYP11B1 haplotype was associated with persistent postoperative hypertension in Chinese patients undergoing adrenalectomy with APA ($P = .006$). Specifically, the rs4539 (AA) polymorphism was associated with persistent postoperative hypertension ($P = .002$). Multivariate logistic regression revealed the common haplotypes H1 (AGACT), H2 (AGAWT), and H3 (AGAWC) were associated with the persistent postoperative hypertension ($P = .01$, 0.03, 0.005 after Bonferroni correction). Additional predictors of persistent postoperative hypertension included duration of hypertension ($P < .0005$), family history of hypertension ($P = .001$), and elevated systolic blood pressure ($P = .015$).

Conclusions.—The rs4539 (AA), H1, H2, and H3 are genetic predictors for postoperative persistence of hypertension for Chinese patients treated by adrenalectomy with APA. DNA polymorphisms at CYP11B2/B1 locus may confer susceptibility to postoperative hypertension of patients with APA.

▶ Ever since the first series of patients with primary aldosteronism underwent resection of an aldosterone-secreting adrenocortical adenoma, it was learned that aldosterone levels decrease and serum potassium normalizes shortly after surgery. While blood pressure usually improves and the number of drugs required for control decreases, many patients continue to exhibit hypertension. Several factors have been blamed for the persistence of hypertension, including the duration of hypertension and the level of control, height of aldosterone levels, and the presence of underlying renal disease as a consequence of the high aldosterone levels. Wang et al studied a Chinese cohort of 93 patients with aldosterone-producing adrenocortical adenomas for evidence of a genetic defect among those with persistent hypertension. CYP11B2 and CYP11B1, 2 critical enzymes in aldosterone synthesis, were assessed for polymorphism. A rs4539 (AA) polymorphism was associated with postoperative hypertension. Thus, rs459 (AA), H1, H2, H3 were found to be genetic predictors for persistent hypertension. A possible mechanism by which these mutations cause the hypertension may be altered 11β-hydroxylase activity in the contralateral remaining gland, which, through increased adrenocorticotropic hormone drive, would lead to further dysregulation of aldosterone synthesis and blood pressure. Thus, these patients would have a bilateral adrenal synthesis defect, and, perhaps, they would respond to suppression with corticosteroids like patients with congenital adrenal hyperplasia.

D. E. Schteingart, MD

Aldosterone Synthase Inhibition With LCI699: A Proof-of-Concept Study in Patients With Primary Aldosteronism

Amar L, Azizi M, Menard J, et al (Université Paris Descartes, France; et al)
Hypertension 56:831-838, 2010

We report the first administration of an orally active aldosterone synthase inhibitor, LCI699, to 14 patients with primary aldosteronism. After a 2-week placebo run-in, patients received oral LCI699 (0.5 mg BID) for 2 weeks, LCI699 (1.0 mg BID) for 2 weeks, and placebo for 1 week. We assessed changes in hormone concentrations, plasma potassium levels, and 24-hour ambulatory systolic blood pressure and safety. The supine plasma aldosterone concentration decreased from 540 pmol/L (95% CI: 394 to 739 pmol/L) to 171 pmol/L (95% CI: 128 to 230 pmol/L) after 0.5 mg of LCI699 (-68%; $P < 0.0001$) and to 133 pmol/L (95% CI: 100 to 177 pmol/L) after 1.0 mg of LCI699 (-75%; $P < 0.0001$). Plasma 11-deoxycorticosterone concentrations increased by 710% after 0.5 mg of LCI699 ($P < 0.0001$) and by 1427% after 1.0 mg of LCI699 ($P < 0.0001$). The plasma potassium concentration increased from 3.27 ± 0.31 to 4.03 ± 0.33 mmol/L ($P < 0.0001$) after only 1 week on 0.5 mg of LCI699. Twenty-four—hour ambulatory systolic blood pressure decreased by −4.1 mm Hg (95% CI: −8.1 to −0.1 mm Hg) after 4 weeks of treatment ($P = 0.046$). Basal plasma cortisol concentrations remained unchanged, whereas plasma adrenocorticotropic hormone concentrations increased by 35% after 0.5 mg of LCI699 ($P = 0.08$) and by 113% after 1.0 mg of LCI699 ($P < 0.0001$), and the plasma cortisol response to an adrenocorticotropic hormone test was blunted. All of the variables except plasma 11-deoxycorticosterone concentration returned to initial levels after the placebo. LCI699 was well tolerated. In conclusion, the administration of LCI699, up to 1.0 mg BID, effectively and safely inhibits aldosterone synthase in patients with primary aldosteronism. This 4-week treatment corrected the hypokalemia and mildly decreased blood pressure. The effects on the glucocorticoid axis were consistent with a latent inhibition of cortisol synthesis.

▶ The treatment of choice for patients with primary aldosteronism secondary to an aldosterone-secreting adenoma is adrenalectomy, while patients with bilateral hyperplasia benefit the most from medical treatment with mineralocorticoid receptor antagonists such as spironolactone and eplerenone. While these drugs are generally effective, both have potential side effects, including allergic reactions and hypokalemia if not carefully monitored. Amar et al introduce proof of concept for the use of aldo synthase inhibitors as a specific treatment for patients with primary aldosteronism. In a clinical trial of patients with aldosterone-secreting adenomas, 14 patients were selected from a large cohort of potential subjects for an open-label trial. Many of the other patients did not meet inclusion criteria or refused to participate. After a 2-week placebo lead-in period, patients received a low dose of drug for 2 weeks, followed by a high dose for 2 weeks and placebo for 1 week. As shown in Fig 1 in the original article, LC1699 caused a sustained dose-dependent decrease in plasma and urinary aldosterone concentration, increase in plasma 11-deoxycorticosterone, increase in serum potassium, and improvement of hypertension. The main target of this drug appears to be CYP11B2, but some effect is also anticipated on CYP11B1 because as also shown in Fig 1 in the original article, patients developed increases in plasma 11-deoxycortisol and adrenocorticotropic hormone (ACTH) levels, most likely as a result of partial suppression of CYP11B1. This is an important study because of the potential application of a drug like LC1699 to patients with primary aldosteronism secondary to bilateral hyperplasia as well as to patients with cardiac or renal disease in whom aldosterone excess may lead to fibrotic complications. Phase 3, comparative, controlled randomized clinical trials should follow. The future of this drug rests on whether it impairs cortisol secretion sufficiently to limit its usefulness as an aldosterone inhibitor. The data presented here suggest that the partial block is compensated by a feedback increase in ACTH secretion and maintenance of normal cortisol levels.

D. E. Schteingart, MD

Glucocorticoid Receptors/Glucocorticoid Sensitivity

Glucocorticoids in the prefrontal cortex enhance memory consolidation and impair working memory by a common neural mechanism
Barsegyan A, Mackenzie SM, Kurose BD, et al (Univ of Groningen, The Netherlands; Univ of California, Irvine)
Proc Natl Acad Sci U S A 107:16655-16660, 2010

It is well established that acute administration of adrenocortical hormones enhances the consolidation of memories of emotional experiences and, concurrently, impairs working memory. These different glucocorticoid effects on these two memory functions have generally been considered to be independently regulated processes. Here we report that a glucocorticoid receptor agonist administered into the medial prefrontal cortex (mPFC) of male Sprague-Dawley rats both enhances memory consolidation and impairs working memory. Both memory effects are mediated by activation of a membrane-bound steroid receptor and depend on noradrenergic activity within the mPFC to increase levels of cAMP-dependent protein kinase. These findings provide direct evidence that glucocorticoid effects on both memory consolidation and working memory share a common neural influence within them PFC.

▶ Glucocorticoids (GCs) have direct brain effects and have been shown to induce hippocampal structure and function changes affecting memory in both experimental animals and people on corticosteroid therapy, endogenous Cushing syndrome, and depression. GCs can affect other brain areas such as the prefrontal cortex and cause alteration in different types of memory in a complex manner. For example, GCs impair working memory but enhance memory consolidation. Barsegyan et al dissected the mechanism of this effect of GCs on the prefrontal cortex in male rats and show that the changes in these 2 types of memory are linked by common nongenomic mechanisms involving activation of a noradrenergic and protein kinase A (PKA) signaling pathway. While these observations suggest that GC antagonists, β-adrenoceptor antagonists, and PKA inhibitors may be used to treat prefrontal cortex cognitive dysfunction during chronic stress, aging, or other pathological conditions, the fact the 2 types of memory are interdependent and in opposite directions could result in further impairment of cognitive function.

D. E. Schteingart, MD

Cushing's Disease: Diagnosis and Treatment

Systematic Analysis of G Protein-Coupled Receptor Gene Expression in Adrenocorticotropin-Independent Macronodular Adrenocortical Hyperplasia Identifies Novel Targets for Pharmacological Control of Adrenal Cushing's Syndrome

Assie G, Louiset E, Sturm N, et al (Université Paris Descartes, France; Univ of Rouen, Mont Saint Aignan, France; Centre Hospitalier Universitaire Albert Michallon, Grenoble, France; et al)

J Clin Endocrinol Metab 95:E253-E262, 2010

Context.—Stimulation of cortisol secretion through abnormally expressed G protein-coupled receptors (GPCRs) is a frequent feature of ACTH-independent macronodular adrenal hyperplasia (AIMAH). This has opened a pharmacological strategy that targets GPCRs for the treatment of Cushing's syndrome in AIMAH. However, only few drugs are available for the presently described GPCRs.

Objective.—The objective of the study was to identify new GPCR targets for the pharmacological treatment of adrenal Cushing's syndrome.

Design and Patients.—We designed a cDNA chip containing 865 nucleotidic sequences of GPCRs. mRNAs were extracted from three normal adrenals, 18 AIMAHs, four adrenals from Cushing's disease patients, and 13 cortisol-secreting adenomas. A set of GPCR mRNAs that showed significantly higher or lower expression in AIMAH than in normal adrenal were studied by quantitative RT-PCR analysis. Analysis of protein expression and function were performed on selected GPCRs.

Setting.—The study was conducted at a tertiary care center and basic research laboratories.

Results.—The ACTH MC2 receptor showed a low expression in 15 of 18 AIMAHs samples, whereas several previously undescribed GPCR genes were found highly expressed in a subset of AIMAH, such as the receptors for motilin (MLNR; three of 18 AIMAHs) and γ-aminobutyric acid (GABBR1; five of 18 AIMAHs), and the α2A adrenergic receptor (ADRA2A; 13 of 18 AIMAHs), on which we focused our attention. Western blot and immunochemistry analyses showed expression of ADRA2A protein in AIMAH but not in normal adrenal cortex. The ADRA2A agonist clonidine enhanced both basal and stimulated cortisol production. Clonidine-induced increase in basal cortisol levels was blocked by the ADRA2A antagonist yohimbine.

Conclusion.—ADRA2A is a potential target for pharmacological treatment of Cushing's syndrome linked to AIMAH.

▶ Patients with Cushing syndrome secondary to adrenocorticotropic hormone (ACTH)-independent macronodular adrenocortical hyperplasia (AIMAH) have expression of G protein-coupled ectopic receptors in their adrenal glands. Ligands to these receptors have been shown to regulate cortisol secretion independently of ACTH. While bilateral adrenalectomy is the definitive treatment for those patients, some patients have been treated pharmacologically with drugs that inhibit the specific receptor. Assie et al conducted a systematic analysis of G protein-coupled receptor gene expression using specially designed gene chips in 18 adrenal glands with AIMAH and compared them with 3 normal adrenals, 4 adrenals from patients with pituitary ACTH-dependent Cushing, and 13 cortisol-secreting adenomas. They found receptors for motilin and γ-aminobutyric acid in the AIMAH adrenals, and specifically α2A adrenergic receptors. These receptors were exclusively overexpressed in AIMAH and not in the glands used as control. The importance of this finding is the possibility of treatment of these patients with adrenergic receptor blockers.

D. E. Schteingart, MD

Glucocorticoid-Induced Autophagy in Osteocytes
Xia X, Kar R, Gluhak-Heinrich J, et al (Univ of Texas Health Science Ctr, San Antonio; et al)
J Bone Miner Res 25:2479-2488, 2010

Glucocorticoid (GC) therapy is the most frequent cause of secondary osteoporosis. In this study we have demonstrated that GC treatment induced the development of autophagy, preserving osteocyte viability. GC treatment resulted in an increase in autophagy markers and the accumulation of autophagosome vacuoles in vitro and in vivo promoted the onset of the osteocyte autophagy, as determined by expression of autophagy markers in an animal model of GC-induced osteoporosis. An autophagy inhibitor reversed the protective effects of GCs. The effects of GCs on osteocytes were in contrast to tumor necrosis factor α (TNF-α), which induced apoptosis but not autophagy. Together this study reveals a novel mechanism for the effect of GC on osteocytes, shedding new insight into mechanisms responsible for bone loss in patients receiving GC therapy.

▶ Osteoporosis is a frequent complication of long-term corticosteroid therapy or severe Cushing disease. The mechanism for the loss of bone mineral density is complex and involves a loss of bone matrix because of the protein catabolic effect of glucocorticoids (GCs), interference with calcium absorption because of the inhibitory effect of GC on vitamin D intestinal action, and direct GC effects on osteoblasts and osteocytes, possibly inducing apoptosis. Xia et al show in an elegant study that GC can induce autophagy as a means of protecting osteocytes, but, ultimately, this mechanism leads to destruction of osteocytes. Autophagy is a basic biological response essential for cell growth, survival, differentiation, development, and homeostasis. It can protect cells from apoptosis by removing oxidatively damaged organelles, but excessive autophagy can lead to cell death. Using osteocyte cell cultures, they showed that dexamethasone decreases cell number or proliferation, and this effect is not mediated by significant apoptosis but by induction of formation of mature autophagic vacuoles. Autophagy may have an initial protective effect on oste-ocytes, but, with chronic GC exposure, autophagy leads to cell death and loss of bone mass.

D. E. Schteingart, MD

Pheochromocytomas: Diagnosis and Treatment

Functional and Oncologic Outcomes of Partial Adrenalectomy for Pheochromocytoma in Patients With von Hippel-Lindau Syndrome After at Least 5 Years of Followup
Benhammou JN, Boris RS, Pacak K, et al (Natl Insts of Health, Bethesda, MD)
J Urol 184:1855-1859, 2010

Purpose.—Although the safety and feasibility of partial adrenalectomy in patients with von Hippel-Lindau syndrome have been established, long-term outcomes have not been examined. In this study we evaluate the recurrence and functional outcomes in a von Hippel-Lindau syndrome cohort treated for pheochromocytoma with partial adrenalectomy with a followup of at least 5 years.

Materials and Methods.—We reviewed the records of patients with von Hippel-Lindau syndrome treated with partial adrenalectomy for pheo-chromocytoma at the National Cancer Institute. Demographic, germline mutation status, surgical indication, oncologic and functional outcome data were collected. Local recurrence was defined as radiographic evidence of recurrent tumor on the ipsilateral side of partial adrenalectomy. Patients were considered steroid dependent if they required steroids at most recent followup.

Results.—A total of 36 partial adrenalectomies for pheochromocytoma were performed in 26 patients with von Hippel-Lindau syndrome between September 1995 and December 2003. Of these cases 23 were performed open and 13 were performed laparoscopically. Prior surgical history was obtained for all patients. At a median followup of 9.25 years (range 5 to 46) metastatic pheochromocytoma had not developed in any patients. In 3 patients (11%) there were 5 local recurrences treated with surgical extirpation or active surveillance. All recurrences were asymptomatic and detected by radiographic imaging on followup. In addition, 3 of 26 patients (11%) subse-quently required partial adrenalectomy for pheochromocytoma on the contra-lateral adrenal gland. In the entire cohort only 3 patients became steroid dependent (11%).

Conclusions.—Outcomes of partial adrenalectomy in patients with von Hippel-Lindau syndrome with pheochromocytoma are encouraging at long-term followup and should be recommended as a primary surgical approach whenever possible. Adrenal sparing surgery can obviate the need for steroid replacement in the majority of patients. Local recurrence rates appear to be infrequent and can be managed successfully with subsequent observation or intervention.

▶ Patients with von Hippel-Lindau (VHL) syndrome often have bilateral pheochromocytoma requiring bilateral adrenalectomy. The result is adrenal insufficiency requiring permanent steroid replacement. A possible alternative is partial adrenalectomy preserving part of the adrenal cortex, but there remains the possibility that the adrenal cortex will not be fully functional. Benhammou et al from the National Institutes of Health review the results of 36 partial adrenalectomies for pheochromocytoma in 26 patients with VHL syndrome. Surgery was performed laparoscopically in about half of the cases. Long-term steroid replacement was required in only 11%. One of the concerns in this type of patient is recurrence if the primary resection is not complete. Again, only 11% of the patients had recurrences requiring total adrenalectomy. It appears that adrenal sparing surgery in these patients can be effective in preserving adrenal cortical function with minimal risk of recurrent disease.

D. E. Schteingart, MD

Autoimmunity and Addison's Disease

Addison's Disease in Women Is a Risk Factor for an Adverse Pregnancy Outcome

Björnsdottir S, Cnattingius S, Brandt L, et al (Karolinska Institutet, Stockholm, Sweden; et al)
J Clin Endocrinol Metab 95:5249-5257, 2010

Context.—Autoimmune Addison's disease (AAD) tends to affect young and middle-aged women. It is not known whether the existence of undiagnosed or diagnosed AAD influences the outcome of pregnancy.

Objective.—The aim of the study was to compare the number of children and pregnancy outcomes in individuals with AAD and controls.

Design and Setting.—We conducted a population-based historical cohort study in Sweden.

Patients.—Through the Swedish National Patient Register and the Total Population Register, we identified 1,188 women with AAD and 11,879 age-matched controls who delivered infants between 1973 and 2006.

Main Outcome Measures.—We measured parity and pregnancy outcome.

Results.—Adjusted odds ratios (ORs) for infants born to mothers with deliveries 3 yr or less before the diagnosis of AAD were 2.40 [95% confidence interval (CI), 1.27−4.53] for preterm birth ($\leq$37 wk), 3.50 (95% CI, 1.83−6.67) for low birth weight (<2500 g), and 1.74 (95% CI, 1.02−2.96) for cesarean section. Compared to controls, women who gave birth after their AAD diagnosis were at increased risk of both cesarean delivery (adjusted OR, 2.35; 95% CI, 1.68−3.27) and preterm delivery (adjusted OR, 2.61; 95% CI, 1.69−4.05). Stratifying by isolated AAD and concomitant type 1 diabetes and/or autoimmune thyroid disease in the mother did not essentially influence these risks. There were no differences in risks of congenital malformations or infant death. Women with AAD had a reduced overall parity compared to controls ($P < 0.001$).

Conclusion.—Clinically undiagnosed and diagnosed AAD both entail increased risks of unfavorable pregnancy outcomes. AAD also influences the number of childbirths.

▶ Taking advantage of a comprehensive register, Bjornsdottir et al examined all the patients in Sweden with autoimmune Addison disease (AAD) between 1973 and 2006 for evidence of adverse pregnancy outcomes. They identified 1188 women with AAD and compared them with 11 879 age-matched controls who delivered during that period. Adjusted odds ratios for women who delivered 3 or less years before diagnosis were 2.4 for preterm birth, 3.5 for low-birth weight, 1.7 for cesarean section and for those who delivered after diagnosis, 2.6 for preterm birth, and 2.3 for cesarean section. The data are impressive in terms of the number of patients examined but leave many questions the registry is unable to answer. The health status of women who became pregnant prior to diagnosis and the adequacy of treatment of those whose diagnosis had already been established. These are limitations of the registry. The management of patients with AAD has evolved over the 40 years the data was collected, and most pregnant women with those conditions are currently being followed up in high-risk pregnancy clinics where replacement is monitored and adjusted on an ongoing basis. Perhaps preterm birth and cesarean section can be avoided in these patients with better endocrine care.

D. E. Schteingart, MD

Miscellaneous

Insulin resistance and metabolic syndrome in patients with nonfunctioning adrenal incidentalomas: a cause-effect relationship?

Peppa M, Boutati E, Koliaki C, et al (Attikon Univ Hosp, Athens, Greece)
Metabolism 59:1435-1441, 2010

The objective of the study was to assess insulin resistance (IR) and metabolic syndrome (MS) in patients with nonfunctioning adrenal incidentalomas (NFAIs). Among a total cohort of 46 patients with adrenal incidentalomas, we studied 29 patients with NFAIs (mean age, 54 ± 9 years; body mass index, 29 ± 3 kg/m^2) and 37 age-, sex-, and body mass index—matched healthy controls. Besides the endocrine workup, IR was evaluated using fasting glucose and insulin concentrations, homeostasis model assessment of IR, and quantitative insulin sensitivity check index. In a subgroup of patients undergoing an oral glucose tolerance test, Matsuda index and total area under the curve for glucose and insulin were also evaluated. Total cholesterol, high-density lipoprotein, low-density lipoprotein, triglycerides, and other biochemical parameters were measured with standard techniques. Body composition was determined with dual-energy x-ray absorptiometry. Patients with NFAIs exhibited higher fasting glucose, insulin, and homeostasis model assessment of IR values; decreased quantitative insulin sensitivity check index and Matsuda index; and an increased—although not statistically significant—area under the curve for glucose and insulin compared with controls ($P < .05$). In addition, they exhibited higher systolic and diastolic blood pressure, triglycerides, and γ-glutamyltransferase and lower high-density lipoprotein cholesterol levels compared with controls ($P < .05$). Patients with NFAIs were all obese with a central type of fat accumulation and increased appendicular lean mass. Indices of IR showed a positive correlation with indices of MS ($P < .05$), but no correlation with markers of hormonal activity. Nonfunctioning adrenal incidentalomas are characterized by IR, hypertension, dyslipidemia, and fatty liver disease, all of them being components of MS. Thus, patients with NFAIs should be screened for MS during their initial workup to identify those at cardiometabolic risk and implement the appropriate interventions.

▶ The main concern about incidentally discovered adrenal masses is whether they are malignant or hormone secreting. Some of these masses present with subclinical syndromes, the result of autonomous hormone secretion by the tumor. There is general agreement that malignant or functioning masses should be surgically removed. The question is the significance of so-called nonfunctioning adrenal masses, that is, if they are truly nonfunctioning, or whether it's a matter of how one defines function and if they are associated with clinical or metabolic comorbidities that may be reversed by adrenalectomy. Peppa et al from Athens studied insulin sensitivity and features of the metabolic syndrome in 29 patients with nonfunctioning adrenal incidentalomas. They found that these patients had higher fasting glucose and insulin levels and decreased insulin sensitivity values, in addition to higher systolic and diastolic blood pressures and triglyceride levels and lower high-density lipoprotein cholesterol levels than age-, sex-, and body mass index-matched controls. Of interest is that these patients had normal hormonal profiles, but the metabolic changes resolved after adrenalectomy. The possibility that the nonfunctioning masses may produce subclinically abnormal levels of cortisol and aldosterone was previously suggested by another group from Athens in an article we reviewed in the 2010 edition of YearBooks. Piaditis et al[1] established new cutoff limits for the testing of adrenal function and concluded that many patients with nonfunctioning incidentalomas had excessive cortisol and aldosterone secretions. These studies raise an interesting and provocative proposition with potential implication in the management of nonfunctioning incidentally discovered adrenal masses. Should these patients undergo adrenalectomy?

D. E. Schteingart, MD

Reference

1. Piaditis GP, Kaltsas GA, Androulakis II, et al. High prevalence of autonomous cortisol and aldosterone secretion from adrenal adenomas. *Clin Endocrinol (Oxf)*. 2009;71:772-778.

7 Reproductive Endocrinology

Introduction

This year's selections include many citations related to menopause, aging, metabolic syndrome, hypogonaidism in men, and hormonal influences on bone metabolism.

In the articles on pediatric reproductive endocrinology, Coutani et al provide evidence for distinguishing delayed puberty from constitutional delay using inhibin B and anti-Mullerian hormone. An approach for diagnosing constitutional delay or hypogonadotrophic hypogonadism was proposed by Grinspon.

Female reproductive endocrinology is introduced with an article in which diagnosing ovarian reserve with the use of inhibin B, anti-Mullerian hormone (AMH), and FSH has potential for assessment of fertility and can be made particularly with AMH, according to Sowers et al. Hagen et al also provide evidence for AMH for assessing ovarian reserve in women with PCOS and Turner's syndrome. The relative influences of estradiol-17β and raloxifene on the response of growth hormone replacement therapy was investigated by Birzniece et al.

In the first of 2 articles on bone health, Eisman et al showed benefits of osteoporosis in women treated with odanacatib, but the benefits were reversed in 1 year after discontinuing therapy. The study by Modder et al confirmed that estrogen produced from testosterone suppresses bone resorption.

The topic of polycystic ovary syndrome (PCOS) includes 6 studies. Ovulation induction was investigated by Partagni et al to determine the beneficial influence of finasteride, a 5ħ-reductase inhibitor, on FSH and hCG induced ovulation. Both nonclassical adrenal hyperplasia from 21-hydroxylase deficiency and PCOS are common. Pall et al suggest that measurement of 17-hydroxyprogesterone during the follicular phase of the menstrual cycle has merit in diagnosing nonclassical adrenal hyperplasia. Alterations in glucose metabolism and impaired insulin responsiveness are common in PCOS. Karakas et al provide evidence that patients with both impaired fasting glucose and impaired glucose tolerance have both hepatic and peripheral insulin resistance. Candidate genes for PCOS have evaded investigators, but Ewers et al suggest they are closing in on the genes causing PCOS. Women with PCOS are usually not estrogen deficient and have excess androgens compared to normal women. Kassanos et al provide evidence that women with PCOS have better bone quality and more protection from osteoporosis. While it is well known that women with PCOS have elevated androgens beginning with menarche, less is known about persistence of elevated androgen during menopause. The study by Markopulos et al confirms that hyperandrogenism persists with menopause.

In the male reproductive function and prostate disease section, men with lower serum testosterone concentration were associated with higher risk of mortality, but the causal relationship was not determined. The prostate is an androgen-responsive organ, but Linstrom et al did not find a significant relationship between CAG repeats and prostate cancer. Prolactin is locally made in the prostate and Rouet et al showed that in a mouse model a prolactin-receptor antagonist inhibited early stages of prostate cancer development. Bonde et al found an association between BMI and lower serum testosterone, sex hormone binding globulin, and inhibin concentrations. In contrast to other studies, semen quality was not compromised by BMI. Serum estrogen concentrations are higher in obese compared with normal-weight men. Hammound et al observed that aromatase polymorphism modulated the relationship between body weight and serum estradiol concentrations in obese men. Birth weight was positively associated with serum testosterone concentrations in adults independent of adult weight or fat mass, based on the study of Vanbillemont et al.

While testosterone replacement therapy benefits depressed mood, depression, low energy, depressed libido, and sense of well-being, Pope et al were able to confirm benefits in many but not all men.

A. Wayne Meikle, MD

Pediatric Reproductive Endocrinology

Baseline Inhibin B and Anti-Mullerian Hormone Measurements for Diagnosis of Hypogonadotropic Hypogonadism (HH) in Boys with Delayed Puberty

Coutant R, Biette-Demeneix E, Bouvattier C, et al (Angers Univ Hosp, France; General Hosp, Frejus, France; St Vincent de Paul Hosp and René Descartes Univ, Paris, France)

J Clin Endocrinol Metab 95:5225-5232, 2010

Context.—The diagnosis of isolated hypogonadotropic hypogonadism (IHH) in boys with delayed puberty is challenging, as may be the diagnosis of hypogonadotropic hypogonadism (HH) in boys with combined pituitary hormone deficiency (CPHD). Yet, the therapeutic choices for puberty induction depend on accurate diagnosis and may influence future fertility.

Objective.—The aim was to assess the utility of baseline inhibin B (INHB) and anti-Mullerian hormone (AMH) measurements to discriminate HH from constitutional delay of puberty (CDP). Both hormones are produced

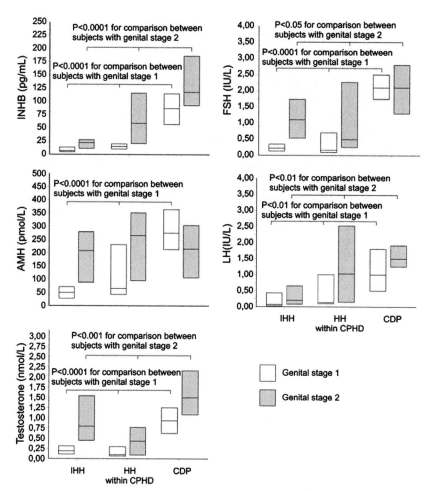

FIGURE 1.—Median and interquartile ranges for INHB (*left upper panel*), AMH (*left middle panel*), T (*left lower panel*), FSH (*right upper panel*), and LH (*right lower panel*) according to the genital stage. Genital stage 1 (testis < 3 ml), *white boxes*. Genital stage 2 (testis, 3–6 ml), *gray boxes*. Comparisons between IHH, HH within CPHD, and CDP were performed according to the genital stage using Kruskal-Wallis tests for multiple groups comparison. For T, to convert to nanograms per milliliter, divide by 3.47; for AMH, to convert to nanograms per milliliter, divide by 7.14. For interpretation of the references to color in this figure legend, the reader is referred to web version of this article. (Reprinted from Coutant R, Biette-Demeneix E, Bouvattier C, et al. Baseline inhibin B and anti-Mullerian hormone measurements for diagnosis of hypogonadotropic hypogonadism (HH) in boys with delayed puberty. *J Clin Endocrinol Metab*. 2010;95:5225-5232. Copyright © [2010], The Endocrine Society.)

by Sertoli cells upon FSH stimulation. Moreover, prepubertal AMH levels are high as a reflection of Sertoli cell integrity.

Patients.—We studied 82 boys aged 14 to 18 yr with pubertal delay: 16 had IHH, 15 congenital HH within CPHD, and 51 CDP, as confirmed by follow-up. Subjects were genital stage 1 (testis volume <3 ml; 9 IHH, 7 CPHD, and 23 CDP) or early stage 2 (testis volume, 3–6 ml; 7 IHH, 8 CPHD, and 28 CDP).

Results.—Age and testis volume were similar in the three groups. Compared with CDP subjects, IHH and CPHD subjects had lower INHB, testosterone, FSH, and LH concentrations ($P < 0.05$), whereas AMH concentration was lower only in IHH and CPHD subjects with genital stage 1, likely reflecting a smaller pool of Sertoli cells in profound HH. In IHH and CPHD boys with genital stage 1, sensitivity and specificity were 100% for INHB concentration of 35 pg/ml or less. In IHH and CPHD boys with genital stage 2, sensitivities were 86 and 80%, whereas specificities were 92 and 88%, respectively, for an INHB concentration of 65 pg/ml or less. The performance of testosterone, AMH, FSH, and LH measurements was lower. No combination or ratio of hormones performed better than INHB alone.

Conclusion.—Discrimination of HH from CDP with baseline INHB measurement was excellent in subjects with genital stage 1 and fair in subjects with genital stage 2 (Fig 1).

▶ Delayed puberty occurs in approximately 2% of boys at 14 years of age. Distinguishing between constitutional delay of puberty (CDP) and isolated hypogonadotropic hypogonadism (IHH) in boys is difficult, and these disorders exhibit comparable baseline serum testosterone and gonadotropins. Several tests to distinguish them have been met with variable success, including lutenising hormone (LH) and prolactin responses to gonadotropin-releasing hormone (GnRH), testosterone responses to human chorionic gonadotropin, and daily urinary excretion of follicle-stimulating hormone (FSH) and LH. Coutant et al used inhibin B (from the Sertoli cell), testosterone and anti-Mullerian hormone, which are secreted by the Leydig cells, and LH and FSH in an attempt to correctly diagnose these 2 disorders. As shown in Fig 1, there was no overlap of inhibin B concentrations in boys with CDP during genital stage 1 when compared with boys with IHH and hypogonadotropic hypogonadism with combined pituitary hormone deficiency. The distinction of concentration of inhibin B in boys at genital stage 2 with CDP was less precise but still good in leading to a correct diagnosis of CDP. These observations require confirmation, but the testing with inhibin B would be most welcome and greatly simplify correctly diagnosing CDP.

A. W. Meikle, MD

Basal Follicle-Stimulating Hormone and Peak Gonadotropin Levels after Gonadotropin-Releasing Hormone Infusion Show High Diagnostic Accuracy in Boys with Suspicion of Hypogonadotropic Hypogonadism
Grinspon RP, Ropelato MG, Gottlieb S, et al (Hospital de Niños R. Gutiérrez, Buenos Aires, Argentina)
J Clin Endocrinol Metab 95:2811-2818, 2010

Context.—Differential diagnosis between hypogonadotropic hypogonadism (HH) and constitutional delay of puberty in boys is challenging.

Most tests use an acute GnRH stimulus, allowing only the release of previously synthesized gonadotropins. A constant GnRH infusion, inducing *de novo* gonadotropin synthesis, may allow a better discrimination.

Objective.—We evaluated the diagnostic accuracy of basal and peak gonadotropins after GnRH infusion, measured by ultrasensitive assays, to confirm the diagnosis in boys with suspected HH.

Design and Setting.—We conducted a validation study following Standards for Reporting of Diagnostic Accuracy criteria at a tertiary public hospital.

Patients and Methods.—A GnRH iv infusion test was performed in 32 boys. LH and FSH were determined by immunofluorometric assay at 0—120 min.

Diagnosis Ascertainment.—The following diagnoses were ascertained: complete HH (n = 19; testes < 4 ml at 18 yr), partial HH (n = 6; testes enlargement remained arrested for ≥1 yr or did not reach 15 ml), and constitutional delay of puberty (n = 7; testes ≥ 15 ml at 18 yr).

Main Outcome Measures.—Sensitivity, specificity, positive and negative predictive values, and diagnostic efficiency were assessed.

Results.—Basal FSH less than 1.2 IU/liter confirmed HH with specificity of 1.00 (95% confidence interval = 0.59—1.00), rendering GnRH infusion unnecessary. In patients with basal FSH of at least 1.2 IU/liter, the coexistence of peak FSH less than 4.6 IU/liter and peak LH less than 5.8 IU/liter

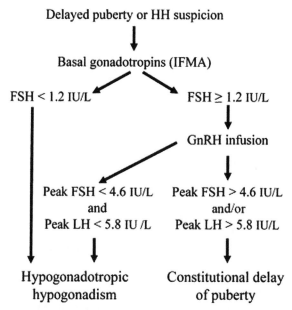

FIGURE 4.—Algorithm proposed for the evaluation of male patients with delayed puberty or suspicion of HH. (Reprinted from Grinspon RP, Ropelato MG, Gottlieb S, et al. Basal follicle-stimulating hormone and peak gonadotropin levels after gonadotropin-releasing hormone infusion show high diagnostic accuracy in boys with suspicion of hypogonadotropic hypogonadism. *J Clin Endocrinol Metab.* 2010;95:2811-2818. Copyright © 2010, The Endocrine Society.)

after GnRH infusion had high specificity (1.00; 95% confidence interval = 0.59—1.00) and diagnostic efficiency (76.9%) for HH.

Conclusions.—Basal FSH less than 1.2 IU/liter confirms HH, which precludes from further testing, reducing patient discomfort and healthcare system costs. In patients with basal FSH of at least 1.2 IU/liter, a GnRH infusion test has a high diagnostic efficiency (Fig 4).

▶ Pubertal delay in boys is at approximately age 14 years and affects about 2.5%. Constitutional delay of puberty (CDP) is not a pathological disorder and requires distinction from hypogonadotropic hypogonadism (HH) caused by pathological conditions. The differential diagnosis between HH and CDP is difficult, and basal gonadotropin and serum testosterone measurements usually do not resolve the issue. The study used the measurement of luteinizing hormone (LH) and follicle-stimulating hormone (FSH) following an infusion of gonadotropin releasing hormone (GnRH). They reported that a basal FSH of <1.2 IU/L confirmed HH, and further testing was not required. If the basal FSH was >1.2 IU/L with a peak FSH <4.6 IU/L and LH <5.8 IU/L after the GnRH infusion, the results strongly favored HH. While the distinction between CDP and HH the clinical outcome is the gold standard and any misdiagnoses are determined by the clinical outcome, there are social issues with boys with either HH or CDP that are critical for the child and the parents. Having a test with high reliability for this distinction will benefit both the clinician and child as well as parents.

A. W. Meikle, MD

Female Reproductive Function and Menopause

Anti-Müllerian hormone and inhibin B variability during normal menstrual cycles
Sowers M, McConnell D, Gast K, et al (Univ of Michigan, Ann Arbor)
Fertil Steril 94:1482-1486, 2010

Objective.—To describe anti-Müllerian hormone (AMH) variation across normal menstrual cycles.

Design.—Cohort study.

Setting.—Academic environment.

Patient(s).—Twenty regularly menstruating women.

Intervention(s).—Serum AMH and inhibin B assayed daily during one normal menstrual cycle.

Main Outcome Measure(s).—Intracycle variability of AMH and inhibin B.

Result(s).—Data were classified into quartiles of AMH area-under-the-curve (AUCs). Mean AMH AUC was 15.7 ng/mL for quartile 1 versus 43.5, 80.9 and 144.9 ng/mL for quartiles 2, 3, and 4. Mean AMH levels (ng/mL) were 0.67, 1.71, 3.02, and 5.33, respectively. There was no variation in quartile 1 AMH rate of change from stochastic modeling, but in quartiles 2 to 4, there were increased rates of change in days 2 to 7. Women in

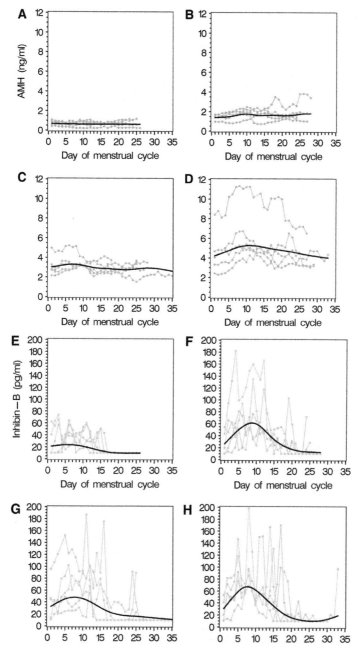

FIGURE 1.—Mean AMH (top panel, **A–D**) and inhibin B (bottom panel, **E–H**) across the menstrual cycle in 20 women, according to quartiles of their AMH AUC. Black solid line is the spline smoothed mean values and the cyan dashed lines are individual profiles. (Reprinted from Sowers M, McConnell D, Gast K, et al. Anti-Müllerian hormone and inhibin B variability during normal menstrual cycles. *Fertil Steril.* 2010;94:1482-1486, with permission from American Society for Reproductive Medicine.)

quartile 1 had the lowest mean inhibin B (24.2 pg/mL vs. 44.3, 43.2, and 42.2 pg/mL), and had shorter menstrual cycles (24.6 days) than women in quartiles 3 and 4 (28.2 and 28.4 days).

Conclusion(s).—There were two menstrual cycle patterns of AMH. The "aging ovary" pattern included low AMH levels with little variation, lower inhibin B, and shorter cycle lengths. The "younger ovary" pattern included higher AMH levels with significant variation days 2 to 7, suggesting that for women with AMH > 1 ng/mL, the interpretation of AMH levels is contingent upon the day of the menstrual cycle on which the specimen is obtained (Fig1).

▶ Ovarian reserve is used clinically to assess potential fertility and treatment as well as approach of ovarian failure. Follicle stimulating hormone, inhibin B, and anti-Müllerian hormone (AMH) have been the main biomarkers in the assessment. Of these, AMH has emerged as the most promising because it has less menstrual cycle variability and declines with age. Sowers et al indicated that based on these biomarkers, there were 2 menstrual cycle patterns of AMH. One was an aging pattern with lower AMH and inhibin B and a short cycle length. The younger ovary pattern was characterized by higher AMH with more variation during days 2 to 7 of the cycle. Their findings are in agreement with other reports that women with low AMH are approaching menopause, despite continued regular cycles. Further observation is needed to apply AMH and inhibin B in clinical practice to assess the fertility potential, treatment guides, and approach of menopause in women.

A. W. Meikle, MD

Serum Levels of Anti-Müllerian Hormone as a Marker of Ovarian Function in 926 Healthy Females from Birth to Adulthood and in 172 Turner Syndrome Patients

Hagen CP, Aksglaede L, Sørensen K, et al (Copenhagen Univ Hosp, Denmark; et al)
J Clin Endocrinol Metab 95:5003-5010, 2010

Context.—In adult women, anti-Müllerian hormone (AMH) is related to the ovarian follicle pool. Little is known about AMH in girls.

Objective.—The objective of the study was to provide a reference range for AMH in girls and adolescents and to evaluate AMH as a marker of ovarian function.

Setting.—The study was conducted at a tertiary referral center for pediatric endocrinology.

Main Outcome Measures.—We measured AMH in 926 healthy females (longitudinal values during infancy) as well as in 172 Turner syndrome (TS) patients according to age, karyotype (A: 45,X; B: miscellaneous karyotypes; C: 45,X/46,XX), and ovarian function (1: absent puberty; 2: cessation of ovarian function; 3: ongoing ovarian function).

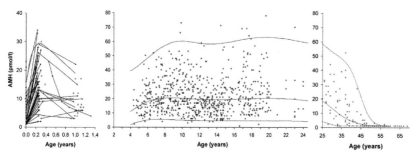

FIGURE 1.—Serum AMH (picomoles per liter) in 926 healthy infants, girls, adolescents, and adult women. Longitudinal values during infancy are connected with *black lines*. The *red curves* represent the median, the 2.5th percentile, and the 97.5th percentile. For interpretation of the references to color in this figure legend, the reader is referred to web version of this article. (Reprinted from Hagen CP, Aksglaede L, Sørensen K, et al. Serum levels of anti-Müllerian hormone as a marker of ovarian function in 926 healthy females from birth to adulthood and in 172 turner syndrome patients. *J Clin Endocrinol Metab.* 2010;95:5003-5010. Copyright © [2010], The Endocrine Society.)

Results.—AMH was undetectable in 54% (38 of 71) of cord blood samples (<2; <2—15 pmol/liter) (median; 2.5th to 97.5th percentile) and increased in all (37 of 37) infants from birth to 3 months (15; 4.5—29.5 pmol/liter). From 8 to 25 yr, AMH levels were stable (19.9; 4.7—60.1 pmol/liter), with the lower level of the reference range clearly above the detection limit. AMH levels were associated with TS-karyotype groups (median A *vs.* B: <2 *vs.* 3 pmol/liter, $P = 0.044$; B *vs.* C: 3 *vs.* 16 pmol/liter, $P < 0.001$) as well as with ovarian function (absent puberty *vs.* cessation of ovarian function: <2 *vs.* 6 pmol/liter, $P = 0.004$; cessation of ovarian function *vs.* ongoing ovarian function: 6 *vs.* 14 pmol/liter, $P = 0.001$). As a screening test of premature ovarian failure in TS, the sensitivity and specificity of AMH less than 8 pmol/liter was 96 and 86%, respectively.

Conclusion.—AMH seems to be a promising marker of ovarian function in healthy girls and TS patients (Fig 1).

▶ Anti-Mullerian hormone (AMH) is synthesized by primary and preantral ovarian follicles. Evidence supports AMH as an assessment of follicle reserve and follicle mass in women with polycystic ovary syndrome. The study by Hagen et al was unique in that it evaluated AMH in females from birth to adulthood and also in patients with Turner syndrome who have ovarian dysfunction resulting from having complete or partial absence of the second X chromosome. Other markers of ovarian reserve have included follicle-stimulating hormone (FSH) and inhibin, but AMH has been shown to be a better predictor. They confirmed that AMH is a sensitive indicator of ovarian failure. In addition to predicting ovarian reserved in postpubertal and premenopausal normal females, they observed for the first time a marked increase in AMH in girls from birth to 3 months of age. They hypothesize that the rising levels of AMH during the minipuberty might be an ovarian response to prevent FSH-induced follicle growth when further differentiation of follicles would be unwanted. AMH levels did not change in childhood and adolescence but did show large fluctuation in concentrations between females of comparable age.

A. W. Meikle, MD

Modulatory Effect of Raloxifene and Estrogen on the Metabolic Action of Growth Hormone in Hypopituitary Women

Birzniece V, Meinhardt U, Gibney J, et al (St Vincent's Hosp, Sydney, New South Wales, Australia; et al)
J Clin Endocrinol Metab 95:2099-2106, 2010

Context.—The metabolic action of GH is attenuated by estrogens administered via the oral route. Selective estrogen receptor modulators lower IGF-I to a lesser degree than 17β-estradiol in GH-deficient women, and their effect on fat and protein metabolism is unknown.

Objective.—The aim of the study was to compare the modulatory effects of 17β-estradiol and raloxifene, a selective estrogen receptor modulator, on the metabolic action of GH.

Design.—We conducted an open-label, two-group, randomized, two-period crossover study.

Patients and Intervention.—Ten hypopituitary women received GH therapy alone (0.5 mg/d) and GH plus 17β-estradiol (E_2; 2 mg/d). Eleven hypopituitary women received GH therapy alone and GH plus raloxifene (R; 60 mg/d). The treatment duration was 1 month, with a 4-wk washout period.

Main Outcome Measures.—IGF-I, IGFBP-3, resting energy expenditure, and fat oxidation were quantified by indirect calorimetry. We measured whole body leucine turnover from which leucine rate of appearance and leucine incorporation into protein were estimated.

Results.—GH significantly stimulated all outcome measures. During GH treatment, addition of R significantly reduced mean IGF-I but not IGFBP-3, whereas E_2 reduced both IGF-I and IGFBP-3 levels. Cotreatment with R but not E_2 significantly attenuated the stimulatory effects of GH on fat oxidation. There was a strong trend ($P = 0.08$) toward a greater reduction in leucine incorporation into protein after R compared to E_2 cotreatment.

Conclusions.—The modulatory effects of E_2 and R at therapeutic doses on GH action are different. R during GH therapy exerts a greater inhibitory effect on lipid oxidation and protein anabolism compared to E_2 (Fig 2).

▶ Growth hormone (GH) deficiency in postpubertal persons results in a reduction in muscle and bone mass and an increase in body fat by reducing fat oxidation. These adverse metabolic effects are reversed by GH replacement therapy. Orally administered estrogen suppresses serum insulin-like growth factor 1 (IGF-1) concentrations by reducing the liver's production in response to GH and reduces body fat oxidation and protein synthesis. The study by Birzniece et al compared the effects of oral estradiol-17β with raloxifene, a selective

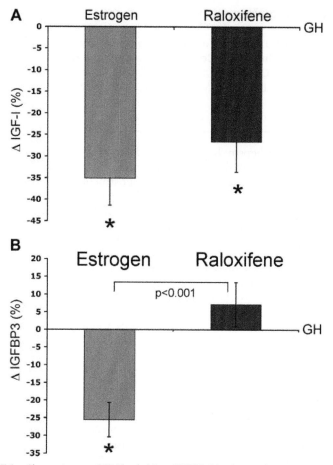

FIGURE 2.—Changes in serum IGF-I levels (A) and IGFBP-3 levels (B) in hypopituitary women after 4 wk of GH (0.5 mg/d) cotreatment with 17β-estradiol (2 mg/d) and raloxifene (60 mg/d). Data are presented as percentage change from GH treatment alone and expressed as means ± SEM. *, $P < 0.01$ compared with GH treatment alone using paired comparison. Between-group differences were analyzed using unpaired comparison. (Reprinted from Birzniece V, Meinhardt U, Gibney J, et al. Modulatory effect of raloxifene and estrogen on the metabolic action of growth hormone in hypopituitary women. *J Clin Endocrinol Metab*. 2010;95:2099-2106. Copyright © [2010], The Endocrine Society.

estrogen receptor modulator, in women with hypopituitarism on IGF-1, IGF binding protein-3 (IGFBP3), resting energy expenditure, and fat oxidation on the actions of GH therapy. Estradiol-17β reduced the IGF-1 and IGFBP-3 responses to GH therapy, and raloxifene only reduced IGF-1 but not IGFBP-3. Raloxifene but not estradiol-17β suppressed the fat oxidation stimulation of GH. Thus, raloxifene would not appear to have an advantage over estradiol-17β for estrogen therapy in GH-deficient women receiving GH therapy. In addition, fat accumulation over longer periods of time would be expected to be greater in women receiving raloxifene versus estradiol-17β.

A. W. Meikle, MD

Osteoporosis in Women

Odanacatib in the Treatment of Postmenopausal Women With Low Bone Mineral Density: Three-Year Continued Therapy and Resolution of Effect

Eisman JA, Bone HG, Hosking DJ, et al (Univ of New South Wales, Sydney, Australia; Michigan Bone and Mineral Clinic, Detroit; Nottingham City Hosp, UK; et al)

J Bone Miner Res 26:242-251, 2011

The selective cathepsin K inhibitor odanacatib (ODN) progressively increased bone mineral density (BMD) and decreased bone-resorption markers during 2 years of treatment in postmenopausal women with low BMD. A 1-year extension study further assessed ODN efficacy and safety and the effects of discontinuing therapy. In the base study, postmenopausal women with BMD T-scores between -2.0 and -3.5 at the lumbar spine or femur received placebo or ODN 3, 10, 25, or 50 mg weekly. After 2 years, patients ($n = 189$) were rerandomized to ODN 50 mg weekly or placebo for an additional year. Endpoints included BMD at the lumbar spine (primary), total hip, and hip subregions; levels of bone turnover markers; and safety assessments. Continued treatment with 50 mg of ODN for 3 years produced significant increases from baseline and from year 2 in BMD at the spine (7.9% and 2.3%) and total hip (5.8% and 2.4%). Urine cross-linked N-telopeptide of type I collagen (NTx) remained suppressed at year 3 (-50.5%), but bone-specific alkaline phosphatase (BSAP) was relatively unchanged from baseline. Treatment discontinuation resulted in bone loss at all sites, but BMD remained at or above baseline. After ODN discontinuation at month 24, bone turnover markers increased transiently above baseline, but this increase largely resolved by month 36. There were similar overall adverse-event rates in both treatment groups. It is concluded that 3 years of ODN treatment resulted in progressive increases in BMD and was generally well tolerated. Bone-resorption markers remained suppressed, whereas bone-formation markers returned to near baseline. ODN effects were reversible: bone resorption increased transiently and BMD decreased following treatment discontinuation (Fig 2).

▶ Osteoporosis is clinically significant in approximately 30% of postmenopausal women in the United States and Europe, and it uses considerable health care resources. Currently, therapy includes bisphosphonates, estrogens, selective estrogen receptor modulator, calcitonin, and teriparatide. These agents, except for teriparatide, reduce bone resorption and suppress markers of bone resorption but do not improve bone formation markers, such as P1NP. Teriparatide increases bone mineral density and both bone formation and bone resorption markers. Odanacatib (ODN) is an orally active selective inhibitor of cathepsin K (catK). ODN decreases bone resorption by inhibiting proteolysis of matrix protein by catK and only transiently suppresses bone formation markers. The overall effect of ODN was to increase bone mineral density

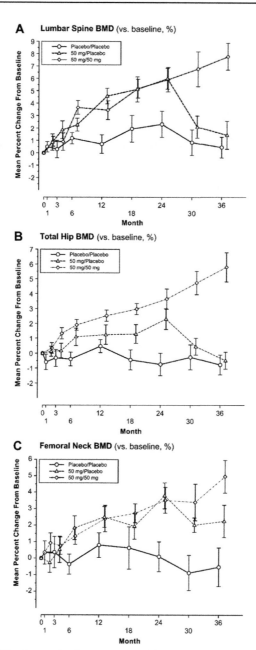

FIGURE 2.—BMD endpoints. Graphic presentation of the mean percentage change from baseline over 3 years in BMD at the specified site for the 50-mg/50-mg (ODN/ODN), 50-mg/placebo (ODN/Pbo), and placebo/placebo (Pbo/Pbo) treatment groups in the per-protocol extension population: (*A*) lumbar spine, (*B*) total hip, (*C*) femoral neck. (Reproduced from Eisman JA, Bone HG, Hosking DJ, et al. Odanacatib in the treatment of postmenopausal women with low bone mineral density: three-year continued therapy and resolution of effect. *J Bone Miner Res.* 2011;26:242-251, with permission from American Society for Bone and Mineral Research.)

(BMD) of the lumbar spine and proximal femur in postmenopausal women treated for 3 years. The benefits on BMD were largely reversed within a year of discontinuation of ODN. It was generally well tolerated, and observations on reducing fracture risk await further investigation.

A. W. Meikle, MD

Bone Health in Men

Regulation of Circulating Sclerostin Levels by Sex Steroids in Women and in Men

Mödder UI, Clowes JA, Hoey K, et al (Mayo Clinic, Rochester, MN)
J Bone Miner Res 26:27-34, 2011

Sex steroids are important regulators of bone turnover, but the mechanisms of their effects on bone remain unclear. Sclerostin is an inhibitor of Wnt signaling, and circulating estrogen (E) levels are inversely associated with sclerostin levels in postmenopausal women. To directly test for sex steroid regulation of sclerostin levels, we examined effects of E treatment of postmenopausal women or selective withdrawal of E versus testosterone (T) in elderly men on circulating sclerostin levels. E treatment of postmenopausal women ($n = 17$) for 4 weeks led to a 27% decrease in serum sclerostin levels [versus + 1% in controls ($n = 18$), $p < .001$]. Similarly, in 59 elderly men, we eliminated endogenous E and T production and studied them under conditions of physiologic T and E replacement, and then following withdrawal of T or E, we found that E, but not T, prevented increases in sclerostin levels following induction of sex steroid deficiency. In both sexes, changes in sclerostin levels correlated with changes in bone-resorption, but not bone-formation, markers ($r = 0.62$, $p < .001$, and $r = 0.33$, $p = .009$, for correlations with changes in serum C-terminal telopeptide of type 1 collagen in the women and men, respectively). Our studies thus establish that in humans, circulating sclerostin levels are reduced by E but not by T. Moreover, consistent with recent data indicating important effects of Wnts on osteoclastic cells, our findings suggest that in humans, changes in sclerostin production may contribute to effects of E on bone resorption (Fig 3).

▶ Sex steroids are regulators of bone turnover and formation. Testosterone can be converted to estrogen, which is known to suppress bone resorption by inhibiting osteoclast development and activity. Sclerostin is a Wnt signaling inhibitor, and C-terminal telopeptide of type 1 collagen (CTX) is also a marker of bone resorption. The study by Mödder et al was designed to determine the effects of testosterone and estrogen on circulating sclerostin and CTX in men treated with estrogen or testosterone or both and women treated with estrogen. In men, the conversion of testosterone to estrogen was prevented by treatment with an aromatase inhibitor. They observed that both circulating sclerostin and CTX were inhibited by estrogen but not directly by testosterone. It remains to be determined if estrogen regulates the production of sclerostin or its degradation.

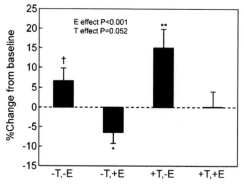

FIGURE 3.—Percent change from baseline in serum sclerostin levels in the subjects in study B. The p values for the E and T effects are based on the two-factor ANOVA model described under "Methods." Briefly, this compares changes in the +E versus −E groups for the E effect and changes in the +T versus the −T groups for the T effect. $*p < .05$, $**p < .01$, and $^{\dagger}p = .051$ for significance of change from baseline. (Reproduced from Mödder UI, Clowes JA, Hoey K, et al. Regulation of circulating sclerostin levels by sex steroids in women and in men. *J Bone Miner Res.* 2011;26:27-34, with permission from American Society for Bone and Mineral Research.)

Their findings suggest that estrogen has a role in maintaining bone formation by affecting sclerostin. They also support the use of testosterone, which can be converted to estrogen rather than androgen that cannot be converted to estrogen.

A. W. Meikle, MD

PCOS

Effect of finasteride on ovulation induction in nonresponder (hyperandrogenic) polycystic ovary syndrome (PCOS) women

Tartagni M, Cicinelli E, De Pergola G, et al (Univ of Bari, Italy)
Fertil Steril 94:247-249, 2010

Objective.—To evaluate whether the addition of finasteride (a 5⟨-reductase inhibitor) to conventional protocol of ovarian stimulation with gonadotropin can improve ovarian follicular growth in polycystic ovary syndrome (PCOS) women who did not respond to previous stimulation with gonadotropin alone.

Design.—Double-blind randomized study.

Setting.—Outpatient in an academic research environment.

Patient(s).—Thirty-six PCOS patients in whom the previous multifollicular stimulation protocols with gonadotropin failed.

Intervention(s).—The patients were randomly assigned to two treatment groups: group 1 underwent ovarian stimulation with recombinant FSH (rFSH) plus finasteride, and group 2 received rFSH alone. When the dominant follicle reached a mean diameter of 18 mm, hCG was administered and finasteride withdrawn.

Main Outcome Measure(s).—Ovulation rate in women with PCOS.

TABLE 2.—Serum Hormonal Profiles at Cycle Day 1 and at hCG Administration Day in the Two Groups of Patients

	Normal Range Follicular Phase	Group 1 Cycle Day 1	Group 1 hCG Administration Day	Group 2 Cycle Day 1	Group 2 hCG Administration Day	P Value
FSH, mIU/mL	3.2–12.2	6.3 ± 1.60	/	6.69 ± 1.40	/	
LH, mIU/mL	1.4–15.3	14.26 ± 3.93	/	14.90 ± 3.6	/	
T, ng/dL	14.0–76.0	77.0 ± 3.06	77.4 ± 2.6	77.7 ± 1.46	77.9 ± 1.98	
DHT ng/dL	11.6–42	41.9 ± 3.00	38.9 ± 2.6^a	41.9 ± 2.35	42.0 ± 2.54^a	$<.001^a$
A, ng/mL	0.6–3.0	3.65 ± 0.56	3.79 ± 0.75	3.80 ± 0.23	3.85 ± 0.16	
E_2, pg/mL	11–165	55.8 ± 5.80	155.08 ± 6.01^b	55.9 ± 7.15	58.46 ± 8.60^b	$<.001^b$

Note: Values are mean ± SD. DHT = dihydroxytestosterone.
[a]DHT at the end of ovarian stimulation: $P < .001$ (Student t test) vs. group 2.
[b]E_2 at the end of ovarian stimulation: $P < .001$ (Student t test) vs. group 2.

Result(s).—Follicular growth and ovulation occurred in eight patients in group 1, whereas no cases were detected in group 2.

Conclusion(s).—This study confirms that hyperandrogenism interferes with follicular growth and suggests that administration of finasteride during ovarian stimulation with rFSH improves ovulation rate in selected hyperandrogenic anovulatory women (Table 2).

▶ Induction of ovulation in women with polycystic ovary syndrome (PCOS) produces variable responses. PCOS is associated with hyperandrogenism, anovulatory infertility, and androgen suppression of follicular growth. Often, the luteinizing hormone is inappropriately elevated, resulting in excessive ovarian production of androgens. In addition, 5-alpha-reductase activity is elevated and converts testosterone to dihydrotestosterone (DHT). These observations led Tartagni et al to determine whether inhibition of DHT formation with finasteride, a 5-alpha-reductase inhibitor, would improve the success of ovulation induction in women with PCOS compared with non-PCOS women. Thirty-eight percent of women with PCOS ovulated in response to follicle-stimulating hormone plus finasteride followed by human chorionic gonadotropin compared with none in the non-PCOS group. While the success of ovulation induction was modest in these women with PCOS who had failed ovulation induction previously, the results do support an androgen component for poor ovulation induction. Further study is needed to establish the mechanism for poor ovulation induction and the influence of androgens.

A. W. Meikle, MD

The phenotype of hirsute women: a comparison of polycystic ovary syndrome and 21-hydroxylase–deficient nonclassic adrenal hyperplasia

Pall M, Azziz R, Beires J, et al (Cedars-Sinai Med Ctr, Los Angeles, CA; Hosp S. João, Porto, Portugal; et al)

Fertil Steril 94:684-689, 2010

Objective.—To test the hypothesis that women with polycystic ovary syndrome (PCOS) are distinguishable from those with 21-hydroxylase–deficient nonclassic adrenal hyperplasia on the basis of having polycystic ovaries and metabolic dysfunction.

Design.—Prospective observational.

Setting.—Tertiary care center.

Patient(s).—Fifty-two lean and 54 obese women with PCOS according to the 1990 National Institutes of Health criteria, 23 women with nonclassic adrenal hyperplasia, and 27 controls.

Intervention(s).—History and physical examination, blood sampling, ovarian sonography, oral glucose tolerance, and acute adrenocorticotropin stimulation testing.

Main Outcome Measure(s).—The frequency of clinical, biochemical, and metabolic features.

Result(s).—Women with PCOS had a higher frequency of oligomenorrhea or amenorrhea than those with nonclassic adrenal hyperplasia. Mean androstenedione and DHEAS levels were highest in nonclassic adrenal hyperplasia. The degree of metabolic dysfunction was greatest in obese women with PCOS; women with nonclassic adrenal hyperplasia and lean women with PCOS did not differ in degree of metabolic dysfunction. Women with nonclassic adrenal hyperplasia had a lower prevalence of polycystic ovaries than those with PCOS. The proportion of patients with an LH/FSH ratio >2 was greater in women with PCOS, compared with those with nonclassic adrenal hyperplasia. Basal 17-hydroxyprogesterone levels >2 ng/mL were found in 87%, 25%, 20%, and 7% of women with nonclassic adrenal hyperplasia, lean women with PCOS, obese women with PCOS, and controls, respectively.

Conclusion(s).—Nonclassic adrenal hyperplasia should be excluded in all women presenting with hirsutism, with use of a basal follicular phase 17-hydroxyprogesterone level, regardless of the presence of polycystic ovaries or metabolic dysfunction; however, women with nonclassic adrenal hyperplasia have a higher prevalence of normal ovulation and lower likelihood of having an LH/FSH ratio >2 or polycystic ovaries (Table 3).

▶ Hirsutism is common in women and is caused by excess androgen secretion. There are several disorders that are associated with androgenism, including polycystic ovary syndrome (PCOS), nonclassic adrenal hyperplasia from 21-hydroxylase deficiency, and androgen-secreting tumors. Both nonclassic adrenal hyperplasia from 21-hydroxylase deficiency and PCOS are common. There is variability in the clinical presentation in these patients, and the

TABLE 3.—Biochemical Features of Subjects

	Obese Patients with PCOS	Lean Patients with PCOS	Patients with NCAH	Controls
No. of subjects	54	52	23	27
FT (pg/mL)	3.60 ± 1.41^{a}	2.64 ± 1.17^{b}	3.53 ± 2.12^{a}	1.35 ± 0.48^{b}
Total T (ng/mL)	0.78 ± 0.33	0.73 ± 0.28	0.91 ± 0.47	0.43 ± 0.13^{b}
A (ng/mL)	3.67 ± 1.16	3.56 ± 1.21	4.71 ± 2.54^{b}	2.20 ± 0.67^{b}
DHEAS (ng/mL)	$2,717 \pm 1,305$	$2,487 \pm 1,167$	$3,220 \pm 1,220^{c}$	$2,356 \pm 827$
SHBG (mg/L)	19 ± 11	26 ± 18	20 ± 15	52 ± 18^{b}
LH/FSH	1.36 ± 0.89	1.88 ± 1.85^{c}	1.28 ± 1.97	0.94 ± 0.52
LH/FSH >2 (%)	$12/54\ (22)^{c}$	$15/52\ (29)^{c}$	$2/23\ (9)$	$1/27\ (4)$
17-OHP (ng/mL)	1.56 ± 0.72	1.54 ± 0.64	14.9 ± 24^{b}	1.26 ± 0.50
17-OHP >3 ng/mL (%)	$1/54\ (2)$	$0/52\ (0)$	$17/23\ (74)^{b}$	$0/27\ (0)$
17-OHP 2–3 ng/mL (%)	$10/54\ (19)$	$13/52\ (25)$	$3/23\ (13)$	$2/27\ (7)$

Note: Values are expressed as mean ± SD.
[a] $P<.05$ compared with lean patients with PCOS and controls.
[b] $P<.05$ compared with all other groups.
[c] $P \leq .05$ compared with controls.

manifestation might include hirsutism, acne, alopecia, and ovulatory dysfunction. The study by Pall et al has proposed criteria for diagnosis of nonclassic adrenal hyperplasia from 21-hydroxylase deficiency with the measurement of 17-hydroxyprogesterone at baseline during the follicular phase of the menstrual cycle. While there is some overlap in values, the criteria would appear useful in making the diagnosis. It might provide a guide for management of androgen excess. It is critical that specific sensitive assay methods are used with appropriate reference intervals. Genotyping is another approach for the diagnosis of nonclassic adrenal hyperplasia from 21-hydroxylase deficiency.

A. W. Meikle, MD

Determinants of Impaired Fasting Glucose Versus Glucose Intolerance in Polycystic Ovary Syndrome

Karakas SE, Kim K, Duleba AJ (Univ of California, Davis; Univ of California at Davis)
Diabetes Care 33:887-893, 2010

Objective.—To determine insulin resistance and response in patients with polycystic ovary syndrome (PCOS) and normal glucose tolerance (NGT), impaired fasting glucose (IFG), impaired glucose tolerance, and combined glucose intolerance (CGI).

Research Design and Methods.—In this cross-sectional study, 143 patients with PCOS (diagnosed on the basis of National Institutes of Health criteria) underwent oral glucose tolerance testing (OGTT), and 68 patients also had frequently sampled intravenous glucose tolerance tests. Changes in plasma glucose, insulin, cardiovascular risk factors, and androgens were measured.

Results.—Compared with patients with NGT, those with both IFG and CGI were significantly insulin resistant (homeostasis model assessment 3.3 ± 0.2 vs. 6.1 ± 0.9 and 6.4 ± 0.5, $P < 0.0001$) and hyperinsulinemic (insulin area under the curve for 120 min 973 ± 69 vs. 1,470 ± 197 and 1,461 ± 172 pmol/l, $P < 0.0001$). Insulin response was delayed in patients with CGI but not in those with IFG (2-h OGTT, insulin 1,001 ± 40 vs. 583 ± 45 pmol/l, $P < 0.0001$). Compared with the NGT group, the CGI group had a lower disposition index (1,615 ± 236 vs. 987 ± 296, $P < 0.0234$) and adiponectin level (11.1 ± 1.1 vs. 6.2 ± 0.8 ng/ml, $P < 0.0096$). Compared with the insulin-resistant tertile of the NGT group, those with IFG had a reduced insulinogenic index (421 ± 130 vs. 268 ± 68, $P < 0.05$). Compared with the insulin-sensitive tertile of the NGT group, the resistant tertile had higher triglyceride and high-sensitivity C-reactive protein (hs-CRP) and lower HDL cholesterol and sex hormone–binding globulin (SHBG). In the entire population, insulin resistance correlated directly with triglyceride, hs-CRP, and the free androgen index and inversely with SHBG.

Conclusions.—Patients with PCOS develop IFG and CGI despite having significant hyperinsulinemia. Patients with IFG and CGI exhibit similar insulin resistance but very different insulin response patterns. Increases in cardiac risk factors and free androgen level precede overt glucose intolerance.

▶ Women with polycystic ovary syndrome (PCOS) often exhibit glucose intolerance, type 2 diabetes, and gestational diabetes. Compared with weight-matched controls, women with PCOS have high insulin concentrations, which can be improved with the administration of insulin sensitizers. Ovarian function, insulin sensitivity, and hyperandrogenism improve. Impaired fasting glucose (IFG, 100-125 mg/dL) is the result of hepatic insulin resistance, and impaired glucose tolerance (IGT, >140 mg/dL) at 2 hours postglucose tolerance test results from peripheral insulin resistance. If they have both defects, it is called combined glucose intolerance. Those with IFG had an increased response to oral glucose tolerance test compared with those with IGT, who exhibited a delayed insulin response. After 60 minutes, the insulin response changed so that those with IGT had higher insulin values than those with IFG. Patients with combined glucose intolerance have both hepatic and peripheral insulin resistance. The authors propose that IFG might precede IGT and combined glucose intolerance. In either case, improving insulin sensitivity will benefit patients with PCOS.

A. W. Meikle, MD

Family-Based Analysis of Candidate Genes for Polycystic Ovary Syndrome

Ewens KG, Stewart DR, Ankener W, et al (Univ of Pennsylvania School of Medicine, Philadelphia; Natl Insts of Health, Bethesda, MD; et al)

J Clin Endocrinol Metab 95:2306-2315, 2010

Context.—Polycystic ovary syndrome (PCOS) is a complex disorder having both genetic and environmental components. A number of association studies based on candidate genes have reported significant association, but few have been replicated. D19S884, a polymorphic marker in fibrillin 3 (*FBN3*), is one of the few association findings that has been replicated in independent sets of families.

Objective.—The aims of the study are: 1) to genotype single nucleotide polymorphisms (SNPs) in the region of D19S884; and 2) to follow up with an independent data set, published results reporting evidence for PCOS candidate gene associations.

Design.—The transmission disequilibrium test (TDT) was used to analyze linkage and association between PCOS and SNPs in candidate genes previously reported by us and by others as significantly associated with PCOS.

Setting.—The study was conducted at academic medical centers.

Patients or Other Participants.—A total of 453 families having a proband with PCOS participated in the study. Sisters with PCOS were also included. There was a total of 502 probands and sisters with PCOS.

Intervention(s).—There were no interventions.

Main Outcome Measure(s).—The outcome measure was transmission frequency of SNP alleles.

Results.—We identified a six-SNP haplotype block spanning a 6.7-kb region on chromosome 19p13.2 that includes D19S884. SNP haplotype allele-C alone and in combination with D19S884-allele 8 is significantly associated with PCOS: haplotype-C TDT $\chi^2 = 10.0$ ($P = 0.0016$) and haplotype-C/A8 TDT $\chi^2 = 7.6$ ($P = 0.006$). SNPs in four of the other 26 putative candidate genes that were tested using the TDT were nominally significant (*ACVR2A*, *POMC*, *FEM1B*, and *SGTA*). One SNP in POMC (rs12473543, $\chi^2 = 9.1$; $P_{corrected} = 0.042$) is significant after correction for multiple testing.

Conclusions.—A polymorphic variant, D19S884, in *FBN3* is associated with risk of PCOS. *POMC* is also a candidate gene of interest (Fig 1).

▶ Polycystic ovary syndrome (PCOS) affects 5% to 10% of reproductive age women and is characterized by anovulation, hyperandrogenemia, infertility, and often type 2 diabetes, cardiovascular disease, and obesity. Familial aggregation of traits of PCOS has been documented and has prompted study of a genetic contribution to the disorder. Candidate genes have evaded investigators. In the study of Ewens and associates, the candidate region of D19S884 was a focus of investigation. They concluded from their investigation that the D19S884 region of *FBN3* was associated with a risk of PCOS, and *POMC* was also a candidate gene of interest. The *POMC* gene encodes a polypeptide

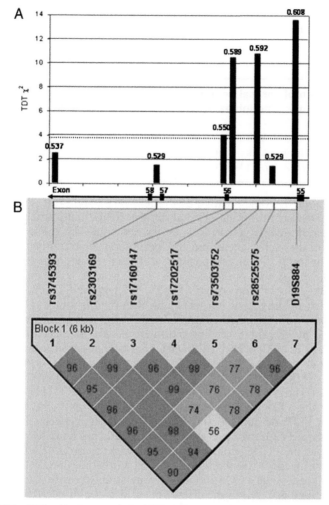

FIGURE 1.—TDT and haplotype analysis of SNPs in the region of D19S884. A, Individual TDT results are shown for six SNPs and D19S884 located between exons 55 and 59 of *FBN3* (*number above each bar* represents transmission frequency, and *dashed line* represents nominally significant $\chi^2 = 3.84$). Also shown are the positions of the markers relative to the exons. B, Pairwise LD plot showing D' values (percent) in the PCOS families. For construction of haplotypes in Haploview, D19S884 was coded as a two-allele system: allele 8 or not-8. (The x-axis displays location of chromosome 19: 8049164-8056141.) (Reprinted from Ewens KG, Stewart DR, Ankener W, et al. Family-based analysis of candidate genes for polycystic ovary syndrome. *J Clin Endocrinol Metab*. 2010;95:2306-2315. Copyright © 2010, The Endocrine Society.)

hormone that can be cleaved to yield 10 different polypeptides including forms of melanocyte-stimulating hormone, lipotropin, adrenocorticotropic hormone, and β-endorphin. This is particularly of interest for an influence in the pathogenesis of PCOS because these hormones are involved in steroidogenesis, energy metabolism, obesity, and lipolysis. We must await further genetic analysis of PCOS, but this study is a step closer.

A. W. Meikle, MD

Augmentation of cortical bone mineral density in women with polycystic ovary syndrome: a peripheral quantitative computed tomography (pQCT) study
Kassanos D, Trakakis E, Baltas CS, et al (Univ of Athens, Greece; General Hosp of Athens 'G.Gennimatas', Greece)
Hum Reprod 25:2107-2114, 2010

Background.—Women with polycystic ovary syndrome (PCOS) may have increased cortical bone mineral density (BMD) and probably higher bone material quality as well as better resistance in the compression strength of the tibia, measured by peripheral quantitative computed tomography (pQCT), in comparison with that of age-matched healthy subjects.

Methods.—Thirty women with PCOS, (15 lean and 15 obese) and 15 age-matched healthy controls were enrolled in this study. The clinical, biochemical and ultrasound characteristics of the two groups were evaluated. Using pQCT, the following parameters were measured: volumetric cortical density (CBD) and volumetric trabecular density (TBD) BMD, total bone cross-sectional area (ToA), cortical area (CoA), cortical thickness (CRT-THK-C) and finally the strength-strain index (SSI).

Results.—The geometrical parameters (CoA, ToA, CRT-THK-C), the SSI as well as the TBD were increased in the PCOS women; however, these differences did not achieve statistical significance between lean PCOS women, obese PCOS women, and controls. Conversely, CBD was significantly higher in PCOS women compared with controls ($P < 0.000$) and furthermore in lean PCOS women compared with obese ones ($P < 0.01040$).

Conclusions.—The PCOS women of our study seem to have a higher quality of bone material in the distal tibia and probably a better resistance of bone in the compression strength without alterations in bone mass and geometry (especially the lean PCOS women), indicating that our oligomenorrheic and hyperandrogonemic PCOS women may be protected from the development of osteoporosis and fracture risk later in life (Table 3).

▶ Polycystic ovary syndrome (PCOS) affects up to 15% of women of the reproductive age. It is characterized by oligomenorrhea and hyperandrogenism with or without polycystic ovaries demonstrated on ovarian ultrasound. Peak bone mass is achieved in women between late teens and early 30s. Ovarian deficiency might adversely affect peak bone mass during these years and lead to early osteoporosis, but women with PCOS are generally not estrogen deficient. Kassanos et al determined cortical bone mineral density using peripheral quantitative computed tomography in women with PCOS and controls. The improved cortical bone density in women with PCOS compared with controls

TABLE 3.—pQCT Parameters in the Distal Tibia of PCOS Women and Controls Studied

	Controls	Lean PCOS Women	Obese PCOS Women
TBD	209 ± 20.66 (185–256)	218.5 ± 42.2 (166–278)	232.6 ± 28 (191–261)
CBD	1143.6 ± 29.69[a] (1081–1183)	1194 ± 17[b] (1175–1227)	1171 ± 24.72[c] (1145–1202)
CoA	261.13 ± 31.60 (207–305)	255 ± 39.7 (210–310)	272 ± 23.8 (248–298)
ToA	1022.66 ± 99 (865–1258)	1027 ± 123 (874–1261)	1055 ± 25 (989–1096)
SSI	1227.3 ± 188.6 (1030–1565)	1299 ± 291 (1060–1881)	1262.3 ± 274.59 (1118–1519)
CRT-THK-C	3.096 ± 0.226 (2.69–3.4)	3.4 ± 0.60 (2.5–4.3)	3.28 ± 0.756 (2.5–4.1)

TBD, trabecular density; CBD, cortical density; CoA, cortical area; ToA, cross-sectional area; SSI, strength strain index; CRT-THK-C, cortical thickness.
[a,b]$P < 0.00001$; [b,c]$P = 0.00604$; [a,c]$P < 0.010$.

suggests better bone quality and more protection from osteoporosis and cortical bone fractures. It is unclear from the study whether the combination of higher androgens or mild hypoestrogenemia benefits cortical bone in PCOS patients. Long-term follow-up will be needed to determine benefits of these hormonal and bone alterations observed in younger women.

A. W. Meikle, MD

Hyperandrogenism in Women with Polycystic Ovary Syndrome Persists after Menopause

Markopoulos MC, Rizos D, Valsamakis G, et al (Aretaieion Hosp, Athens, Greece; et al)
J Clin Endocrinol Metab 96:623-631, 2011

Context.—Ovarian and adrenal hyperandrogenism characterize premenopausal women with polycystic ovary syndrome (PCOS). Androgens decline with age in healthy and PCOS women.

Objective.—The objective of the study was to investigate hyperandrogenism in PCOS after menopause.

Design.—This was a case-control, cross-sectional study.

Setting.—The study was conducted at a university hospital endocrinology unit.

Patients.—Twenty postmenopausal women with PCOS and 20 age- and body mass index-matched controls participated in the study.

Interventions.—Serum cortisol, 17-hydroxyprogesterone (17-OHP), Δ_4- androstenedione (Δ_4A), dehydroepiandrosterone sulfate (DHEAS), total testosterone (T), and free androgen index (FAI) levels were measured at baseline, after ACTH stimulation, and after 3-d dexamethasone suppression. The ACTH and cortisol levels were measured during the CRH test.

Main Outcome Measures.—Androgen profile at baseline, after ACTH stimulation, and 3-d dexamethasone suppression tests were the main outcome measures.

Results.—Postmenopausal PCOS women had higher 17-OHP, Δ_4A, DHEAS, total T, FAI ($P < 0.05$) and lower SHBG ($P < 0.05$) baseline levels than control women. ACTH and cortisol responses during the CRH test were similar in the two groups. After ACTH stimulation, Δ_4A, DHEAS, and total T levels were equally increased in both groups. After dexamethasone suppression, LH levels did not change in either group; 17-OHP-, Δ_4A-, and FAI-suppressed levels remained higher in PCOS than in control women ($P < 0.05$), whereas total T and DHEAS levels were suppressed to similar values in both groups.

Conclusions.—In postmenopausal PCOS women, ACTH and cortisol responses to CRH are normal. Androgen levels at baseline are higher in PCOS than control women and remain increased after ACTH stimulation. The dexamethasone suppression results in postmenopausal PCOS women suggest that DHEAS and total T are partially of adrenal origin. Although the ovarian contribution was not fully assessed, increased Δ_4A production suggests that the ovary also contributes to hyperandrogenism in postmenopausal PCOS women. In conclusion, postmenopausal PCOS women are exposed to higher adrenal and ovarian androgen levels than non-PCOS women.

▶ A high percentage of women with polycystic ovary syndrome (PCOS) exhibit hyperandrogenism, often beginning with menarche.[1-4] The hyperandrogenism is a consequence of increased testosterone production from ovarian thecal cells and dehydroepiandrosterone (DHEA) and DHEA sulfate from the adrenal cortex. Androstenedione is elevated from both ovarian and adrenal sources.[2,3] Transition to menopause greatly affects ovarian function. However, both the ovary and adrenal contribute substantially to androgen status after menopause. It is estimated that after menopause, the ovary contributes approximately 50% to total testosterone and 30% of total Δ_4-androstenedione.[1,4] The remaining production of the androgen is derived from the adrenal cortex and metabolism of precursors in fat cells. There is much less information about the androgen status in postmenopausal women with PCOS. Markopoulos et al provide evidence that hyperandrogenism persists in postmenopausal women with PCOS compared with unaffected women after menopause. The hyperandrogenism in postmenopausal women is responsive to both adrenal suppression with dexamethasone and stimulation with adrenocorticotropic hormone.

A. W. Meikle, MD

References

1. Puurunen J, Piltonen T, Jaakkola P, Ruokonen A, Morin-Papunen L, Tapanainen JS. Adrenal androgen production capacity remains high up to menopause in women with polycystic ovary syndrome. *J Clin Endocrinol Metab.* 2009;94:1973-1978.
2. Rizzo M, Berneis K, Spinas G, Rini GB, Carmina E. Long-term consequences of polycystic ovary syndrome on cardiovascular risk. *Fertil Steril.* 2009;91:1563-1567.
3. Pasquali R, Gambineri A. Polycystic ovary syndrome: a multifaceted disease from adolescence to adult age. *Ann N Y Acad Sci.* 2006;1092:158-174.

4. Ireland K, Child T. Polycystic ovary syndrome and the postmenopausal woman. *J Br Menopause Soc.* 2006;12:143-148.

Hypogonadism and Aging

Low serum testosterone levels are associated with increased risk of mortality in a population-based cohort of men aged 20–79

Haring R, Völzke H, Steveling A, et al (Ernst Moritz Arndt Univ Greifswald, Germany; et al)

Eur Heart J 31:1494-1501, 2010

Aims.—Although the association of low serum testosterone levels with mortality has gained strength in recent research, there are few population-based studies on this issue. This study examined whether low serum testosterone levels are a risk factor for all-cause or cause-specific mortality in a population-based sample of men aged 20–79.

Methods and Results.—We used data from 1954 men recruited for the prospective population-based Study of Health in Pomerania, with measured serum testosterone levels at baseline and 195 deaths during an average 7.2-year follow-up. A total serum testosterone level of less than 8.7 nmol/L (250 ng/dL) was classified as low. The relationships of low serum testosterone levels with all-cause and cause-specific mortality were analysed by Cox proportional hazards regression models. Men with low serum testosterone levels had a significantly higher mortality from all causes than men with higher serum testosterone levels (HR 2.24; 95% CI 1.41–3.57). After adjusting for waist circumference, smoking habits, high-risk alcohol use, physical activity, renal insufficiency, and levels of dehydroepiandrosterone sulfate, low serum testosterone levels continued to be associated with increased mortality (HR 2.32; 95% CI 1.38–3.89). In cause-specific analyses, low serum testosterone levels predicted increased risk of death from cardiovascular disease (CVD) (HR 2.56; 95% CI 1.15–6.52) and cancer (HR 3.46; 95% CI 1.68–6.68), but not from respiratory diseases or other causes.

Conclusion.—Low serum testosterone levels were associated with an increased risk of all-cause mortality independent of numerous risk factors. As serum testosterone levels are inversely related to mortality due to CVD and cancer, it may be used as a predictive marker (Table 3).

▶ It is well documented that serum testosterone concentrations decline in men at 1% to 2% per year with aging, and many health issues have been attributed to the decline, including hypertension, abdominal obesity, insulin resistance, decreased bone mineral density, decreased libido and energy, and chronic fatigue. The risk of mortality has more recently been associated with low serum testosterone as reported by Haring et al. They observed that low serum testosterone was associated with all-cause mortality even after control for independent risk factors. The low testosterone was not related to a single etiology and was strongly associated with cardiovascular disease and cancer deaths.

TABLE 3.—Hazard Ratios for Low Serum Testosterone Levels Associated with All-Cause Mortality Adjusted for Potential Mediators

	Testosterone Level <8.7 nmol/L (250 ng/dL) HR (95% CI)
Model 3[†]	2.32 (1.38; 3.89)[**]
+ Hypertension	2.36 (1.50; 3.71)[***]
+ Diabetes mellitus	2.23 (1.38; 3.59)[**]
+ Metabolic syndrome	2.36 (1.49; 4.06)[***]
+ Myocardial infarction	2.37 (1.45; 3.87)[**]
+ Renal insufficiency	2.06 (1.19; 3.53)[**]
+ Hyperlipidaemia	2.40 (1.49; 3.85)[***]
+ Cohabitation	2.41 (1.53; 3.79)[***]
+ Educational level	2.31 (1.48; 3.61)[***]
+ Stroke	2.41 (1.50; 3.89)[***]
+ DHEAS	2.77 (1.68; 4.58)[***]
+ Blood sampling time	2.13 (1.37; 3.90)[**]

Covariables were added one at a time to model 3. HR, hazard ratio; CI, 95% confidence interval; DHEAS, dehydroepian-drosterone sulfate; WC, waist circumference.
*P < 0.05.
[†]Model 3: adjusted for age, WC, smoking (three categories), high-risk alcohol use, and physical activity.
**P < 0.01.
***P < 0.001.

Their study does not clarify the cause and effect relationship of low serum testosterone and mortality. Many associated factors, such as hypertension, abdominal obesity, and insulin resistance, might be implicated as risks for cardiovascular disease mortality, but it would not account for cancer mortality. Currently, it might be considered a marker of mortality and not a specific cause.

A. W. Meikle, MD

A Large Study of *Androgen Receptor* Germline Variants and Their Relation to Sex Hormone Levels and Prostate Cancer Risk. Results from the National Cancer Institute Breast and Prostate Cancer Cohort Consortium

Lindström S, Ma J, Altshuler D, et al (Harvard School of Public Health, Boston, MA; Brigham and Women's Hosp and Harvard Med School, Boston, MA; Broad Inst of Massachusetts Inst of Technology (MIT) and Harvard, Cambridge; et al)
J Clin Endocrinol Metab 95:E121-E127, 2010

Background.—Androgens are key regulators of prostate gland maintenance and prostate cancer growth, and androgen deprivation therapy has been the mainstay of treatment for advanced prostate cancer for many years. A long-standing hypothesis has been that inherited variation in the androgen receptor (*AR*) gene plays a role in prostate cancer initiation. However, studies to date have been inconclusive and often suffered from small sample sizes.

Objective and Methods.—We investigated the association of *AR* sequence variants with circulating sex hormone levels and prostate cancer

TABLE 2.—Association Between *AR* CAG Repeats and Plasma Hormone Levels

Hormone	Controls	Cases	Mean Difference (95% CI)[a]	r² (%)[b]	P value[c]
Androstanediol	2452	2167	1.86 (−3.84, 7.89)	0.0089	0.52
Estradiol	1059	898	8.89 (3.99, 13.8)	0.7167	0.0002
SHBG	2435	2142	3.51 (−0.68, 8.14)	0.0616	0.10
Testosterone	2419	2121	8.39 (4.23, 12.7)	0.3725	$4.73 \times 10{-5}$

[a]Percentage increase in levels per 10 repeat increase in CAG length.
[b]Percentage variance in trait explained by CAG repeat length.
[c]P value from linear regression, adjusted for cohort, batch (within cohort), prostate cancer case-control status, and age in 5-yr intervals.

risk in 6058 prostate cancer cases and 6725 controls of Caucasian origin within the Breast and Prostate Cancer Cohort Consortium. We genotyped a highly polymorphic CAG microsatellite in exon 1 and six haplotype tagging single nucleotide polymorphisms and tested each genetic variant for association with prostate cancer risk and with sex steroid levels.

Results.—We observed no association between *AR* genetic variants and prostate cancer risk. However, there was a strong association between longer CAG repeats and higher levels of testosterone $(P = 4.73 \times 10^{-5})$ and estradiol $(P = 0.0002)$, although the amount of variance explained was small (0.4 and 0.7%, respectively).

Conclusions.—This study is the largest to date investigating *AR* sequence variants, sex steroid levels, and prostate cancer risk. Although we observed no association between *AR* sequence variants and prostate cancer risk, our results support earlier findings of a relation between the number of CAG repeats and circulating levels of testosterone and estradiol (Table 2).

▶ Development, growth, and maintenance of the prostate are produced in response to androgens. A major form of therapy for prostate hyperplasia or cancer is to blunt androgen responsiveness. Both testosterone and dihydrotestosterone bind to an androgen receptor in the prostate and activate androgen-responsive genes. There has been controversy pertaining to CAG repeat length and serum testosterone concentrations. Some studies have found an association between CAG repeat length and others have not. The study by Lindstrom and associates did not find a significant association between CAG repeats and prostate cancer, but they did find a marked association between CAG repeats and serum concentrations of testosterone and estradiol. This large study included 6058 prostate cancer patients and 6725 controls of Caucasian origin. Their study suggests that inherited variation at the androgen receptor locus is not a risk for prostate cancer. Their findings do not support a direct role of circulating testosterone and estradiol in the development of prostate cancer.

A. W. Meikle, MD

Local prolactin is a target to prevent expansion of basal/stem cells in prostate tumors

Rouet V, Bogorad RL, Kayser C, et al (Université Paris Descartes, Neckersite, France; et al)

Proc Natl Acad Sci U S A 107:15199-15204, 2010

Androgen-independent recurrence is the major limit of androgen ablation therapy for prostate cancer. Identification of alternative pathways promoting prostate tumor growth is thus needed. Stat5 has been recently shown to promote human prostate cancer cell survival/proliferation and to be associated with early prostate cancer recurrence. Stat5 is the main signaling pathway triggered by prolactin (PRL), a growth factor whose local production is also increased in high-grade prostate cancers. The first aim of this study was to use prostate-specific PRL transgenic mice to address the mechanisms by which local PRL induces prostate tumorogenesis. We report that (*i*) Stat5 is the major signaling cascade triggered by local PRL in the mouse dorsal prostate, (*ii*) this model recapitulates prostate tumorogenesis from precancer lesions to invasive carcinoma, and (*iii*) tumorogenesis involves dramatic accumulation and abnormal spreading of p63-positive basal cells, and of stem cell antigen-1—positive cells identified as a stem/progenitor-like subpopulation. Because basal epithelial stem cells are proposed to serve as tumor-initiating cells, we challenged the relevance of local PRL as a previously unexplored therapeutic target. Using a double-transgenic approach, we show that Δ 1−9-G129R-hPRL, a competitive PRL-receptor antagonist, prevented early stages of prostate tumorogenesis by reducing or inhibiting Stat5 activation, cell proliferation, abnormal basal-cell pattern, and frequency or grade of intraepithelial neoplasia. This study identifies PRL receptor/Stat5 as a unique pathway, initiating prostate tumorogenesis by altering basal-/stem-like cell subpopulations, and strongly supports the importance of further developing strategies to target locally overexpressed PRL in human prostate cancer (Fig 4).

▶ Prostate cancer is the most common cancer affecting aging men, and palliative therapy with androgen ablation most often results in relapse. Alternate pathways for regulation of prostate cancer growth in tumors unresponsive to hormonal ablation are needed. Prolactin belongs to the prolactin/growth hormone/placental lactogen family of hormones. While prolactin is best known for milk production from the breast, it has many other hormonal actions and is produced locally in human prostate epithelium. Stat5 is the major signaling cascade promoted by local prolactin production. Human prostate cancer specimens have been shown to express immune-detectable concentrations of prolactin that correlated positively with Stat5 activation and Gleason score. Rouet et al used a mouse model with a double-transgenic construct and showed that a competitive prolactin-receptor antagonist inhibited early stages of prostate cancer development by blocking Stat5 activation. This approach to androgen hormone suppression unresponsiveness would appear

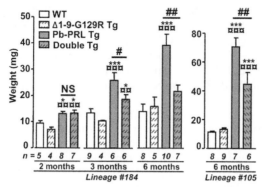

FIGURE 4.—Δ1—9-G129R—hPRL reduces prostate tumor growth induced by local PRL. The wet weights of dorsal prostate lobes harvested from WT, Met-Δ1—9-G129R—hPRL Tg, Pb-PRL Tg, and double Tg littermates (#184 and #105 line-ages) were measured as a function of age. Values represent mean lobe-pair weights ± SEM. Symbols are as follows: *versus WT; □versus Δ1—9-G129R-hPRL; #versus Pb-PRL. One symbol (*, □, or #), P < 0.05; two symbols, P < 0.01; three symbols, P < 0.001; NS, not significant. (Reprinted from Rouet V, Bogorad RL, Kayser C, et al. Local prolactin is a target to prevent expansion of basal/stem cells in prostate tumors. *Proc Natl Acad Sci U S A*. 2010;107:15199-15204. Copyright (2010) National Academy of Sciences, U.S.A.)

to have promise in treatment of these patients. Other approaches are also needed to control prostate cancer disease in refractory prostate cancers.

A. W. Meikle, MD

Metabolic Syndrome and Hypogonadism

Semen quality and reproductive hormones according to birthweight and body mass index in childhood and adult life: two decades of follow-up
Ramlau-Hansen CH, Hansen M, Jensen CR, et al (Aarhus Univ Hosp, Denmark; et al)
Fertil Steril 94:610-618, 2010

Objective.—To investigate the association between childhood body mass index (BMI), birth weight, and adulthood BMI, and adult semen quality and level of reproductive hormones.

Design.—Follow-up study.

Setting.—From a pregnancy cohort established in 1984—1987.

Patient(s).—347 out of 5,109 sons were selected for a study conducted 2005 to 2006.

Intervention(s).—Semen and blood samples were related to information on BMI in boys (5—8 years), birth weight, and adult BMI.

Main Outcome Measure(s).—Semen characteristics and reproductive hormones.

Result(s).—Neither childhood BMI, birth weight, nor adulthood BMI were significantly associated with semen quality. Men with the 33% highest childhood BMI had 15% lower sex hormone binding globulin, 8% lower testosterone, and 16% lower FSH than men with the 33%

lowest childhood BMI. Men with high adulthood BMI had 14% lower testosterone, 9% lower inhibin B, 31% lower sex hormone binding globulin, and 20% higher estradiol than men with low adulthood BMI.

Conclusion(s).—The results do not indicate an effect of childhood BMI, birth weight, or adult BMI on semen quality, but the exposure contrast in our study was limited. The hormonal status was affected by adult BMI.

▶ Semen quality is associated with body mass index (BMI) in adults but not consistently. Obese men have lower concentration of testosterone, sex hormone binding globulin (SHBG), and inhibin but higher serum concentrations of estradiol with slightly lower serum concentrations of gonadotropins. There is less known about the effects of birth weight and BMI in childhood and follow-up in adult life. Sertoli cells in the testes increase during fetal and neonatal life in boys and then proliferate during puberty to reach adult numbers, and inhibin also reaches adult levels. In prepubertal boys, obesity does not affect inhibin B, but obesity might affect inhibin at puberty. Although they did not find an effect of BMI on semen quality in young adult men, it did have a lowering effect on hormone concentrations including follicle-stimulating hormone, testosterone, SHBG, inhibin, and elevating estradiol. These results vary somewhat with other studies that have shown at least in obese adults that semen quality is compromised.

A. W. Meikle, MD

An aromatase polymorphism modulates the relationship between weight and estradiol levels in obese men

Hammoud A, Carrell DT, Meikle AW, et al (Univ of Utah, Salt Lake City; Univ of Utah School of Medicine, Salt Lake City)
Fertil Steril 94:1734-1738, 2010

Objective.—To describe the influence of the TTTA aromatase polymorphism (TTTAn) on the relation between obesity and plasma estradiol (E_2) in obese men.

Design.—A 2-year cohort study.

Setting.—Clinical research center.

Patient(s).—Severely obese men (31 who had had gastric bypass surgery and 118 controls).

Intervention(s).—Men were genotyped for the TTTAn CYP19A1 polymorphism. Anthropomorphic measures, plasma E_2, and other hormonal levels were determined at baseline and 2-year follow-up.

Main Outcomes Measure(s).—Relationships between weight and changes in weight and plasma E_2 were examined in relation to the TTTAn polymorphism.

Result(s).—The mean age was 46.5 ± 10.82 years, and mean body mass index was 47.1 ± 8.46 kg/m². The most common repeats were 7 and 11. TTTAn number did not correlate with plasma E_2 in the univariate analysis.

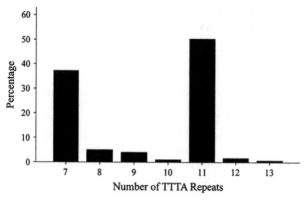

FIGURE 1.—Distribution of the different alleles with different numbers of TTTAn repeats. (Reprinted from Hammoud A, Carrell DT, Meikle AW, et al. An aromatase polymorphism modulates the relationship between weight and estradiol levels in obese men. *Fertil Steril.* 2010;94:1734-1738, with permission from American Society for Reproductive Medicine.)

When patients were stratified per weight group, the correlation between plasma E_2 and weight was seen only among men with a higher TTTA repeat at baseline and 2 years. Similarly, only men with higher TTTA exhibited reduced E_2 levels after weight loss.

Conclusion(s).—A higher TTTA repeat is associated with a strengthened relationship between obesity and E_2. The well-established effect of increased weight on plasma E_2 appears to be absent in men with low TTTA numbers (Fig 1).

▶ Elevated serum estradiol concentrations are observed in obese men as a result of increased conversion of androgens to estrogen by aromatase. Both free and total serum testosterone concentrations are often subnormal in obese men with or without diabetes, and the suppressed values are improved with substantial weight loss. There have been mixed findings of the polymorphism of aromatase polymorphism associated with breast cancer and endometriosis in women and osteoporosis in both men and women. In the study by Hammoud et al, aromatase polymorphism was shown to modulate the relationship between weight and serum estradiol concentrations in obese men. The aromatase enzyme has several tissue-specific promoters, and the expression is regulated by cytokines and glucocorticoids. They concluded that various allelic forms of the TTTA aromatase (TTTAn) polymorphism account for different effects of body weight on serum estradiol concentrations. However, a direct influence of the TTTAn polymorphism on transcriptional or posttranscriptional aromatase requires further study.

A. W. Meikle, MD

Birth Weight in Relation to Sex Steroid Status and Body Composition in Young Healthy Male Siblings

Vanbillemont G, Lapauw B, Bogaert V, et al (Ghent Univ Hosp, Belgium; et al)

J Clin Endocrinol Metab 95:1587-1594, 2010

Context.—Sex steroid concentrations have a strong genetic determination, but environmental factors and body composition play an important role. From studies in children with intrauterine growth restriction, low birth weight has been associated with altered gonadotropin concentrations.

Objective.—We aim to investigate sex steroid concentrations in healthy young brothers in relation to birth weight (normal gestational age), body composition, and parental steroid concentrations.

Design and Setting.—We conducted a cross-sectional, population-based sibling pair study with inclusion of parental data.

Participants.—A total of 677 men (25–45 yr old) were included in this study, with 296 independent pairs of brothers and 122 fathers.

Main Outcomes.—We measured testosterone, estradiol, leptin, adiponectin, IGF-I (immunoassays), and free steroid hormones (calculated) in relation to birth weight and changes in body composition (dual-energy x-ray absorptiometry).

Results.—Birth weight was associated with serum testosterone ($P = 0.0004$) and SHBG ($P = 0.0001$), independent from weight, age, or fat mass, whereas no association with (free) estradiol, LH, or FSH was found. Paternal testosterone ($P = 0.02$), estradiol ($P = 0.04$), and SHBG ($P = 0.0004$) were associated with the respective sex steroid concentrations in the brothers. Weight increase (population rank) during life, was associated with lower testosterone (-15%; $P < 0.001$), independent from current weight and with higher free estradiol concentrations ($+8\%$; $P = 0.002$), whereas weight decrease was associated with higher testosterone ($+13\%$; $P < 0.001$).

Conclusion.—Birth weight and paternal steroid concentrations are associated with testosterone concentrations, independent from adult weight. These findings support the concept of *in utero* programming across the range of birth weight (Fig 1).

▶ Studies in twins and sib pairs have documented that genetic and nongenetic factors are determinants of serum sex steroid concentrations in adult men. Genes have been shown to contribute also to body composition and serum sex steroid concentrations. Elevated body fat mass tends to lower serum testosterone, sex hormone-binding globulin, and luteinizing hormone and elevate serum estradiol. Fetal growth and development of obesity has been observed to be influenced by intrauterine life and might impair gonadal function in adult life. Vanbillemont et al investigated the relationship between birth weight as a parameter of intrauterine life and adult sex steroid status in sib pairs controlling for adult body composition and parental data. Birth weight was positively associated with serum testosterone concentrations independent of

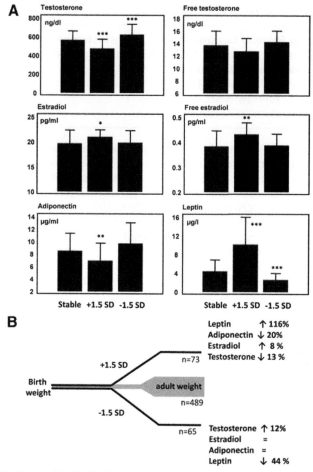

FIGURE 1.—Sex steroid and adipokine concentrations according to changes in weight distribution in our population at birth and young adulthood. A, Sex steroid and adipokine concentrations in subjects who maintained weight (stable), gained (+1.5 SD), or lost (−1.5 SD) weight in relation to their birth weight. B, A schematic representation of the relative difference in hormonal concentrations between subjects who gained or lost weight, compared with weight-stable subjects. (***, $P \le 0.001$; **, $P \le 0.01$; *, $P \le 0.05$ (*bars* indicate median, *error bars* indicate 25% to 75% confidence interval). (Reprinted from Vanbillemont G, Lapauw B, Bogaert V, et al. Birth weight in relation to sex steroid status and body composition in young healthy male siblings. *J Clin Endocrinol Metab.* 2010;95:1587-1594. Copyright 2010, The Endocrine Society.)

adult weight or fat mass. In addition, healthy young men have testosterone concentrations that are associated with paternal steroid concentrations.

A. W. Meikle, MD

Male Hormone Replacement

Parallel-Group Placebo-Controlled Trial of Testosterone Gel in Men With Major Depressive Disorder Displaying an Incomplete Response to Standard Antidepressant Treatment

Pope HG Jr, Amiaz R, Brennan BP, et al (McLean Hosp, Belmont, MA; Chaim Sheba Med Ctr, Tel Hashomer, Israel; et al)
J Clin Psychopharmacol 30:126-134, 2010

Exogenous testosterone therapy has psychotropic effects and has been proposed as an antidepressant augmentation strategy for depressed men. We sought to assess the antidepressant effects of testosterone augmentation of a serotonergic antidepressant in depressed, hypogonadal men. For this study, we recruited 100 medically healthy adult men with major depressive disorder showing partial response or no response to an adequate serotonergic antidepressant trial during the current episode and a screening total testosterone level of 350 ng/dL or lower. We randomized these men to receive testosterone gel or placebo gel in addition to their existing antidepressant regimen. The primary outcome measure was the Hamilton Depression Rating Scale (HDRS) score. Secondary measures included the Montgomery-Asberg Depression Rating Scale, the Clinical Global Impression Scale, and the Quality of Life Scale. Our primary analysis, using a mixed effects linear regression model to compare rate of change of scores between groups on the outcome measures, failed to show a significant difference between groups (mean [95% confidence interval] 6-week change in HDRS for testosterone vs placebo, -0.4 [-2.6 to 1.8]). However, in one exploratory analysis of treatment responders, we found a possible trend in favor of testosterone on the HDRS. Our findings, combined with the conflicting data from earlier smaller studies, suggest that testosterone is not generally effective for depressed men. The possibility remains that testosterone might benefit a particular subgroup of depressed men, but if so, the characteristics of this subgroup would still need to be established (Fig 2).

▶ Testosterone deficiency in men has been associated with depressed mood, depression, low energy, depressed libido, and well-being. Correction of testosterone deficiency using androgen replacement therapy with various preparations of testosterone has been associated with improvement of many of these symptoms. In this study, men with major depressive disorders showing partial or no response to standard antidepressant therapy were treated with testosterone or placebo to determine whether the therapy would affect depression. The study suggests that men with depression without hypogonadism should not be treated routinely with testosterone therapy. Even in men with documented testosterone deficiency, testosterone replacement therapy does not correct all symptoms attributed to hypogonadism. In men with depression without hypogonadism, further study might identify a subpopulation of men who benefited with testosterone therapy, with resistance to standard antidepressive therapy. Any use of

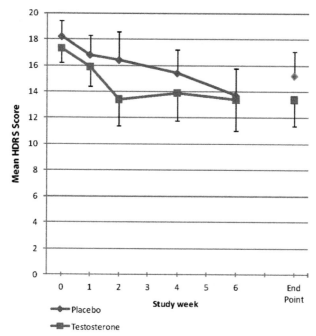

FIGURE 2.—Mean HDRS scores at each study week and at endpoint (LOCF) in participants receiving testosterone and placebo. (Reprinted from Pope HG Jr, Amiaz R, Brennan BP, et al. Parallel-group placebo-controlled trial of testosterone gel in men with major depressive disorder displaying an incomplete response to standard antidepressant treatment. *J Clin Psychopharmacol.* 2010;30:126-134.)

testosterone obviously requires a benefit-risk assessment, and until such time when benefits of relieving depression in a subgroup of men are established, testosterone is not recommended.

A. W. Meikle, MD

8 Neuroendocrinology

Introduction

The neuroendocrine literature (spanning various subtopics) published over the past year was reviewed. Twenty articles were selected for summary and review here. These articles were selected for a variety of reasons, including their potential impact on the practice of medicine, the breadth of the audience to which they apply, and the strength of their investigational rigor. I believe these reports address fundamental issues in neuroendocrinology and are likely to have an important bearing on how we manage pituitary disease. Obviously, many outstanding and significant works were not discussed in this limited overview of the literature.

In the first section, 6 articles were selected in the area of growth hormone (GH) disorders; 4 articles were selected on GH deficiency, and 2 were selected on acromegaly. The first 2 papers by Attanasio et al and Webb et al contribute additional evidence for the physiologic effect of GH deficiency in different clinical settings. The third paper, by Sondergaard et al, addresses a potentially new therapeutic option of a long-acting GH product. The fourth paper, by Yuen et al, looks at the option of using glucagon testing as a GH stimulation test. The final 2 papers in this section focus on GH excess (acromegaly). The paper by Chahal et al identifies AIP mutation in a family of Irish giants (a newly identified form of familial acromegaly). The study by Sandret at al is a meta-analysis of papers looking at the efficacy of cabergoline in the treatment of acromegaly.

The second section reviews 3 studies focusing on the management of hyperprolactinemia. The first paper, by Melmed et al, is a new and updated practice guideline for the treatment of acromegaly. The second paper, by Lebbe et al, looks at the safety of cabergoline treatment in pregnant women with prolactinomas. The third paper, by Barber et al, addresses the role of dopamine agonist withdrawal in patients with prolactin-producing pituitary tumors.

Five articles are reviewed in the third section on hypercortisolemia. The first 2 papers, by Pedroncelli and Castinetti et al, provide reviews of 2 potential new medical treatment options for hypercortisolemia. The third article by Anurag et al addresses a novel PET scan-mediated imaging system for identifying potential adrenal rest tissue in adrenalectomized patients with persistent Cushing's. The fourth paper, by Lindsay et al, looks at different postoperative testing algorithms for optimally determining those patients with postsurgical cure of Cushing's disease. The last paper in this section (by Almeida et al) correlates the size of adrenal nodules in macronodular adrenocortical hyperplasia with the propensity for activation of oncogenic pathways.

The fourth and final section contains 6 articles in general neuroendocrinology. The first 2 papers, both by Sheehan et al, respectively address medical (temozolamide) and radiosurgical therapies for the treatment of pituitary adenomas. The third and fourth articles, by Maio et al and Eboli et al, focus on neurosurgical advances in the treatment of pituitary lesions. The fifth paper, by Freda et al, is a new practice guideline for the treatment of pituitary incidentalomas. The sixth paper, by Zada et al, addresses the clinical characteristics of atypical pituitary adenomas.

William H. Ludlam, MD, PhD

Growth Hormone

Prevalence of Metabolic Syndrome in Adult Hypopituitary Growth Hormone (GH)-Deficient Patients Before and After GH Replacement

Attanasio AF, on behalf of the International Hypopituitary Control and Complications Study Advisory Board (Cascina del Rosone, Agliano Terme, Italy; et al)
J Clin Endocrinol Metab 95:74-81, 2010

Context and Objective.—Metabolic and body compositional consequences of GH deficiency (GHD) in adults are associated with a phenotype similar to the metabolic syndrome (MetS).

Patients.—We assessed MetS prevalence in adult GHD patients (n = 2531) enrolled in the Hypopituitary Control and Complications Study. Prevalence was assessed at baseline and after 3 yr of GH replacement in a subset of 346 adult-onset patients.

Results.—Baseline MetS crude prevalence was 42.3%; age-adjusted prevalence in the United States and Europe was 51.8 and 28.6% ($P < 0.001$), respectively. In the United States, age-adjusted prevalence was significantly higher ($P < 0.001$) than in a general population survey. Increased MetS risk at baseline was observed for age 40 yr or older (adjusted relative risk 1.34, 95% confidence interval 1.17−1.53, $P < 0.001$), females (1.15, 1.05−1.25, $P = 0.002$), and adult onset (1.77, 1.44−2.18, $P < 0.001$). In GH-treated adult-onset patients, MetS prevalence was not changed after 3 yr (42.5−45.7%, $P = 0.172$), but significant changes were seen for waist circumference (62.1−56.9%, $P = 0.008$), fasting glucose (26.0−32.4%, $P < 0.001$), and blood pressure (59.8−69.7%, $P < 0.001$). Significantly increased risk of MetS at yr 3 was associated with baseline MetS (adjusted relative risk 4.09, 95% confidence interval 3.02−5.53, $P < 0.001$) and body mass index 30 kg/m^2 or greater (1.53, 1.17−1.99, $P = 0.002$) and increased risk (with a P value < 0.1) for GH dose 600 μg/d or greater (1.18, 95% confidence interval 0.98−1.44, $P = 0.088$).

Conclusion.—MetS prevalence in GHD patients was higher than in the general population in the United States and higher in the United States than Europe. Prevalence was unaffected by GH replacement, but baseline MetS status and obesity were strong predictors of MetS after GH treatment.

▶ Growth hormone deficiency (GHD) in adults leads to a constellation of effects, including central weight gain, fatigue, lack of vigor, memory deficits, bone loss, and lipid abnormalities. This constellation of symptomatic and physical complaints is often referred to as the adult GHD syndrome. Many of the consequences of GHD on body composition are similar to that seen in metabolic syndrome. These authors evaluated data for 2531 adults with GHD followed in the Hypopituitary Control and Complications Study and assessed parameters of metabolic syndrome in a subset of 346 of these patients who were treated with GH for 3 years. They found that the incidence of metabolic syndrome was higher in patients with GHD than in the general population and was higher in the United States than in Europe. They noted that the overall prevalence of metabolic syndrome was unaffected by GH replacement (some parameters such as central obesity significantly improved, while other parameters worsened). These authors conclude that the treatment of both GHD and non-GHD risk factors must be addressed for patients to have a significant reduction in the overall presentation of the metabolic syndrome.

W. H. Ludlam, MD, PhD

Metabolic, Cardiovascular, and Cerebrovascular Outcomes in Growth Hormone-Deficient Subjects with Previous Cushing's Disease or Non-Functioning Pituitary Adenoma

Webb SM, on behalf of the International HypoCCS Advisory Board (Hosp Sant Pau, Barcelona, Spain; et al)
J Clin Endocrinol Metab 95:630-638, 2010

Context.—Previous exposure to hypercortisolism due to Cushing's disease (CD) may adversely affect long-term metabolic and cardiovascular outcomes. In particular, metabolic and cardiovascular outcomes of patients with previous CD who require GH replacement have not been fully established.

Objective.—The aim of the study was to compare the prevalence and incidence of metabolic syndrome (Adult Treatment Panel III criteria), diabetes mellitus, cardiovascular disease, and cerebrovascular disease in GH-treated subjects with previous CD with GH-treated subjects with previous nonfunctioning pituitary adenoma (NFPA).

Design.—We conducted post hoc analysis of the observational Hypopituitary Control and Complications Study conducted at 362 international centers (1995–2006).

Subjects.—We studied adult-onset GH-deficient subjects with previous CD (n = 160) or NFPA (n = 879). All subjects received GH replacement therapy and were GH naive at enrollment. Multiple pituitary deficits were prevalent in both groups.

Main Outcome Measures.—We measured the prevalence and incidence of metabolic syndrome, diabetes mellitus, cardiovascular disease, and cerebrovascular disease at baseline and at 3 yr, standardized for age and sex differences between groups.

Results.—Compared with subjects with previous NFPA, subjects with previous CD had a significantly greater 3-yr incidence of metabolic syndrome (CD, 23.4%; NFPA, 9.2%; $P = 0.01$), baseline (CD, 6.3%; NFPA, 2.2%; $P < 0.01$) and 3-yr (CD, 7.6%; NFPA, 3.9%; $P = 0.04$) prevalence of cardiovascular disease, and baseline (CD, 6.4%; NFPA, 1.8%; $P = 0.03$) and 3-yr (CD, 10.2%; NFPA, 2.9%; $P = 0.01$) prevalence of cerebrovascular disease.

Conclusions.—Previous hypercortisolism may predispose GH-treated, GH-deficient subjects with prior CD to an increased risk of metabolic syndrome, cardiovascular disease, and cerebrovascular disease.

▶ Patients with a history of Cushing disease (CD; ie, hypercortisolemia as a result of an adrenocorticotropic hormone [ACTH]-producing pituitary tumor) are at high risk for acquiring associated growth hormone deficiency (GHD) secondary to treatment with pituitary surgery or pituitary radiation or because of mass effects of the tumor itself on the pituitary gland. Little is known about the potential impact of the history of long-standing hypercortisolism on the metabolic or cardiovascular effects of GH replacement. These authors conducted a post hoc analysis of data from the observational Hypopituitary Control and Complications Study. They collected data from patients with GHD and either a history of CD (160 patients) or history of nonfunctioning pituitary adenoma (NFPA, 879 patients). They found that, compared with patients with NFPA, the patients with CD had a significantly increased incidence of metabolic syndrome, cardiovascular disease, and cerebrovascular disease. They conclude that prior long-term exposure to glucocorticoid excess may predispose patients with GHD to increased risks of metabolic syndrome, cardiovascular disease, and cerebrovascular disease. This finding may explain the apparent delay in benefit of GH replacement in some posttreatment CD patients.

W. H. Ludlam, MD, PhD

Pegylated Long-Acting Human Growth Hormone Possesses a Promising Once-Weekly Treatment Profile, and Multiple Dosing Is Well Tolerated in Adult Patients with Growth Hormone Deficiency
Søndergaard E, Klose M, Hansen M, et al (Aarhus Univ Hosp, Aarhus C, Denmark; Copenhagen Univ, Denmark; Odense Univ Hosp, Denmark; et al)
J Clin Endocrinol Metab 96:681-688, 2011

Background.—Recombinant human GH (rhGH) replacement therapy in children and adults currently requires daily sc injections for several years or lifelong, which may be both inconvenient and distressing for patients. NNC126-0083 is a pegylated rhGH developed for once-weekly administration.

Objectives.—Our objective was to evaluate the safety, tolerability, pharmacokinetics, and pharmacodynamics of multiple doses of NNC126-0083 in adult patients with GH deficiency (GHD).

Subjects and Methods.—Thirty-three adult patients with GHD, age 20–65 yr, body mass index 18.5–35.0 kg/m^2, and glycated hemoglobin of 8.0% or below. Fourteen days before randomization, subjects discontinued daily rhGH. NNC126-0083 (0.01, 0.02, 0.04, and 0.08 mg/kg) was given sc once weekly for 3 wk (NNC126-0083 for six subjects and placebo for two subjects). Blood samples were collected up to 168 h after the first and up to 240 h after the third dosing. Physical examination, antibodies, and local tolerability were assessed.

Results.—NNC126-0083 was well tolerated with no difference in local tolerability compared with placebo and with no signs of lipoatrophy. A more than dose-proportional exposure was observed at the highest NNC126-0083 dose (0.16 mg protein/kg). Steady-state pharmacokinetics seemed achieved after the second dosing. A clear dose-dependent pharmacodynamic response in circulating IGF-I levels was observed [from a predose mean (SD) IGF-I SD score of −3.2 (1.7) to peak plasma concentration of −0.5 (1.3), 1.6 (1.3), 2.1 (0.5), and 4.4 (0.9) in the four dose groups, respectively].

Conclusion.—After multiple dosing of NNC126-0083, a sustained pharmacodynamic response was observed. NNC126-0083 has the potential to serve as an efficacious, safe, and well-tolerated once-weekly treatment of adult patients with GHD.

▶ Adult growth hormone deficiency syndrome is commonly seen in the context of patients with pituitary tumors and often results from the treatment of the tumor with pituitary surgery or pituitary radiation, or as the result of compressive mass effects of the tumor on the pituitary gland. Because of the relatively short half-life of growth hormone (GH), its replacement is currently given in a once-a-day injection process. The frequency of injections can be tedious for the patients. To address this issue, these authors evaluated a pegylated recombinant human GH (rhGH) (developed for once-weekly injection) for safety, tolerability, pharmacokinetics, and pharmacodynamics. Thirty-three adult patients were evaluated on 4 different doses of the drug ranging from 0.01 to 0.08 mg/kg given as a once-per-week injection for 3 weeks. The drug-treated subjects to placebo-treated subjects ratio was 3:1. The once-weekly pegylated rhGH injections were well tolerated. Steady state pharmacokinetics appeared to be achieved after the second dose. A dose-dependent pharmacodynamic response in insulin-like growth factor 1 was observed. These authors conclude that pegylated rhGH achieved a sustained pharmacodynamic response and appeared to be safe, well tolerated, and efficacious.

W. H. Ludlam, MD, PhD

Is Lack of Recombinant Growth Hormone (GH)-Releasing Hormone in the United States a Setback or Time to Consider Glucagon Testing for Adult GH Deficiency?

Yuen KCJ, Biller BMK, Molitch ME, et al (Oregon Health and Science Univ, Portland; Massachusetts General Hosp, Boston; Northwestern Univ, Chicago, IL)

J Clin Endocrinol Metab 94:2702-2707, 2009

Context.—The use of the combined GHRH and arginine (GHRH-ARG) test has gained increasing acceptance in the United States as a reliable alternative test to the insulin tolerance test (ITT) for diagnosing adult GH deficiency (GHD). In July 2008, the only manufacturer of recombinant GHRH in the United States, EMD Serono, Inc., announced the discontinuation of Geref, thus raising the question of which reliable alternative GH stimulation test should practicing endocrinologists be considering in place of the GHRH-ARG test. In this article, we review the existing published data and consensus guidelines and provide recommendations for alternative stimulation tests to the GHRH-ARG test.

Evidence Acquisition.—The major source of data acquisition included PubMed search strategies and personal experience of the authors from clinical experience.

Evidence Synthesis.—Previous consensus guidelines and previous data assessing the reliability and discriminatory value of the GHRH-ARG, glucagon, ARG, and GH secretagogues on assessing GH reserve are discussed. Our recommendations for performing the glucagon stimulation test, potential drawbacks in conducting this test, and caveats in interpreting this test are also discussed.

Conclusions.—The ITT should remain the test of choice in diagnosing adult GHD. However, when the ITT is not desirable and recombinant GHRH remains unavailable in the United States, we recommend the alternative to the GHRH-ARG test to be the glucagon stimulation test, based on its reliability and availability. Nevertheless, further studies into alternative GH stimulation tests that are available in the United States, comparable, and simpler to perform than the ITT in diagnosing adult GHD are still needed.

▶ Adult growth hormone deficiency (AGHD) syndrome is characterized by fatigue, loss of vigor, central weight gain, memory impairment, bone loss, and distortion of lipid profile. The insulin tolerance test (ITT) has historically been the gold standard for diagnosing AGHD, but the arginine/growth-hormone-releasing hormone (GHRH) test became widely used when it was shown to have a similar sensitivity and specificity to the ITT. However, with the current unavailability of GHRH in the United States, alternate testing methods for diagnosing AGHD are needed. To help characterize alternative testing methods to the ITT, these authors review existing published data discussing various GH stimulation tests. Of all the tests that have been historically performed to assess for AGHD, they note that the glucagon stimulation test (GST) is an excellent test based on its accuracy and reliability, availability, reproducibility, safety,

and lack of being influenced by body mass index, gender, or presence of hypothalamic causes of AGHD. They conclude that the GST is an excellent test for
diagnosing AGHD as long as GHRH continues to not be available in the United
States and when the ITT is contraindicated or not desirable.

W. H. Ludlam, MD, PhD

Prolactin

Place of Cabergoline in Acromegaly: A Meta-Analysis

Sandret L, Maison P, Chanson P (Hôpital de Bicêtre, Le Kremlin Bicêtre,
France; Université Paris Est Créteil, France; Université Paris-Sud, Le Kremlin
Bicêtre, France)
J Clin Endocrinol Metab 96:1327-1335, 2011

Context.—Cabergoline is widely considered to be poorly effective in
acromegaly.

Objective.—The aim of this study was to obtain a more accurate picture
of the efficacy of cabergoline in acromegaly, both alone and in combination with somatostatin analogs.

Design.—We systematically reviewed all trials of cabergoline therapy for
acromegaly published up to 2009 in four databases (PubMed, Pascal,
Embase, and Google Scholar). We identified 15 studies (11 prospective)
with a total of 237 patients; none were randomized or placebo-controlled.
A meta-analysis was conducted on individual data (n = 227).

Results.—Cabergoline was used alone in nine studies. Fifty-one (34%)
of the 149 patients achieved normal IGF-I levels. In multivariate analysis,
the decline in IGF-I was related to the baseline IGF-I concentration
($\beta = 1.16$; $P < 0.001$), treatment duration ($\beta = 0.28$; $P < 0.001$), and baseline prolactin concentration ($\beta = -0.18$; $P = 0.01$), and with a trend
toward a relation with the cabergoline dose ($\beta = 0.38$; $P = 0.07$). In five
studies, cabergoline was added to ongoing somatostatin analog treatment
that had failed to normalize IGF-I. Forty patients (52%) achieved normal
IGF-I levels. The change in IGF-I was significantly related to the baseline
IGF-I level ($\beta = 0.74$; $P < 0.001$) but not to the dose of cabergoline, the
duration of treatment, or the baseline prolactin concentration.

Conclusion.—This meta-analysis suggests that cabergoline single-agent
therapy normalizes IGF-I levels in one third of patients with acromegaly.
When a somatostatin analog fails to control acromegaly, cabergoline
adjunction normalizes IGF-I in about 50% of cases. This effect may
occur even in patients with normoprolactinemia.

▶ Pituitary surgery is typically the first-line treatment for acromegaly. When
surgery is unsuccessful or contraindicated, medications often are able to control
growth hormone (GH) excess. However, the somatostatin analogs (octreotide
and lanreotide) as well as the GH receptor blocker (pegvisomant) are very
expensive and in some cases do not provide good biochemical control of the
somatotrophic tumor. Cabergoline is a relatively cheap medical alternative to

the more expensive drugs but is widely perceived as being ineffective at biochemically controlling GH excess in most cases. To obtain a more accurate assessment of the efficacy of cabergoline in the treatment of acromegaly, these authors reviewed all published trials of acromegalics treated with cabergoline up to 2009. They identified 15 trials (for a total of 237 patients), and a meta-analysis was performed. In the 9 trials where cabergoline was used alone, 51 of 149 patients (34%) achieved biochemical control of insulinlike growth factor 1 (IGF1) levels. Cabergoline was used in combination with somatostatin analogs in 5 trials where initial somatostatin analog therapy alone was unsuccessful. In these studies, 40 patients (52%) with dual therapy achieved control of their IGF1. These authors conclude that cabergoline treatment alone controls GH excess in acromegaly in about one-third of the cases. They note that it also controls GH excess in about one-half of the cases when cabergoline is used in combination with somatostatin therapy after initial somatostatin therapy alone was unsuccessful.

W. H. Ludlam, MD, PhD

Diagnosis and Treatment of Hyperprolactinemia: An Endocrine Society Clinical Practice Guideline
Melmed S, Casanueva FF, Hoffman AR, et al (Cedars Sinai Med Ctr, Los Angeles, CA; Univ of Santiago de Compostela, Spain; VA Palo Alto Health Care System, CA; et al)
J Clin Endocrinol Metab 96:273-288, 2011

Objective.—The aim was to formulate practice guidelines for the diagnosis and treatment of hyperprolactinemia.

Participants.—The Task Force consisted of Endocrine Society-appointed experts, a methodologist, and a medical writer.

Evidence.—This evidence-based guideline was developed using the Grading of Recommendations, Assessment, Development, and Evaluation (GRADE) system to describe both the strength of recommendations and the quality of evidence.

Consensus Process.—One group meeting, several conference calls, and e-mail communications enabled consensus. Committees and members of The Endocrine Society, The European Society of Endocrinology, and The Pituitary Society reviewed and commented on preliminary drafts of these guidelines.

Conclusions.—Practice guidelines are presented for diagnosis and treatment of patients with elevated prolactin levels. These include evidence-based approaches to assessing the cause of hyperprolactinemia, treating drug-induced hyperprolactinemia, and managing prolactinomas in nonpregnant and pregnant subjects. Indications and side effects of therapeutic agents for treating prolactinomas are also presented.

▶ Adult growth hormone deficiency (AGHD) syndrome is characterized by fatigue, loss of vigor, central weight gain, memory impairment, bone loss, and distortion of lipid profile. The insulin tolerance test (ITT) has historically been the gold standard for diagnosing AGHD, but the arginine/growth hormone—releasing hormone (GHRH) test became widely used when it was shown to have a similar sensitivity and specificity to the ITT. However, with the current unavailability of the GHRH in the United States, alternate testing methods for diagnosing AGHD are needed. To help characterize alternative testing methods to the ITT, these authors review existing published data discussing various growth hormone stimulation tests. Of all the tests that have been historically performed to assess for AGHD, they note that the glucagon stimulation test (GST) is an excellent test based on its accuracy and reliability, availability, reproducibility, safety, and lack of being influenced by body mass index, gender, or presence of hypothalamic causes of AGHD. They conclude that the GST is an excellent test for diagnosing AGHD as long as GHRH continues to not be available in the United States and when the ITT is contraindicated or not desirable.

W. H. Ludlam, MD, PhD

Outcome of 100 pregnancies initiated under treatment with cabergoline in hyperprolactinaemic women
Lebbe M, Hubinont C, Bernard P, et al (Université Catholique de Louvain, Brussels, Belgium)
Clin Endocrinol 73:236-242, 2010

Context.—Data concerning the safety for pregnancy of cabergoline treatment in hyperprolactinaemic women are still scarce.

Objective.—To exclude a higher than normal risk for miscarriage and congenital malformation in pregnancies initiated under cabergoline treatment.

Design.—A retrospective study of 100 pregnancies in 72 hyperprolactinaemic women treated with cabergoline at the time of conception and follow-up of the 88 newborn children.

Methods.—Cabergoline was interrupted in 99 pregnancies and continued in one case. Foetal exposure dose to cabergoline was calculated for each pregnancy. Complications of pregnancy and neonatal status were compared to those observed in an age-and delivery time-matched control group of 163 women.

Results.—The mean foetal exposure dose to cabergoline was 3·6 ± 4·7 mg. The rate of spontaneous miscarriages was 10%. Three medical terminations of pregnancy were performed for a foetal malformation (3%). Minor to moderate complications were observed in 31% of the pregnancies, a figure similar to that found in the control group. An increase in tumour size (2—8 mm) was observed in 17/37 evaluated cases, needing reintroduction of cabergoline during pregnancy in five patients. The 84 deliveries resulted in 88 infants, three of them presenting with a malformation (3·4%). Neonatal status was comparable to the control group, where a malformation rate of 6·3% was observed. Postnatal development of the children was normal.

Conclusion.—Cabergoline treatment at the time of conception appears to be safe for both the pregnancy and the neonate, although more data are still needed on a larger number of pregnancies.

▶ Treating hyperprolactinemia with dopamine agonist therapy (with the goal of normalizing ovulation) is often required to restore fertility in patients with prolactin-producing pituitary adenomas. This process often includes treating patients with dopamine agonists until pregnancy is confirmed, at which point the dopamine agonist is discontinued. Although cabergoline is frequently used to treat patients with prolactinomas, much more safety data are available regarding the safety of bromocriptine in the early phases of pregnancy, and clinicians often feel compelled to switch women from cabergoline to bromocriptine when pregnancy is desired. To address whether cabergoline causes any risk to the fetus when used in the early stages of pregnancy (prior to discontinuance), these authors perform a retrospective study of 100 pregnancies in 72 women with prolactinomas. Complications of pregnancy and neonatal health were compared with 163 controls (women with no history of hyperprolactinemia). In the cabergoline-treated group, the rate of spontaneous miscarriage was 10%, and the rate of medical terminations because of fetal abnormalities was 3%. These rates were very close to those found in the control group. The postdelivery development of the children from the cabergoline-treated mothers was normal. These authors conclude that cabergoline treatment at the time of conception is safe for both the mother and the child, although they acknowledge that the number of cases of cabergoline treatment is still far less than the data available for bromocriptine treatment in this setting.

W. H. Ludlam, MD, PhD

Recurrence of hyperprolactinaemia following discontinuation of dopamine agonist therapy in patients with prolactinoma occurs commonly especially in macroprolactinoma

Barber TM, Kenkre J, Garnett C, et al (Churchill Hosp, Headington, Oxford, UK)
Clin Endocrinol 2011 [Epub ahead of print]

Context.—The optimal duration of dopamine agonist (DA) therapy in prolactinoma is unknown. There are concerns that despite low recurrence rates in highly-selected groups, high recurrence rates after DA withdrawal may occur in routine practice.

Objective.—To explore recurrence of hyperprolactinaemia and predictive factors following DA withdrawal in patients with microprolactinoma and macroprolactinoma.

Design.—A retrospective study on adult patients with confirmed prolactinoma attending the Oxford Endocrine Department.

Patients and Measurements.—We identified patients with macroprolactinoma (n=15) and microprolactinoma (n=45) treated with DA therapy for >3 years, with a trial off DA therapy. None had other treatments. Measurements included recurrence of hyperprolactinaemia following DA withdrawal, tumour size (macroprolactinomas), duration of DA therapy, prolactin levels (baseline, during DA therapy, recurrence), and time to recurrence. Data reported as mean (range).

Results.—During DA therapy, prolactin levels suppressed to normal range in all patients with macroprolactinoma and microprolactinoma, and most macroprolactinomas (n=14) had substantial tumour shrinkage. Hyperprolactinaemia recurred in 93% of macroprolactinomas (n=14) at 8.8 months (3-36) and 64% of microprolactinomas (n=29) at 4.8 months (3-12). Duration of DA therapy: macroprolactinomas 7.5 years (4-15); microprolactinomas 4.1 years (3-10). Prolactin levels during DA therapy: macroprolactinomas 144mU/l (7-336); microprolactinomas 278mU/l (30-629). For microprolactinomas, prolactin levels during DA therapy were less suppressed in those with recurrence than in those without recurrence ($P<0.05$).

Conclusions.—In routine practice, hyperprolactinaemia recurs early in most macroprolactinomas (93%) and microprolactinomas (64%) following DA therapy discontinuation. For most macroprolactinomas, cessation of DA cannot be recommended even after 7 years of therapy.

▶ Dopamine agonist (DA) therapy is the mainstay of treatment for prolactinomas. DA treatment in these cases typically leads to reduction in hyperprolactinemia, pituitary tumor shrinkage, and resolution of unwanted effects of prolactin excess. After several years of treatment, DA therapy can be discontinued in some cases with resulting long-term tumor control. However, unwanted return of hyperprolactinemia and tumor growth is often the consequence once DA treatment is discontinued. It is not clear how often tumor recurrence occurs in general practice after stopping DA therapy, but with general concerns about DA side effects such as cardiac valve fibrosis, clinicians often try to minimize prolonged exposure to DA treatment. To address the issue of how frequently DA withdrawal is successful, these authors perform a retrospective analysis of 45 microprolactinomas and 15 macroprolactinomas over a 3-year period and review the recurrence rate of hyperprolactinemia and tumor growth after DA withdrawal. Hyperprolactinemia recurred after DA withdrawal in 93% of macroprolactinomas after 8.8 months and 64% of microprolactinomas at 4.8 months. They conclude that recurrence of hyperprolactinemia occurs more frequently after DA withdrawal in macroprolactinomas. These authors therefore do not recommend DA withdrawal in this patient population even after prolonged therapy.

W. H. Ludlam, MD, PhD

ACTH

Medical Treatment of Cushing's Disease: Somatostatin Analogues and Pasireotide

Pedroncelli AM (Novartis Pharma AG, Basle, Switzerland)
Neuroendocrinology 92:120-124, 2010

Cushing's disease is Cushing's syndrome caused by an adrenocorticotropic hormone-secreting pituitary adenoma and, in the absence of adequate treatment, can be fatal. Cushing's disease represents an unmet medical need, with no approved medical therapies. Pasireotide is a novel multi-receptor- targeted somatostatin analogue with high affinity for $sst_{1,2,3}$ and sst_5. Compared with octreotide, pasireotide has an in vitro binding affinity 40-, 30- and 5-fold higher for sst_5, sst_1 and sst_3, respectively, and 2-fold lower for sst_2. Adrenocorticotropic hormone-secreting pituitary adenomas predominantly express sst_5, followed by sst_2 and sst_1, suggesting that pasireotide may be effective in the treatment of Cushing's disease. In a 15-day phase II trial of pasireotide 600 µg s.c. b.i.d. in patients with de novo or persistent/recurrent Cushing's disease, 22 of 29 patients (76%) achieved reduced urinary free cortisol (UFC) levels, 5 of whom (17%) achieved normalized UFC. Patients who achieved normalized UFC had a significantly greater reduction in serum cortisol than those who did not ($p = 0.04$), and minimum pasireotide plasma concentrations appeared to be higher in responders. Based on these results, a randomized, double-blind phase III study comparing pasireotide 600 µg b.i.d. and 900 µg b.i.d. was initiated and is ongoing. This is the largest ever phase III study in patients with Cushing's disease. The primary end point of this study is normalization of UFC after 6 months of treatment. Finally, preliminary results from a study on 17 patients with Cushing's disease suggest that the combined use of pasireotide, cabergoline and low-dose ketoconazole may have additive beneficial effects in the medical treatment of Cushing's disease.

▶ Cushing disease is caused by an adrenocorticotropic hormone—producing pituitary adenoma. Transsphenoidal pituitary surgery is the first-line treatment but is unsuccessful in 10% to 20% of cases. When surgery is not successful, adjunct treatment is necessary and may include repeat pituitary surgery, bilateral adrenalectomy, or stereotactic radiosurgery. Each of these adjunct treatment options has the potential of improving the hypercortisolemia, but each has significant drawbacks (eg, respectively, pituitary insufficiency, Nelson syndrome, frontal lobe necrosis, or vision damage, etc). The only medical option available at this point that has any significant efficacy are inhibitors steroidogenesis (such as ketoconazole), but these drugs have significant toxicity, including significant gastrointestinal upset and potential liver damage. For this reason, SOM230 (pasireotide) was developed, which is a nonspecific somatostatin receptor analog that has higher affinity for somatostatin receptor subtype 5 than octreotide does (somatostatin receptor subtype 5 is most predominant subtype on Cushing tumors). Early clinical trials, as described in this article, demonstrate that urinary-free cortisols are reduced by half on the doses tested and act as quickly as 2 weeks. Phase III clinical data should be available soon. If the drug is approved for the treatment of Cushing disease, it will be the first centrally acting drug for the treatment of Cushing disease on the market.

W. H. Ludlam, MD, PhD

Medical Treatment of Cushing's Syndrome: Glucocorticoid Receptor Antagonists and Mifepristone

Castinetti F, Conte-Devolx B, Brue T (Hôpital de la Timone, Marseille, France)
Neuroendocrinology 92:125-130, 2010

Mifepristone is the first and only available glucocorticoid receptor antagonist. It was initially mainly considered as a socalled 'contragestive' pill due to its antiprogestin activity. In this review, we summarize the results of mifepristone reported in the literature as a treatment of Cushing's syndrome. Most of the patients were treated due to unsuccessful surgery and/or partially effective anticortisolic drugs. The majority of them presented a rapid decrease of clinical signs of hypercortisolism during the first month of treatment; about half experienced a reduction in their elevated blood pressure, and half of the diabetic patients presented improved blood glucose levels. Mifepristone treatment has 2 main drawbacks: (1) the blockade of glucocorticoid receptors leads to increased ACTH and cortisol levels, making it difficult to adapt the treatment and diagnose adrenal deficiency, and (2) increased cortisol levels can also lead to severe hy pokalemia. Follow-up of efficacy should only be clinical (weight, blood pressure, skin lesions) and biological (regular blood potassium sampling). Dose adjustment will be performed based on these parameters. The lack of a large available prospective cohort of patients on mifepristone, and the scarcity of data on its long-term effects, does not allow recommending it as a first-line drug in the treatment of hypercortisolism. However, as mifepristone is a rapidly effective drug, it can play a role in the management of hypercortisolism. The main indication is the partial efficacy or bad tolerance of other well-known anticortisolic drugs, either by replacement (bad tolerance, lack of effectiveness) or addition (multimodal approach) of mifepristone.

▶ Mifepristone (RU-486) has historically been used as an abortifacient because of its antiprogestin activity. However, it also acts as a glucocorticoid receptor antagonist that offers a potentially promising therapeutic role in the control of hypercortisolemia. Although mifepristone does not lower serum cortisol levels (it actually increases cortisol and corticotropin [ACTH] levels), it acts as a competitive inhibitor of cortisol at the glucocorticoid receptor effectively lowering the physiologic actions of the steroid in the body. In anticipation of the soon to be released results from the recently concluded mifepristone phase III study, these authors review what has been published to date on the role of mifepristone in Cushing syndrome. Most patients in the studies reviewed had marked reduction in the clinical features of hypercortisolemia after treatment with mifepristone, and most had reduction in their elevated blood pressure and blood sugar levels that were secondary to hypercortisolemia. The most significant disadvantages of mifepristone are the following: (1) Because ACTH and cortisol increase with therapy, these biochemical parameters cannot be used for dose titration, and (2) the patients can have hypokalemia secondary to the increased cortisol levels. These authors suggest that mifepristone may have a role in the management of hypercortisolemia.

W. H. Ludlam, MD, PhD

Localization of Remnant and Ectopic Adrenal Tissues with Cosyntropin-Stimulated 18F-FDG-PET/CT in a Patient with Nelson Syndrome with Persistent Hypercortisolism
Lila AR, Malhotra G, Sarathi V, et al (Seth G. S. Med College, Mumbai, India; Tata Memorial Hosp, Parel, Mumbai, India)
J Clin Endocrinol Metab 95:5172-5173, 2010

A 27-yr-old woman with Cushing's disease (CD) had persistent hypercortisolism despite two transsphenoidal operations. She underwent bilateral adrenalectomy (BA) by open surgery, which resulted in temporary remission of the disease. Two years after BA, she had a recurrence of Cushingoid features. Diagnostic evaluation showed hypercortisolism [basal cortisol, 29.1 μg/dl (800.25 nmol/liter); 2-mg 48-h dexamethasone suppression test serum cortisol, 17 μg/dl (467.5 nmol/liter)] and highly elevated basal ACTH [884 pg/ml (194.04 pmol/liter)] with enlargement of the pituitary tumor (8 × 8 mm), suggestive of Nelson syndrome with persistent hypercortisolism.

The patient underwent 2-(^{18}F)-fluoro-2-deoxy-D-glucose positron emission tomography/computed tomography (^{18}F-FDG-PET/CT) to look for the source of cortisol production. FDG hypermetabolism was seen at the right [standard uptake value (SUV), 2.2] and left (SUV, 1.6) suprarenal regions (marked with metallic clips during previous surgery) and at a focus near the left renal hilum (SUV, 2.0). SUV at these sites increased to 6.1, 6.8, and 7.2, respectively, after 30 min of sc administration of 250 μg of cosyntropin (Figs 1 and 2), confirming them to be adrenal tissues. The patient declined a repeat adrenalectomy/pituitary adenomectomy and opted for pituitary radiotherapy.

The prevalence of Nelson syndrome varies between 8 and 29%. Persistent hypercortisolism after BA is rare (1 in 37) in CD patients. It may be due to residual or ectopic adrenal tissues. In a previously reported case of CD with recurrence of Cushing's syndrome after BA, remnant left adrenal tissue was demonstrated using ^{131}I-adosterol (6β-iodomethyl-19-norcholesterol). We report a similar case where remnant and ectopic adrenal tissues were identified with ACTH-stimulated ^{18}F-FDG-PET/CT. This diagnostic modality may be used in clinical practice to localize adrenal tissue.

▶ Bilateral adrenalectomy (BLA) is sometimes performed as a second-line treatment for Cushing disease when pituitary surgery is unsuccessful at achieving biochemical cure. Although BLA is thought to offer definitive cure for Cushing disease in the vast majority of cases, there are times when patients have persistence of Cushing symptoms and detectable serum cortisol levels after BLA consistent with the presence of adrenal rest tissue. Historically, the I-adosterol cholesterol scan was helpful in potentially identifying adrenal rest tissue, but this test is no longer readily available. To address the need for a good imaging technique for the visualization of adrenal rest tissue, these authors used 2-(^{18}F)-fluoro-2-deoxy-D-glucose positron emission tomography/CT in a patient who had symptoms and biochemistry consistent with an ectopic source of cortisol. The study identified several hilar masses that were potential surgical targets. This is a promising technique that can be made available to patients who have signs and symptoms of persistent cortisol levels.

W. H. Ludlam, MD, PhD

The Postoperative Basal Cortisol and CRH Tests for Prediction of Long-Term Remission from Cushing's Disease after Transsphenoidal Surgery

Lindsay JR, Oldfield EH, Stratakis CA, et al (Altnagelvin Area Hosp, Londonderry, UK; Natl Insts of Health, Bethesda, MD)
J Clin Endocrinol Metab 96:2011 [Epub ahead of print]

Context.—Selective adenomectomy via transsphenoidal surgery induces remission of Cushing's disease (CD) in most patients. Although an undetectable postoperative serum cortisol (<2 μg/dl) has been advocated as an index of remission, there is no consensus on predictors of recurrence.

Objective.—We hypothesized that patients with subnormal cortisol (2–4.9 μg/dl) might achieve long-term remission and that postoperative responses to CRH might predict recurrence.

Design, Setting, and Participants.—We prospectively studied CD patients with initial remission after adenomectomy or hemihypophysectomy (n = 14). Long-term recurrence (n = 39) or remission (n = 293) was assigned by laboratory results, glucocorticoid dependence, or patient survey at a mean of 10.6 yr after surgery.

Intervention and Main Outcome Measures.—Postoperatively, morning cortisol was measured on d 3–5, and cortisol and ACTH responses to ovine CRH were assessed around d 10.

Results.—Follow-up duration was median 11 yr (range 1–22.8 yr). Fewer patients achieved a cortisol nadir below 2 μg/dl (87%) than below 5 μg/dl (98%), yet recurrence rates were similar (<2 μg/dl, 9.5%; <5 μg/dl,

10.4%; 2–4.9 μg/dl, 20%; not significant). CRH-stimulated cortisol ($P < 0.002$) and ACTH ($P = 0.04$) values were higher for the recurrence than the remission group. However, no basal or stimulated ACTH or serum or urine cortisol cutoff value predicted all who later recurred.

Conclusions.—A postoperative cortisol below 2 μg/dl predicts long-term remission after transsphenoidal surgery in CD. Remission in those with intermediate d 3–5 postoperative cortisol values (2–4.9 μg/dl) suggests that these patients do not require immediate reoperation. However, because no single cortisol cutoff value excludes all patients with recurrence, all require long-term clinical follow-up.

▶ Cushing disease (caused by a corticotropin-producing pituitary adenoma) can be difficult to cure in 10% to 20% of cases on initial surgery. These surgical failures therefore need additional treatment that may include repeat pituitary surgery, radiation, adrenalectomy, or medical therapy in some cases. For this reason, determining whether a person is cured after pituitary surgery is very important. Many pituitary centers have historically measured serum cortisol levels on the third day after surgery after withdrawing the patient from steroid for 24 hours prior to the draw. This process may potentially suggest erroneously that a patient is not cured from the Cushing disease because their drop in cortisol may not have reached a nadir by the morning of the third day. This could inadvertently lead their doctors to conclude that they are not cured and proceed to another pituitary surgery. To get around this timing issue, some centers now hold all postoperative steroids starting immediately after surgery and then measure serum cortisol every 3 to 6 hours until a cortisol nadir is reached. Postoperative steroids are not given in this scenario until the patient clinically needs them. This is a more accurate way to assess nadir of cortisol after Cushing surgery. To help determine which patients were at highest risk for noncure or recurrence of disease, these authors performed serial postoperative serum cortisol monitoring for several days and then a corticotropin-releasing hormone (CRH) stimulation test around postoperative day 10. Follow-up was for a mean of 10.6 years, and the patients were divided into a recurrence and a remission group depending on their postoperative data. Surprisingly, those patients with an immediate postoperative cortisol of less than 5 μg/dL were as likely to recur as those patients with a postoperative cortisol nadir of less than 2 μg/dL. CRH-stimulated cortisols were higher in the recurrence group. These authors conclude that patients with immediate postoperative cortisols of less than 5 μg/dL do not require reexploration.

W. H. Ludlam, MD, PhD

Integrated Genomic Analysis of Nodular Tissue in Macronodular Adrenocortical Hyperplasia: Progression of Tumorigenesis in a Disorder Associated with Multiple Benign Lesions

Almeida MQ, Harran M, Bimpaki EI, et al (Natl Insts of Health, Bethesda, MD; et al)

J Clin Endocrinol Metab 96:E728-E738, 2011

Context.—Massive macronodular adrenocortical disease or ACTH-independent macronodular adrenal hyperplasia (AIMAH) is a clinically and genetically heterogeneous disorder.

Objective and Design.—Whole-genome expression profiling and oligonucleotide array comparative genomic hybridization changes were analyzed in samples of different nodules from the same patients with AIMAH. Quantitative RT-PCR and staining were employed to validate them RNA array data.

Results.—Chromosomal gains were more frequent in larger nodules when compared with smaller nodules from the same patients. Among the 50 most overexpressed genes, 50% had a chromosomal locus that was amplified in the comparative genomic hybridization data. Although the list of most over-and underexpressed genes was similar between the nodules of different size, the gene set enrichment analysis identified different pathways associated with AIMAH that corresponded to the size; the smaller nodules were mainly enriched for metabolic pathways, whereas p53 signaling and cancer genes were enriched in larger nodules. Confirmatory studies demonstrated that *BCL2, E2F1, EGF, c-KIT,MYB, PRKCA,* and *CTNNB1* were overexpressed in the larger nodules at messenger and/or protein levels. Chromosomal enrichment analysis showed that chromosomes 20q13 and 14q23 might be involved in progression of AIMAH from smaller to larger tumors.

Conclusion.—Integrated transcriptomic and genomic data for AIMAH provides supporting evidence to the hypothesis that larger adrenal lesions, in the context of this chronic, polyclonal hyperplasia, accumulate an increased number of genomic and, subsequently, transcript abnormalities. The latter shows that the disease appears to start with mainly tissue metabolic derangements, as suggested by the study of the smaller nodules, but larger lesions showed aberrant expression of oncogenic pathways.

▶ Cushing syndrome can be caused by corticotropin (ACTH)-dependant causes such as pituitary tumors or ACTH-independent causes such as cortisol-producing adrenal tumors. ACTH-independent macronodular adrenal hyperplasia (AIMAH), also known as massive macronodular adrenal disease, is a rare cause of Cushing syndrome and is characterized by multiple benign adrenal gland lesions of varying sizes. It is a very heterogeneous disorder both clinically and genetically. These authors seek to better characterize the disorder through analysis of whole-genome expression profiling and oligonucleotide array comparative genomic hybridization changes of the nodular tissue. Their data show that the smaller size nodules contain a predominance of metabolic pathway abnormalities, and the larger nodules were associated with pathologic p53 signaling and cancer genes. They conclude that the larger adrenal nodules found in AIMAH contain a large number of genomic and associated transcript abnormalities. The disease appears to start with derangements of tissue metabolism and progress to expression of oncogenic pathways.

W. H. Ludlam, MD, PhD

Pituitary-General

AIP Mutation in Pituitary Adenomas in the 18th Century and Today
Chahal HS, Stals K, Unterländer M, et al (Queen Mary Univ of London, UK; Royal Devon and Exeter Foundation Trust, UK; Johannes Gutenberg Univ, Mainz, Germany; et al)
N Engl J Med 364:43-50, 2011

Gigantism results when a growth hormone—secreting pituitary adenoma is present before epiphyseal fusion. In 1909, when Harvey Cushing examined the skeleton of an Irish patient who lived from 1761 to 1783, he noted an enlarged pituitary fossa. We extracted DNA from the patient's teeth and identified a germline mutation in the aryl hydrocarbon—interacting protein gene (*AIP*). Four contemporary Northern Irish families who presented with gigantism, acromegaly, or prolactinoma have the same mutation and haplotype associated with the mutated gene. Using coalescent theory, we infer that these persons share a common ancestor who lived about 57 to 66 generations earlier.

▶ Although the vast majority of cases of gigantism result from sporadic mutations, there are some rare familial sources such as the *MEN-1* gene mutation. Additionally, it has been long appreciated that there is a likely familial connection (ie, genetic connection) between multiple members of 4 contemporary Northern Irish families that have a high prevalence of gigantism. To study the potential genetic connection between these families, these authors extracted DNA from 2 teeth from the skull of an Irish giant (index patient) who had lived in the 1700s. They compared it with DNA samples from 4 contemporary Northern Irish families also with a history of gigantism. Using polymerase chain reaction, they sequenced DNA of the region flanking the R304 site in each of these patients and noted a similar germ line mutation in the aryl hydrocarbon-interacting protein gene, which was a heterozygous c.910C to T change. These authors conclude that the index patient carried the same founder mutation as that seen in 4 contemporary families with gigantism and, therefore, have identified a new genetic link predisposing for gigantism.

W. H. Ludlam, MD, PhD

Temozolomide-induced inhibition of pituitary adenoma cells

Sheehan J, Rainey J, Nguyen J, et al (Univ of Virginia Health Sciences Ctr, Charlottesville)

J Neurosurg 114:354-358, 2011

Object.—Aggressive pituitary adenomas frequently require multimodality treatment including pituitary-suppressive medications, microsurgery, and radiation therapy or radiosurgery. The effectiveness of temozolomide in terms of growth suppression and decreased hormonal production is evaluated.

Methods.—Three pituitary adenoma cell lines—MMQ, GH3, and AtT20—were used. A dose escalation of temozolomide was performed for each cell line, and inhibition of cell proliferation was assessed using an MTT assay. Concentrations of temozolomide that produced statistically significant inhibition of cell proliferation for each cell type were identified. Extent of apoptosis for each selected temozolomide concentration was studied using TUNEL staining. The effect of temozolomide on prolactin secretion in MMQ and GH3 cells was also measured via ELISA.

Results.—Significant inhibition of cell proliferation was noted for MMQ and GH3 cells at a concentration of 250 μM temozolomide. The AtT20 cells demonstrated statistically significant cell inhibition at a concentration of only 50 μM temozolomide ($p < 0.05$). Apoptosis significantly increased in all cell lines in as little as 24 hours of incubation at the respective temozolomide concentrations ($p < 0.05$). Prolactin secretion in the prolactin secreting MMQ and GH3 cell lines was inhibited by 250 μM temozolomide.

Conclusions.—Temozolomide inhibits cell proliferation and induces apoptotic cell death in aggressive pituitary adenoma cells. A reduction in hormonal secretion in prolactinoma cells was also afforded by temozolomide. Temozolomide may prove useful in the multimodality management of aggressive pituitary adenomas.

▶ Pituitary tumors are typically managed with transsphenoidal surgery, radiation, and in some hormonally active tumors like prolactinomas, medications such as dopamine agonists. Aggressive pituitary lesions can be refractory to these measures and may require additional intervention. Temozolomide is useful in patients with high-grade gliomas, and some clinicians believe that it may be effective in treating aggressive pituitary tumors. To address this question, these authors assessed the effectiveness of temozolomide on the suppression of tumor growth and tumor hormone overproduction in pituitary tumor cell lines. Increasing doses of temozolomide were applied to 3 cell lines (MMQ, GH3 and AtT20), and effects on cell proliferation were assessed. They found that cell proliferation was inhibited and that apoptosis increased in all 3 cell lines. Furthermore, prolactin secretion was inhibited in the cells that produce prolactin. These authors conclude that because temozolomide suppresses tumor growth and hormone production and induces apoptosis in aggress pituitary tumor cells in vitro, it may play a role in the treatment of aggressive pituitary tumors in vivo. Further clinical studies are warranted in this area.

W. H. Ludlam, MD, PhD

Gamma Knife surgery for pituitary adenomas: factors related to radiological and endocrine outcomes

Sheehan JP, Pouratian N, Steiner L, et al (Univ of Virginia Health System, Charlottesville; et al)
J Neurosurg 114:303-309, 2011

Object.—Gamma Knife surgery (GKS) is a common treatment for recurrent or residual pituitary adenomas. This study evaluates a large cohort of patients with a pituitary adenoma to characterize factors related to endocrine remission, control of tumor growth, and development of pituitary deficiency.

Methods.—A total of 418 patients who underwent GKS with a minimum follow-up of 6 months (median 31 months) and for whom there was complete follow-up were evaluated. Statistical analysis was performed to evaluate for significant factors ($p < 0.05$) related to treatment outcomes.

Results.—In patients with a secretory pituitary adenoma, the median time to endocrine remission was 48.9 months. The tumor margin radiation dose was inversely correlated with time to endocrine remission. Smaller adenoma volume correlated with improved endocrine remission in those with secretory adenomas. Cessation of pituitary suppressive medications at the time of GKS had a trend toward statistical significance in regard to influencing endocrine remission. In 90.3% of patients there was tumor control. A higher margin radiation dose significantly affected control of adenoma growth.

New onset of a pituitary hormone deficiency following GKS was seen in 24.4% of patients. Treatment with pituitary hormone suppressive medication at the time of GKS, a prior craniotomy, and larger adenoma volume at the time of radiosurgery were significantly related to loss of pituitary function.

Conclusions.—Smaller adenoma volume improves the probability of endocrine remission and lowers the risk of new pituitary hormone deficiency with GKS. A higher margin dose offers a greater chance of endocrine remission and control of tumor growth.

▶ Pituitary surgery is the treatment of choice for most clinically significant pituitary lesions (other than prolactinomas that are typically treated medically). However, when pituitary surgery is not successful or is contraindicated, adjunct therapy with various forms of radiation may be indicated. Although radiation therapy offers many positive consequences in terms of stopping tumor growth or reducing hormonal activity, it also has the potential of inducing negative sequela such as pituitary damage, frontal lobe necrosis, and vision loss. These authors retrospectively review their own patients at a single institution to assess the positive and negative effects of one form of stereotactic radiosurgery, specifically gamma knife surgery (GKS). These authors reviewed records for 418 patients who underwent GKS with a minimum follow-up of 6 months. They note that the median time to endocrine remission was 48.9 months, that smaller tumors had a shorter time to endocrine remission, and that a higher margin dose led to greater endocrine remission. New endocrine deficiencies were noted in 24.4%. GKS is a safe and effective means of creating control of tumor growth as well as endocrine remission, and it has minimal side effects.

W. H. Ludlam, MD, PhD

Extended endoscopic endonasal approach for selected pituitary adenomas: early experience

Maio SD, Cavallo LM, Esposito F, et al (Univ of British Columbia, Vancouver, Canada; Università degli Studi di Napoli Federico II, Naples, Italy)
J Neurosurg 114:345-353, 2011

Object.—Whereas most pituitary adenomas are removable via the transsphenoidal approach, certain cases, such as dumbbell-shaped or suprasellar adenomas and recurrent and/or fibrous tumors, remain difficult to treat. The authors present their experience with the extended endoscopic endonasal approach to the suprasellar area in managing this subset of tumors, which are classically treated through a transcranial route.

Methods.—From June 1997 to December 2008, 615 patients underwent endoscopic endonasal transsphenoidal surgery for pituitary adenomas in the Department of Neurosurgery of the Universitá degli Studi di Napoli Federico II. Of this group, 20 patients with pituitary adenomas needed an extended endoscopic endonasal transtuberculum/transplanum approach for tumor removal. Two surgical corridors were used during the transsphenoidal approach: 1) the conventional endosellar extraarachnoidal corridor and 2) a suprasellar transarachnoidal corridor.

Results.—The extent of resection was gross total in 12 (60%) of the 20 patients, near total in 4 (20%), subtotal in 3 (15%), and partial in 1 (5%). Postoperative CSF leakage occurred in 1 patient. One patient experienced worsening of temporal hemianopsia.

Conclusions.—The authors' initial results with the extended endoscopic approach to the suprasellar area for selected pituitary adenomas are promising and may justify a widening of the current classical indications for transsphenoidal surgery.

▶ Transsphenoidal adenomectomy (TSA) is the most common neurosurgical approach for removing pituitary adenomas. Historically, this procedure was not considered a safe means of removing complex dumbbell-shaped tumors, giant tumors, or hard lesions such as fibrous tumors, meningiomas, or craniopharyngiomas. As a safe alternative, craniotomies have been performed to give good visibility of the optic apparatus and carotid arteries. The morbidity, prolonged convalescence, and cost associated with craniotomies are significant. In recent years, some surgeons have begun to use a variant of the TSA in which the surgical window at the floor of the sella turcica is given wide exposure, allowing the surgeon to get excellent visibility of the optic chiasm and other vital structures while removing the pituitary lesion from below. To help characterize the positives and negatives of the extended TSA, these authors retrospectively review 615 of their own patients who underwent TSA between 1997 and 2008. They identify 20 patients who had the extended approach performed with the TSA. They note that 12 of the 20 patients (60%) had complete tumor removal and an additional 4 patients (20%) had a near total resection. Postoperatively, 1 patient had a cerebrospinal fluid leak and 1 patient had worsening pituitary-related vision compromise. They conclude that this extended TSA is a promising technique for removing complex pituitary lesions and that the associated morbidity is less than that associated with the traditional craniotomy used in this setting.

W. H. Ludlam, MD, PhD

Intraoperative computed tomography registration and electromagnetic neuronavigation for transsphenoidal pituitary surgery: accuracy and time effectiveness

Eboli P, Shafa B, Mayberg M (Swedish Neuroscience Inst, Seattle, WA)
J Neurosurg 114:329-335, 2011

Object.—The authors assessed the feasibility, anatomical accuracy, and cost effectiveness of frameless electromagnetic (EM) neuronavigation in conjunction with portable intraoperative CT (iCT) registration for transsphenoidal adenomectomy (TSA).

Methods.—A prospective database was established for data obtained in 208 consecutive patients who underwent TSA in which the iCT/EM navigation technique was used. Data were compared with those acquired in a retrospective cohort of 65 consecutive patients in whom fluoroscope-assisted TSA had been performed by the same surgeon. All patients in both groups underwent transnasal removal of pituitary adenomas or neuroepithelial cysts, using identical surgical techniques with an operating microscope. In the iCT/EM technique—treated cases, a portable iCT scan was obtained immediately prior to surgery for registration to the EM navigation system, which did not require rigid head fixation. Preexisting (nonnavigation protocol) MR imaging studies were fused with the iCT scans to enable 3D navigation based on MR imaging data. The accuracy of the navigation system was determined in the first 50 iCT/EM cases by visual concordance of the navigation probe location to 5 preselected bony landmarks. For all patients in both cohorts, total operating room time, incision-to-closure time, and relative costs of imaging and surgical procedures were determined from hospital records.

Results.—In every case, iCT registration was successful and preoperative MR images were fused to iCT scans without affecting navigation accuracy. There was 100% concordance between probe tip location and predetermined bony loci in the first 50 cases involving the iCT/EM technique. Total operating room time was significantly less in the iCT/EM cases (mean 108.9 ± 24.3 minutes [208 patients]) compared with the fluoroscopy group (mean 121.1 ± 30.7 minutes [65 patients]; p < 0.001). Similarly, incision-to-closure time was significantly less for the iCT/EM cases (mean 61.3 ± 18.2 minutes) than for the fluoroscopy cases (mean 71.75 ± 19.0 minutes; p < 0.001). Relative overall costs for iCT/EM technique and intraoperative C-arm fluoroscopy were comparable; increased costs for navigation equipment were offset by savings in operating room costs for shorter procedures.

Conclusions.—The use of iCT/MR imaging–guided neuronavigation for transsphenoidal surgery is a time-effective, cost-efficient, safe, and technically beneficial technique.

▶ Transsphenoidal adenomectomy (TSA) is the surgical treatment choice for clinically significant macroadenomas and hormonally active adenomas (growth hormone and adrenocorticotropic hormone). Many technical advances have been made with regard to the TSA procedure in recent years. These authors discuss the feasibility, accuracy, and cost-effectiveness of using the intraoperative CT (iCT) combined with frameless electromagnetic (EM) navigation technique. Two hundred eight consecutive patients who underwent iCT/EM-guided TSA were compared with 65 consecutive patients who had fluoroscope-assisted TSA performed by the same surgeon. Total time for operating, time for incision to closure, and relative costs of imaging and surgical procedures were determined through chart review. They conclude that there was 100% accuracy with the iCT/EM technique when fused to preoperative iCT images. There was also 100% concordance between probe tip and predetermined bony landmarks. Both total operating time and incision-to-closure time were better with iCT/EM. Relative overall costs were similar for the 2 techniques. These authors conclude that the iCT/EM navigation technique is feasible, accurate, and cost effective.

W. H. Ludlam, MD, PhD

Pituitary Incidentaloma: An Endocrine Society Clinical Practice Guideline
Freda PU, Beckers AM, Katznelson L, et al (Columbia College of Physicians & Surgeons, NY; University of Liége Domaine Universitaire du Sart-Tilman, Belgium; Stanford Univ, CA; et al)
J Clin Endocrinol Metab 96:894-904, 2011

Objective.—The aim was to formulate practice guidelines for endocrine evaluation and treatment of pituitary incidentalomas.

Consensus Process.—Consensus was guided by systematic reviews of evidence and discussions through a series of conference calls and e-mails and one in-person meeting.

Conclusions.—We recommend that patients with a pituitary incidentaloma undergo a complete history and physical examination, laboratory evaluations screening for hormone hypersecretion and for hypopituitarism, and a visual field examination if the lesion abuts the optic nerves or chiasm. We recommend that patients with incidentalomas not meeting criteria for surgical removal be followed with clinical assessments, neuroimaging (magnetic resonance imaging at 6 months for macroincidentalomas, 1 yr for a microincidentaloma, and thereafter progressively less frequently if unchanged in size), visual field examinations for incidentalomas that abut or compress the optic nerve and chiasm (6 months and yearly), and endocrine testing for macroincidentalomas (6 months and yearly) after the initial evaluations. We recommend that patients with a pituitary incidentaloma be referred for surgery if they have a visual field deficit; signs of compression by the tumor leading to other visual abnormalities, such as ophthalmoplegia, or neurological compromise due to compression by the lesion; a lesion abutting the optic nerves or chiasm; pituitary apoplexy with visual disturbance; or if the incidentaloma is a hypersecreting tumor other than a prolactinoma.

▶ Pituitary lesions are often discovered incidentally when head MRIs are performed for reasons unrelated to symptoms of pituitary pathology (ie, headaches, hearing loss, stroke, etc). Knowing how to appropriately manage these incidentally discovered masses can be perplexing to many clinicians. To address this knowledge gap, the Endocrine Society has prepared a clinical guideline with evidence-based recommendations to help in the management of pituitary incidentalomas. Their recommendations include (but are not limited to) that patients with an incidentally discovered pituitary lesion should undergo a complete history, physical, and neuroendocrine evaluation. Those patients meeting the criteria for resection of their pituitary tumor (ie, tumor causing impingement of the vision apparatus, apoplexy with vision disturbance, or hormonal hypersecretion [other than with hyperprolactinemia]) should be referred to an experienced pituitary surgeon. Those patients not meeting the criteria for resection of their pituitary lesion should have a repeat MRI at 6 months for macroadenomas and at 1 year for microadenomas. If the lesion is nongrowing, the interval for subsequent MRIs should be progressively increased. Visual field testing and neuroendocrine testing should be repeated at the 6-month interval for macroadenomas. The guideline will likely be very helpful to many clinicians so that they appropriately react to incidentally found pituitary masses.

W. H. Ludlam, MD, PhD

Atypical pituitary adenomas: incidence, clinical characteristics, and implications

Zada G, Woodmansee WW, Ramkissoon S, et al (Harvard Med School, Boston, MA)

J Neurosurg 114:336-344, 2011

Object.—The 2004 WHO classification of pituitary adenomas now includes an "atypical" variant, defined as follows: MIB-1 proliferative index greater than 3%, excessive p53 immunoreactivity, and increased mitotic activity. The authors review the incidence of this atypical histopathological subtype and its correlation with tumor subtype, invasion, and surgical features.

Methods.—The records of 121 consecutive patients who underwent transsphenoidal surgery for pituitary adenomas during an 18-month period were retrospectively reviewed for evidence of atypical adenomas.

Results.—Eighteen adenomas (15%) met the criteria for atypical lesions; 17 (94%) of the 18 were macroadenomas. On imaging, 15 (83%) demonstrated imaging evidence of surrounding invasion, compared with 45% of typical adenomas (p = 0.004). Atypical tumors occurred in 12 female (67%) and 6 male (33%) patients. Patient age ranged from 16 to 70 years (mean 48 years). Nine patients (50%) had hormonally active tumors, and 9 had nonfunctional lesions. Four (22%) of the 18 patients presented to us with recurrent tumors. Immunohistochemical analysis demonstrated the following tumor subtypes: GH-secreting adenoma with plurihormonal staining (5 patients [28%]); null-cell adenoma (5 patients [28%]); silent ACTH tumor (3 patients [17%]), ACTH-staining tumor with Cushing's disease (2 patients [11%]), prolactinoma (2 patients [11%]), and silent FSH-staining tumor (1 patient [6%]). The MIB-1 labeling index ranged from 3% to 20% (mean 7%).

Conclusions.—Atypical tumors were identified in 15% of resected pituitary adenomas, and they tended to be aggressive, invasive macroadenomas. More longitudinal follow-up is required to determine whether surgical outcomes, potential for recurrence, or metastasis of atypical adenomas vary significantly from their typical counterparts.

▶ Pituitary adenomas have varying degree of aggressiveness, which often affects their clinical course and treatment plan. The World Health Organization recently included a new classification of pituitary tumors, which includes an atypical variant characterized by high p53 immunostaining, increased mitotic activity, and a MIB-1 proliferative index greater than 3%. These authors reviewed records for 121 pituitary surgery patients over an 18-month period at their own institution. They noted that atypical tumors were identified in 15% of the cases and that these tumors tented to be aggressive and invasive. Ninety-four percent of the pituitary tumors were macroadenomas, and 83% showed evidence of invasion into structures such as the cavernous sinuses. The MIB-1 labeling index ranged from 3% to 20% in this group. It was unclear whether these lesions necessarily had a worse long-term course in terms of surgical outcomes, recurrence, and metastases. Further evaluation in larger series over a longer period of time will be necessary to characterize these parameters.

W. H. Ludlam, MD, PhD

9 Pediatric Endocrinology

Introduction

This year's selections address a diverse set of topics that encompass rare disorders as well as those frequently encountered in the pediatric endocrine clinic. Another source of diversity within our specialty stems from the broad age spectrum of our young patients, which ranges from the neonatal period all the way to the cusp of adulthood. While the absolute number of years is hardly notable from the perspective of adult medicine, the magnitude of developmental changes that occur during this time span in children and adolescents is nothing short of breathtaking. Thus, the same endocrinopathy in a toddler has profoundly different implications than when it occurs in an adolescent, and several YEAR BOOK selections this time around include a developmental theme. Indeed, this is one of most enjoyable and challenging aspects of our specialty!

The first selection in this group deals with the treatment of nutritional rickets, and it concludes that vitamin D_2 and vitamin D_3 are equally effective in normalizing 25OHD concentrations. Selection 2 examines the far-less-common scenario of primary hyperparathyroidism, and it provides support for minimally invasive parathyroidectomy for pediatric patients without a family history. The next 2 selections deal with long-term outcomes of different populations of growth hormone (GH) treated patients and are particularly valuable in terms of contributing to our understanding of prognosis when initiating GH therapy. The observation that adult height gains attributable to GH were minimal in patients with Prader Willi syndrome and Turner syndrome should certainly give us pause. More information regarding quality of life in treated as well as untreated subjects is clearly needed. Selection 5 takes us back in time using modern-day sleuthing, with the discovery that a mutation in the gene encoding for the aryl hydrocarbon-interaction protein harbored by 4 Irish families was inherited from an 18th century giant using DNA extracted from his preserved teeth! Selection 6 deals with another exceedingly rare scenario—that of ectopic ACTH syndrome. Although pediatric endocrinologists are highly unlikely to make this diagnosis, it is important to include it in the differential of hypercortisolism, even when imaging studies are normal. In contrast to these unusual entities, selection 7 deals with population based secular changes in the onset of puberty in girls, and adds to the ongoing debate regarding the extent to which such changes are occurring. The prospective, longitudinal nature of this study will undoubtedly continue to yield important information as time goes on. Selection 8 represents a multidisciplinary consensus document on the clinical management of patients with congenital adrenal hyperplasia due to 21-hydroxylase deficiency across the age span. Although much of the guidelines jibe with routine clinical care of children with CAH, they remind us that some practices, such as the use of prenatal dexamethasone and GH, are not substantiated by data and should be considered experimental unless or until evidence to support their use emerges. Another condition that has its "home" in our specialty and has already been mentioned in selection 4 is Turner syndrome (TS). Two additional selections in this year's collection also deal with this relatively common diagnosis. Selection 9 investigated serum levels of anti-mullerian hormone across the age span in both control females and in a cohort with TS, and it represents a preliminary step to potentially be able to utilize this hormone to assess follicular status and ovarian function. A quick and noninvasive method of diagnosis of TS is the focus of selection 11, which evaluated the feasibility of using a high-throughput pyrosequencing system to detect sex chromosome aneuploidy in the clinical setting. An aspect of selection 10 that sets it apart from the others is that it deals with a normal variation of development rather than a pathologic process, which in this case is constitutional delay of growth and puberty. The use of inhibin B could certainly add to our armamentarium in the differentiation of late bloomers from those with hypogonadotropic hypogonadism. Lastly, selection 12 found a troubling association between maternal hypothyroxinemia and cognitive delay in euthyroid offspring, raising several questions that will hopefully lead to additional study.

In summary, this year's YEAR BOOK selections range from the practical to the hypothetical, and encompass new discoveries as well as long-established management challenges. It is my hope that the collection will be of interest to clinicians, researchers, and academicians alike.

Erica Eugster, MD

Bone/Calcium

Comparison of Metabolism of Vitamins D_2 and D_3 in Children With Nutritional Rickets

Thacher TD, Fischer PR, Obadofin MO, et al (Mayo Clinic, Rochester, MN; Jos Univ Teaching Hosp, Nigeria; et al)

J Bone Miner Res 25:1988-1995, 2010

Children with calcium-deficiency rickets may have increased vitamin D requirements and respond differently to vitamin D_2 and vitamin D_3. Our objective was to compare the metabolism of vitamins D_2 and D_3 in rachitic and control children. We administered an oral single dose of vitamin D_2 or D_3 of 1.25 mg to 49 Nigerian children—28 with active rickets and 21 healthy controls. The primary outcome measure was the incremental change in vitamin D metabolites. Baseline serum 25-hydroxyvitamin D [25(OH)D] concentrations ranged from 7 to 24 and 15 to 34 ng/mL in rachitic and control children, respectively ($p < .001$), whereas baseline 1,25-dihydroxy-vitamin D [1,25(OH)$_2$D] values (mean ± SD) were 224 ± 72 and 121 ± 34 pg/mL, respectively ($p < .001$), and baseline 24,25-dihydroxyvitamin D [24,25(OH)$_2$D] values were 1.13 ± 0.59 and 4.03 ± 1.33 ng/mL, respectively ($p < .001$). The peak increment in 25(OH)D was on day 3 and was similar with vitamins D_2 and D_3 in children with rickets (29 ± 17 and 25 ± 11 ng/mL, respectively) and in control children (33 ± 13 and 31 ± 16 ng/mL, respectively). 1,25(OH)$_2$D rose significantly ($p < .001$) and similarly ($p = .18$) on day 3 by 166 ± 80 and 209 ± 83 pg/mL after vitamin D_2 and D_3 administration, respectively, in children with rickets. By contrast, control children had no significant increase in 1,25(OH)$_2$D (19 ± 28 and 16 ± 38 pg/mL after vitamin D_2 and D_3 administration, respectively). We conclude that in the short term, vitamins D_2 and D_3 similarly increase serum 25(OH)D concentrations in rachitic and healthy children. A marked increase in 1,25(OH)$_2$D in response to vitamin D distinguishes children with putative dietary calcium-deficiency rickets from healthy children, consistent with increased vitamin D requirements in children with calcium-deficiency rickets.

▶ Despite having been recognized for centuries, cases of nutritional rickets continue to be recognized throughout the world. Although vitamin D deficiency is typically the culprit in North America and Europe, calcium deficiency is notorious as a cause for nutritional rickets in Africa. Available protocols for the treatment of nutritional rickets are as myriad as its manifestations and include vitamin D_2 and vitamin D_3 given either orally as a prolonged course, intramuscularly as a depot, or in the short-term high-dose oral method known as stoss therapy. Thus, a direct comparison of the metabolism of different vitamin D preparations in rachitic children as compared with controls is particularly welcomed. As the authors point out, their study has some intrinsic limitations. One is that the rachitic children receiving vitamin D_2 were a historic, rather than a prospective control group. Related to this is the fact that several significant differences existed between that group and the rachitic children receiving vitamin D_3. Regardless, the observation that both forms of vitamin D increased 25-hydroxy vitamin D (25[OH]D) to a similar magnitude suggests that either are viable therapeutic options in this population. Additional comparison studies would be helpful to determine whether the slower decline in 25(OH)D observed after vitamin D_3 administration translates in faster resolution of the biochemical and radiographic perturbations characteristic of rickets. The importance of concurrent calcium supplementation is appropriately emphasized.

E. Eugster, MD

What is the optimal treatment for children with primary hyperparathyroidism?

Durkin ET, Nichol PF, Lund DP, et al (Univ of Wisconsin School of Medicine and Public Health, Madison)

J Pediatr Surg 45:1142-1146, 2010

Purpose.—Little information exists regarding the optimal surgical treatment of pediatric primary hyperparathyroidism. We hypothesized that primary hyperparathyroidism in children, in the absence of a family history, is caused by single-gland disease and is amenable to minimally invasive parathyroidectomy (MIP).

Methods.—We reviewed the records of individuals younger than 25 years who underwent parathyroidectomy in a prospectively collected database at a single tertiary hospital from 2003 to 2009.

Results.—Twenty-five patients were identified, with a mean (SD) age of 19 (3.7) years. Sixty percent had single-gland disease (n = 15). Familial disease was present in 6 patients. All of the children younger than 18 years without a family history of disease (9/9) were found to have a single-gland disease (P < .001). Seventy-eight percent of patients without a family history were successfully treated without a bilateral exploration. Average length of stay was less than 1 day with no complications or recurrences.

Conclusions.—Primary hyperparathyroidism in patients younger than 18 years without a family history was uniformly caused by single-gland disease. Minimally invasive parathyroidectomy was successful in these patients and avoided the morbidity of bilateral exploration. We recommend

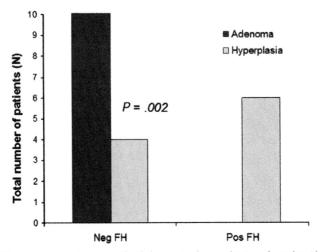

FIGURE 2.—Surgical pathology versus family history. Findings at the time of parathyroidectomy were analyzed based on the presence of a known family history of disease. Data compared using Fischer's Exact test (P =.002). (Reprinted from Durkin ET, Nichol PF, Lund DP, et al. What is the optimal treatment for children with primary hyperparathyroidism. *J Pediatr Surg.* 2010;45:1142-1146, with permission from Elsevier.)

MIP be used in pediatric patients at large referral centers with prior successful institutional experience with the technique (Fig 2).

▶ This retrospective study deals with a condition that is extraordinarily rare in children and adolescents. As the authors point out, less than a dozen case series currently exist in the medical literature, and even these are not limited to the pediatric population. Therefore, whatever information pertaining to optimum management that can be gleaned from a systematic analysis of previous cases is useful. As shown in Fig 2, the fact that all patients with a positive family history had multigland disease while 9/9 of those ≤18 years of age without a family history had single-gland disease (and 60% of those older than 18 years) presents a rather compelling argument for minimally invasive parathyroidectomy in this setting. The associated decreased morbidity from surgical complications that would be expected to result from such an approach makes it even more attractive, especially in pediatric patients. Finally, the authors make the excellent point that the volumes of surgeries performed are directly correlated with outcomes and that all children with primary hyperparathyroidism should be cared for at tertiary care centers with institutional experience in both pediatric and endocrine surgery.

E. Eugster, MD

Growth/Growth Hormone

Long-term effects of growth hormone therapy on patients with Prader-Willi syndrome

Sipilä I, Sintonen H, Hietanen H, et al (Univ of Helsinki, Finland; Diacor Health Services, Helsinki, Finland; et al)
Acta Paediatr 99:1712-1718, 2010

Aim.—To assess the effects of recombinant human growth hormone (rhGH) treatment in children with Prader—Willi syndrome.

Design.—A 1-year study and an observational follow-up visit 10 years later.

Methods.—In 20 patients with Prader—Willi syndrome (PWS): clinical assessment, laboratory tests, body composition analysis by dual energy X-ray absorptiometry, sleep polygraphy, health-related quality of life assessed by 16D.

Results.—Only two patients had normal growth hormone secretion at baseline. All patients were significantly shorter than their expected heights, but experienced catch-up growth during growth hormone treatment. At follow-up, 13 patients had reached adult heights and were markedly taller than historical controls. The cumulative dose of rhGH over 10 years correlated inversely with the total body fat percentage (p = 0.033). However, patients remained severely obese at 10 years. Sleep polygraphy was abnormal in more than half of the patients. Health-related quality of life of the patients remained substantially below that of normal population.

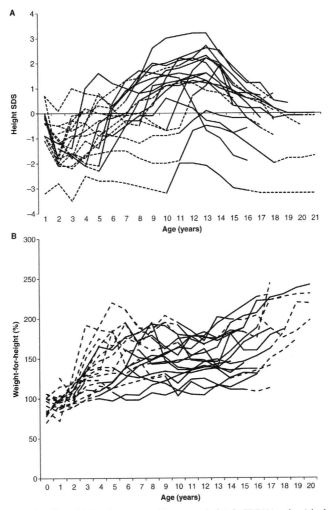

FIGURE 1.—The effect of rhGH therapy over 10 years on the height SDS (A) and weight-for-height (B) of the patients. Dashed lines represent periods without and solid lines periods with rhGH therapy. Missing data are replaced by dashed lines. SDS, standard deviation score; rhGH, recombinant human growth hormone. (Reprinted from Sipilä I, Sintonen H, Hietanen H, et al. Long-term effects of growth hormone therapy on patients with Prader-Willi syndrome. *Acta Paediatr.* 2010;99:1712-1718, with permission from Eli Lilly and Company/Journal Compilation.)

Conclusion.—Growth hormone markedly improved adult height in subjects with PWS when compared to historical data. The cumulative dose of growth hormone correlated with reduction in body fat; nevertheless, patients remained severely obese (Fig 1).

▶ This study highlights the value of obtaining long-term follow-up data in subsets of children receiving recombinant human growth hormone (GH) therapy. In Prader-Willi syndrome (PWS), several aspects of GH treatment are of interest. These include not only stature but also body composition, sleep apnea, and quality of life. Although the lack of a control group is a serious flaw, this article affords us a glimpse of the ultimate outcome of each of these parameters in a real-life fashion in 19 individuals with PWS 10 years after a 1-year trial of GH treatment in all known Finnish children with the disorder at that time (n = 22). As shown in Fig 1, GH increased growth velocity and improved average height standard deviation score (SDS) in the short term. However, the height SDS in the 13 (68%) subjects who were done growing was presumably no different from that at baseline. Although the authors point out that it was significantly higher than in historical controls, the magnitude of improvement is difficult to gauge given that the range of reported heights in untreated individuals with PWS varies widely. Another important finding illustrated in the same figure was that GH did not prevent obesity in these subjects, despite the fact that it is an often-touted benefit of therapy. Similarly, sleep studies at the follow-up visit were abnormal in 61% of the patients, including 3 of 7 still receiving GH therapy. Without baseline or longitudinal assessments, these results add little to the ongoing debate about the relationship between sleep apnea and GH in patients with PWS. Finally, the finding that quality of life at follow-up was poor was disappointing, given the hope that GH treatment might ameliorate some of the problems faced by children and adolescents with PWS. At a minimum, this study serves as a reminder to avoid what may be unrealistic expectations when embarking on long-term GH therapy in patients with PWS. Although not acknowledged by the authors, it also raises questions about the cost/benefit ratio of approximately 8.5 years of daily GH injections in this population. Only large-scale prospective controlled studies to adult height in PWS will enlighten us.

E. Eugster, MD

Growth Hormone plus Childhood Low-Dose Estrogen in Turner's Syndrome

Ross JL, Quigley CA, Cao D, et al (Thomas Jefferson Univ, Philadelphia, PA; Lilly Res Laboratories, Indianapolis, IN; et al)
N Engl J Med 364:1230-1242, 2011

Background.—Short stature and ovarian failure are characteristic features of Turner's syndrome. Although recombinant human growth hormone is commonly used to treat the short stature associated with this syndrome, a randomized, placebo-controlled trial is needed to document whether such treatment increases adult height. Furthermore, it is not known whether childhood estrogen replacement combined with growth hormone therapy provides additional benefit. We examined the independent and combined effects of growth hormone and early, ultralow-dose estrogen on adult height in girls with Turner's syndrome.

Methods.—In this double-blind, placebo-controlled trial, we randomly assigned 149 girls, 5.0 to 12.5 years of age, to four groups: double placebo (placebo injection plus childhood oral placebo, 39 patients), estrogen alone (placebo injection plus childhood oral lowdose estrogen, 40), growth hormone alone (growth hormone injection plus childhood oral placebo, 35), and growth hormone–estrogen (growth hormone injection plus childhood oral low-dose estrogen, 35). The dose of growth hormone was 0.1 mg per kilogram of body weight three times per week. The doses of ethinyl estradiol (or placebo) were adjusted for chronologic age and pubertal status. At the first visit after the age of 12.0 years, patients in all treatment groups received escalating doses of ethinyl estradiol. Growth hormone injections were terminated when adult height was reached.

Results.—The mean standard-deviation scores for adult height, attained at an average age of 17.0 ± 1.0 years, after an average study period of 7.2 ± 2.5 years were −2.81 ± 0.85, −3.39 ± 0.74, −2.29 ± 1.10, and −2.10 ± 1.02 for the double-placebo, estrogen-alone, growth hormone–alone, and growth hormone–estrogen groups, respectively (P<0.001). The overall effect of growth hormone treatment (vs. placebo) on adult height was a 0.78 ± 0.13 increase in the height standard-deviation score (5.0 cm) (P<0.001); adult height was greater in the growth hormone–estrogen group than in the growth hormone–alone group, by 0.32 ± 0.17 standard-deviation score (2.1 cm) (P=0.059), suggesting a modest synergy between childhood low-dose ethinyl estradiol and growth hormone.

Conclusions.—Our study shows that growth hormone treatment increases adult height in patients with Turner's syndrome. In addition, the data suggest that combining childhood ultra-low-dose estrogen with growth hormone may improve growth and provide other potential benefits

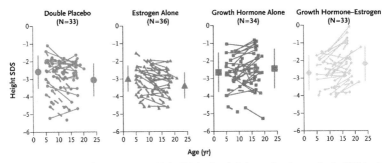

FIGURE 3.—Effects of Treatment on Adult Height. Panel C shows the changes in the SDS for height from baseline to the last available height measurement for individual patients in the intention-to-treat population. Solid lines represent patients with adult-height measurements, and dashed lines patients without adult-height measurements. One patient in the estrogen-alone group who received surreptitious growth hormone during the study is not included. Large symbols represent the group means (± SD) at baseline and at the time of the last height measurement. Mean baseline SDS and end-point SDS in the four groups were as follows: double-placebo group, −2.59 ± 0.96 and −3.08 ± 0.95; estrogen-alone group, −3.01 ± 0.74 and −3.40 ± 0.74; growth hormone–alone group, −2.65 ± 0.91 and −2.45 ± 1.13; and growth hormone–estrogen group, −2.71 ± 0.81 and −2.18 ± 1.00 (P<0.001 for the comparison among the four groups). Individual gains in the height SDS for patients with adult-height measurements (i.e., change in height SDS from baseline to adult height >0) were observed for 15% of patients in the double-placebo group, 32% in the estrogen-alone group, 65% in the growth hormone–alone group, and 79% in the growth hormone–estrogen group (P<0.001 for the comparison among the four groups). (Reprinted from Ross JL, Quigley CA, Cao D, et al. Growth hormone plus childhood low-dose estrogen in turner's syndrome. *N Engl J Med.* 2011;364:1230-1242, Copyright 2011, Massachusetts Medical Society. All rights reserved.)

associated with early initiation of estrogen replacement. (Funded by the National Institute of Child Health and Human Development and Eli Lilly; ClinicalTrials.gov number, NCT00001221.) (Fig 3C).

▶ The focus of this study is hardly new. What is notable is the scope of the project, which was initiated nearly 25 years ago, and its double-blind placebo-controlled design, a stunning feat rare to encounter in research trials involving children. Beyond that, reconciling this rigorous examination with our day-to-day clinical assumptions regarding something as bread and butter as prescribing growth hormone (GH) to girls with Turner syndrome (TS) requires some effort. The relative lack of efficacy of GH in normalizing height in the treated groups is surprising and certainly gives one pause. As the authors point out, there are several potential explanations for this, including the 3 times per week injection regimen and the fact that most previous studies were uncontrolled. It is tempting to speculate that the relatively late age at GH initiation was also a contributing factor and that low-dose estrogen was not as effective as oxandrolone would have been in augmenting ultimate height. Regardless, Fig 3C beautifully illustrates the extreme variation in individual sensitivity to GH among girls with TS, both in terms of direction and degree of responsiveness. This should remind us to temper the implicit expectations engendered during our conversations with parents of girls with TS regarding GH therapy, both in terms of stature and, even more importantly albeit not addressed by this study, outcomes related to quality of life.[1]

E. Eugster, MD

Reference

1. Carel JC, Ecosse E, Bastie-Sigeac I, et al. Quality of life determinants in young women with turner' syndrome after growth hormone treatment: results of the Sta Tur population-based cohort study. *J Clin Endocrinol Metab*. 2005;90:1992-1997.

AIP Mutation in Pituitary Adenomas in the 18th Century and Today

Chahal HS, Stals K, Unterländer M, et al (Queen Mary Univ of London, UK; Royal Devon and Exeter Foundation Trust, UK; Johannes Gutenberg Univ, Mainz, Germany; et al)
N Engl J Med 364:43-50, 2011

Gigantism results when a growth hormone—secreting pituitary adenoma is present before epiphyseal fusion. In 1909, when Harvey Cushing examined the skeleton of an Irish patient who lived from 1761 to 1783, he noted an enlarged pituitary fossa. We extracted DNA from the patient's teeth and identified a germline mutation in the aryl hydrocarbon—interacting protein gene (*AIP*). Four contemporary Northern Irish families who presented with gigantism, acromegaly, or prolactinoma have the same mutation and haplotype associated with the mutated gene. Using coalescent theory, we infer that these persons share a common ancestor who lived about 57 to 66 generations earlier.

▶ This intriguing brief report represents a wonderful blend of medical history, molecular biology, and genetics. Although mutations in the aryl hydrocarbon-interacting protein (*AIP*) gene are not a newly discovered cause of familial somatotropinomas, to confirm that the same mutation and haplotype identified in 4 present-day Irish families were inherited from an 18th century giant who was born in 1761 and died at the age of 22 years using DNA extracted from his preserved teeth is mind boggling indeed! Another fascinating aspect of the study is the use of coalescent simulation to estimate recombination rates, carrier frequency, and population data to derive the number of generations from the most recent common ancestor, which is estimated at 57 to 66 generations. Compelling as the conclusions are, we are left with several questions. Carriers of the heterozygous mutation were 3.6 times as likely to be asymptomatic as to be affected, leading one to speculate about potential modifier genes that impact the rate of penetrance of the *AIP* mutation. We cannot avoid speculating as well about the young giant's short yet notorious life and the circumstances in which he passed along the genetic lineage that would amazingly be discovered so many years later.

E. Eugster, MD

Miscellaneous

Ectopic ACTH Syndrome in Children and Adolescents

More J, the Groupe Français des Tumeurs Endocrines (GTE) (Univ Hosp of Bordeaux, Pessac, France; et al)
J Clin Endocrinol Metab 96:2011 [Epub ahead of print]

Context.—Ectopic ACTH syndrome (EAS) in youngsters has seldom been reported and is poorly known.

Setting.—We conducted a multicenter retrospective study involving 18 French tertiary hospitals. Cases of EAS presenting Cushing's syndrome before the age of 20 during the period from 1985 to 2008 were analyzed.

Patients.—Ten patients aged 14 to 20 yr were identified and compared to 20 age-matched patients with Cushing's disease diagnosed during the same period.

Main Outcome Measures.—Etiologies, clinical, biochemical and radiological features, prognosis, and treatment were described.

Results.—Seven patients had well-differentiated neuroendocrine tumors (five bronchial carcinoids, one mediastinal lymph node, and one thymic), one had a poorly differentiated thymic carcinoma, one had a pleural Ewing's sarcoma, and one had a liver nested stromal epithelial tumor. At presentation, seven tumors were identified with computed tomography scanning and somatostatin receptor scintigraphy, and one with fluoro-18-L-dihydroxyphenylalanine positron emission tomography scan. Two carcinoids were occult and were identified during follow-up. Cushing's syndrome was more intense in EAS, but the clinical and biological spectrum overlapped with that of Cushing's disease. No dynamic test achieved 100% accuracy, whereas petrosal sinus sampling provided correct diagnosis in all patients tested. Medical treatment of hypercortisolism was successful in six of the eight patients with whom it was attempted, and bilateral adrenalectomy had to be performed in only two cases. Prognosis was good; nine patients with curative resection of the tumor were alive and cured (median followup, 6.5 yr), whereas one patient died.

Conclusions.—EAS in youngsters displays many similarities to that described in adults. The diagnostic and therapeutic algorithms recommended in adults can be used in this population.

▶ The topic of this retrospective review is extraordinarily rare, which is emphasized by the fact that only 10 subjects could be gleaned from 23 years and 18 centers' worth of experience! Moreover, 3 of the featured cases have already been published elsewhere. Nonetheless, the comparison between ectopic adrenocorticotropic hormone syndrome (EAS) and Cushing disease in similar-aged cohorts, as well as between these cases and their adult counterparts, provides important new information that will undoubtedly prove useful in the clinical setting. Several findings are worth noting. Although the title of the article includes the term children, the youngest of the subjects with EAS was 15 years, suggesting that pediatric EAS predominantly occurs in older adolescents. Another striking feature of the cases was the fact that the diagnosis was far from straightforward, with 2 patients with undetectable tumors and 3 with an initially negative CT. Lastly, the accuracy of the diagnostic studies and observed outcomes was similar to that reported in adult patients. In conclusion, while we are unlikely to encounter cases of EAS in our young patients, it is important to remember that this entity exists, that it often requires significant diagnostic detective work, and that we can look to our adult colleagues for guidance in testing, treatment, and prognosis.

E. Eugster, MD

Pubertal Assessment Method and Baseline Characteristics in a Mixed Longitudinal Study of Girls

Biro FM, Galvez MP, Greenspan LC, et al (Cincinnati Children's Hosp Med Ctr, OH; Mount Sinai School of Medicine, NY; Kaiser Permanente, San Francisco, CA; et al)
Pediatrics 126:e583-e590, 2010

Objectives.—The objective of this study was to describe the assessment methods and maturation status for a multisite cohort of girls at baseline recruitment and at ages 7 and 8 years.

Methods.—The method for pubertal maturation staging was developed collaboratively across 3 sites. Girls at ages 6 to 8 years were recruited at 3 sites: East Harlem, New York; greater Cincinnati metropolitan area; and

San Francisco Bay area, California. Baseline characteristics were obtained through interviews with caregivers and anthropometric measurements by trained examiners; breast stage 2 was defined as onset of pubertal maturation. The κ statistic was used to evaluate agreement between master trainers and examiners. Logistic regression models were used to identify factors that are associated with pubertal maturation and linear regression models to examine factors that are associated with height velocity.

Results.—The baseline cohort included 1239 girls. The proportion of girls who had attained breast stage 2 varied by age, race/ethnicity, BMI percentile, and site. At 7 years, 10.4% of white, 23.4% of black non-Hispanic, and 14.9% of Hispanic girls had attained breast stage $\geq$2; at 8 years, 18.3%, 42.9%, and 30.9%, respectively, had attained breast stage $\geq$2. The prime determinant of height velocity was pubertal status.

Conclusions.—In this multisite study, there was substantial agreement regarding pubertal staging between examiners across sites. The proportion of girls who had breast development at ages 7 and 8 years, particularly among white girls, is greater than that reported from studies of girls who were born 10 to 30 years earlier.

▶ This study generated significant media attention both nationally and within my own metropolitan area. One reason may be because it was conducted by the Breast Cancer and the Environment Research Centers consortium, which has as its focus a better understanding of the interplay between earlier pubertal maturation in girls and increased risk of breast cancer. Another is likely because of the implication in the article that environmental endocrine disruptors may be causing alterations in pubertal timing, although precisely what exposures are responsible is unclear. At any rate, this study certainly adds to the ongoing discussion of whether secular changes in pubertal timing are occurring and if so, in whom and to what extent. Despite a multitude of publications on this topic, the subject is far from resolved. Although the methods described in the article are highly reassuring regarding the accuracy of the observations made in this cohort, additional analyses would have been helpful. In particular, segregating the girls into those with a normal versus abnormal body mass index (BMI), as has been done in other studies,[1,2] would have potentially illuminated the likely central role of obesity in apparently earlier breast development in some girls. The authors' conclusions that girls are experiencing breast enlargement earlier than they were a decade ago may be a bit overstated because they had nearly 16 000 fewer subjects than the seminal 1997 article cited.[3] Regardless, the continued longitudinal assessments of the girls in this prospective study will be crucial in determining the significance of the findings in terms of age of menarche, BMI trajectories, and associated genetic and environmental factors.

E. Eugster, MD

References

1. Kaplowitz PB. Link between body fat and the timing of puberty. *Pediatrics.* 2008; 121:S208-S217.

2. Rosenfield RL, Lipton RB, Drum ML. Thelarche, pubarche and menarche attainment in children with normal and elevated body mass index. *Pediatrics.* 2009;123: 84-88.
3. Herman-Giddens ME, Slora EJ, Wasserman RC, et al. Secondary sexual characteristics and menses in young girls seen in office practice: a study from the Pediatric Research in Office Settings Network. *Pediatrics.* 1997;99:505-512.

Congenital Adrenal Hyperplasia Due to Steroid 21-Hydroxylase Deficiency: An Endocrine Society Clinical Practice Guideline

Speiser PW, Azziz R, Baskin LS, et al (Cohen Children's Med Ctr of New York and Hofstra Univ School of Medicine, New Hyde Park; Cedars-Sinai Med Ctr, Los Angeles, CA; Univ of California San Francisco; et al)
J Clin Endocrinol Metab 95:4133-4160, 2010

Objective.—We developed clinical practice guidelines for congenital adrenal hyperplasia (CAH).

Participants.—The Task Force included a chair, selected by The Endocrine Society Clinical Guidelines Subcommittee (CGS), ten additional clinicians experienced in treating CAH, a methodologist, and a medical writer. Additional experts were also consulted. The authors received no corporate funding or remuneration.

Consensus Process.—Consensus was guided by systematic reviews of evidence and discussions. The guidelines were reviewed and approved sequentially by The Endocrine Society's CGS and Clinical Affairs Core Committee, members responding to a web posting, and The Endocrine Society Council. At each stage, the Task Force incorporated changes in response to written comments.

Conclusions.—We recommend universal newborn screening for severe steroid 21-hydroxylase deficiency followed by confirmatory tests. We recommend that prenatal treatment of CAH continue to be regarded as experimental. The diagnosis rests on clinical and hormonal data; genotyping is reserved for equivocal cases and genetic counseling. Glucocorticoid dosage should be minimized to avoid iatrogenic Cushing's syndrome. Mineralocorticoids and, in infants, supplemental sodium are recommended in classic CAH patients. We recommend against the routine use of experimental therapies to promote growth and delay puberty; we suggest patients avoid adrenalectomy. Surgical guidelines emphasize early single-stage genital repair for severely virilized girls, performed by experienced surgeons. Clinicians should consider patients' quality of life, consulting mental health professionals as appropriate. At the transition to adulthood, we recommend monitoring for potential complications of CAH. Finally, we recommend judicious use of medication during pregnancy and in symptomatic patients with nonclassic CAH.

▶ The development of consensus statements and clinical practice guidelines creates useful opportunities for careful and comprehensive evaluation of the extant scientific evidence that may be used to support or refute specific aspects of routine clinical care. As we well know, clinical management is rife with habits that have trickled down through a variety of channels but for which rigorous scientific substantiation is lacking. Thus, concrete recommendations such as those presented here serve as an important reminder of which parameters of clinical management are firmly rooted in data and which should be considered experimental until more information is available. As is typically the case, what the task force determined should not be considered routine clinical practice is as important as what they determined should be viewed as standard of care. A few specifics are worth noting. Notwithstanding widespread availability of molecular genetic analysis, the guidelines remind us that the diagnosis of 21-hydroxylase deficiency still rests on clinical and hormonal grounds. Despite ongoing controversy, the guidelines take the clear position that prenatal therapy of fetuses potentially affected with congenital adrenal hyperplasia (CAH) be considered experimental. Similarly, approaches aimed at increasing adult stature, including the use of growth hormone and gonadotropin-releasing hormone analog therapy, are strongly discouraged outside of Institutional Review Board (IRB)-approved experimental trials. Lastly, the panel determined that routine evaluation of bone mineral density in children with CAH is not warranted. Of course, each of these complex areas is rich with unanswered questions that should form the basis for large-scale, prospective, controlled trials. It is only by going back to basics and pursuing well-designed collaborative research studies will the care of patients with CAH truly be advanced.

E. Eugster, MD

Serum Levels of Anti-Müllerian Hormone as a Marker of Ovarian Function in 926 Healthy Females from Birth to Adulthood and in 172 Turner Syndrome Patients

Hagen CP, Aksglaede L, Sørensen K, et al (Copenhagen Univ Hosp, Denmark; et al)
J Clin Endocrinol Metab 95:5003-5010, 2010

Context.—In adult women, anti-Müllerian hormone (AMH) is related to the ovarian follicle pool. Little is known about AMH in girls.

Objective.—The objective of the study was to provide a reference range for AMH in girls and adolescents and to evaluate AMH as a marker of ovarian function.

Setting.—The study was conducted at a tertiary referral center for pediatric endocrinology.

Main Outcome Measures.—We measured AMH in 926 healthy females (longitudinal values during infancy) as well as in 172 Turner syndrome (TS) patients according to age, karyotype (A: 45,X; B: miscellaneous karyotypes; C: 45,X/46,XX), and ovarian function (1: absent puberty; 2: cessation of ovarian function; 3: ongoing ovarian function).

Results.—AMH was undetectable in 54% (38 of 71) of cord blood samples (<2; <2−15 pmol/liter) (median; 2.5th to 97.5th percentile) and

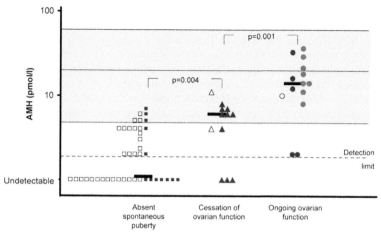

FIGURE 3.—AMH levels and ovarian function at time of AMH measurement in patients with TS, aged 12–25 yr. The reference range is marked by the *hatched area*, and *lines* represent the median, the 2.5th percentile, and the 97.5th percentile. *Dotted line* represents the detection limit of the assay. *Squares,* Patients with absent puberty; *triangles,* patients with cessation of ovarian function; *circles,* patients with ongoing ovarian function. *Thick black bars,* Median of AMH. *Black,* Patients with 45,X; *blue,* miscellaneous karyotypes; *red,* 45,X/46,XX. For interpretation of the references to color in this figure legend, the reader is referred to web version of this article. (Reprinted from Hagen CP, Aksglaede L, Sørensen K, et al. Serum levels of anti-müllerian hormone as a marker of ovarian function in 926 healthy females from birth to adulthood and in 172 turner syndrome patients. *J Clin Endocrinol Metab.* 2010;95:5003-5010, Copyright © [2010], The Endocrine Society.)

increased in all (37 of 37) infants from birth to 3 months (15; 4.5–29.5 pmol/liter). From 8 to 25 yr, AMH levels were stable (19.9; 4.7–60.1 pmol/liter), with the lower level of the reference range clearly above the detection limit. AMH levels were associated with TS-karyotype groups (median A *vs.* B: <2 *vs.* 3 pmol/liter, $P = 0.044$; B *vs.* C: 3 vs. 16 pmol/liter, $P < 0.001$) as well as with ovarian function (absent puberty *vs.* cessation of ovarian function: <2 *vs.* 6 pmol/liter, $P = 0.004$; cessation of ovarian function *vs.* ongoing ovarian function: 6 *vs.* 14 pmol/liter, $P = 0.001$). As a screening test of premature ovarian failure in TS, the sensitivity and pecificity of AMH less than 8 pmol/liter was 96 and 86%, respectively.

Conclusion.—AMH seems to be a promising marker of ovarian function in healthy girls and TS patients (Fig 3).

▶ The utility of measuring serum Müllerian inhibiting substance (MIS), also known as anti-Müllerian hormone, in infants with disorders of sex development in whom a Y chromosome–containing cell line is present is well established. This is because of the excellent correlation between MIS concentration and the presence and integrity of testicular tissue. Thus, the results of this test in such patients can aid in both differential diagnosis and management. In contrast, MIS has not traditionally been measured in the clinical setting in genetic females, and the value of doing so has not been determined. This study, however, represents a definite step in that direction. The value of the results is twofold. Firstly, the serial measurements in infants and cross-sectional values in hundreds of healthy girls and women define normative references ranges for MIS across the lifespan. Particularly intriguing is the robust change in infants concurrent with the minipuberty of infancy and the extremely wide variability of MIS levels in 8- to 25-year olds. While neither of these observations is likely to translate into an immediate application to clinical care, these data certainly advance our knowledge of normal ovarian follicular physiology. The other aspect of this study that clearly does have the potential to be applicable to patient care is the demonstration that MIS levels are related to both karyotype and ovarian function in girls and women aged 12 to 25 years with Turner syndrome (TS). As shown in Fig 3, a clear separation was noted between patients with complete premature ovarian failure, those with cessation of ovarian function, and those with ongoing ovarian function. What is needed next is an investigation of longitudinal changes in serum gonadotropin levels (particularly follicle-stimulating hormone) and MIS in relation to karyotype and ultimate ovarian function in order to truly enhance our ability to provide prognostic information to our patients with TS.

E. Eugster, MD

Baseline Inhibin B and Anti-Mullerian Hormone Measurements for Diagnosis of Hypogonadotropic Hypogonadism (HH) in Boys with Delayed Puberty

Coutant R, Biette-Demeneix E, Bouvattier C, et al (Angers Univ Hosp, France; General Hosp, Frejus, France; St Vincent de Paul Hosp and René Descartes Univ, Paris, France)
J Clin Endocrinol Metab 95:5225-5232, 2010

Context.—The diagnosis of isolated hypogonadotropic hypogonadism (IHH) in boys with delayed puberty is challenging, as may be the diagnosis of hypogonadotropic hypogonadism (HH) in boys with combined pituitary hormone deficiency (CPHD). Yet, the therapeutic choices for puberty induction depend on accurate diagnosis and may influence future fertility.

Objective.—The aim was to assess the utility of baseline inhibin B (INHB) and anti-Mullerian hormone (AMH) measurements to discriminate HH from constitutional delay of puberty (CDP). Both hormones are produced by Sertoli cells upon FSH stimulation. Moreover, prepubertal AMH levels are high as a reflection of Sertoli cell integrity.

Patients.—We studied 82 boys aged 14 to 18 yr with pubertal delay: 16 had IHH, 15 congenital HH within CPHD, and 51 CDP, as confirmed by follow-up. Subjects were genital stage 1 (testis volume <3 ml; 9 IHH, 7 CPHD, and 23 CDP) or early stage 2 (testis volume, 3–6 ml; 7 IHH, 8 CPHD, and 28 CDP).

Results.—Age and testis volume were similar in the three groups. Compared with CDP subjects, IHH and CPHD subjects had lower INHB, testosterone, FSH, and LH concentrations $(P < 0.05)$, whereas AMH concentration was lower only in IHH and CPHD subjects with genital stage 1, likely reflecting a smaller pool of Sertoli cells inprofound HH. In IHH and CPHD boys with genital stage 1, sensitivity and specificity were 100% for INHB concentration of 35 pg/ml or less. In IHH and CPHD boys with genital stage 2, sensitivities were 86 and 80%, whereas specificities were 92% and 88%, respectively, for an INHB concentration of 65 pg/ml or less. The performance of testosterone, AMH, FSH, and LH measurements was lower. No combination or ratio of hormones performed better than INHB alone.

Conclusion.—Discrimination of HH from CDP with baseline INHB measurement was excellent in subjects with genital stage 1 and fair in subjects with genital stage 2.

▶ In boys presenting with delayed puberty, pediatric endocrinologists have long resorted to a wait-and-see policy to differentiate constitutional delay of growth and puberty (CDGP) from permanent hypogonadotropic hypogonadism (HH). This is because of the high degree of overlap in gonadotropins and sex steroids between the 2 conditions. While numerous hormonal stimulation schemes have been proposed throughout the years, none have panned out to have perfect reliability. Thus, patients, parents, and physicians have traditionally relied on the passage of time to reveal whether spontaneous puberty would ensue. Thus, a fresh approach to dealing with this common clinical dilemma is welcome. In particular, the finding that a single baseline inhibin B concentration in prepubertal boys had the best sensitivity and specificity is of particular value, as this simple measure could easily be incorporated into practice. Although the sample size of the CDGP group was quite good, the study would have benefited from a larger number of boys with isolated HH because gonadotropin deficiency will already be highly suspected in patients with anosmia, hypopituitarism, and history of cryptorchidism. A notable strength of the study is that the definitive diagnosis of HH was made by reassessment of the need for testosterone replacement years after pubertal development was completed. In conclusion, while additional investigation will be needed to validate these results, this study has the potential to significantly contribute to the management of boys with delayed puberty.

E. Eugster, MD

A Highly Sensitive, High-Throughput Assay for the Detection of Turner Syndrome
Rivkees SA, Hager K, Hosono S, et al (Yale Child Health Res Ctr, New Haven, CT; JS Genetics, New Haven, CT; et al)
J Clin Endocrinol Metab 96:699-705, 2011

Objective.—Turner syndrome (TS) occurs when an X-chromosome is completely or partially deleted or when X-chromosomal mosaicism is present. Girls with TS benefit from early diagnosis and treatment with GH; however, many girls with TS are not detected until after 10 yr of age, resulting in delayed evaluation and treatment.

Methods.—We developed a high-throughput test for TS, based on a quantitative method of genotyping to detect X-chromosome abnormalities. This test uses pyrosequencing to quantitate relative allele strength (RAS) from single-nucleotide polymorphisms using 18 informative single-nucleotide polymorphisms markers that span the X-chromosome and one marker for the detection of Y-chromosome material.

Results.—Cutoff ranges for heterozygous, homozygous, or out-of-range RAS values were established from a cohort of 496 males and females. Positive TS scoring criteria were defined as the presence of homozygosity for all 18 markers or the presence of at least one out-of-range RAS value. To determine the validity of this rapid test for TS detection, we undertook a large-scale study using DNA from 132 females without TS and 74 females with TS for whom karyotypes were available. TS was identified with 96.0% sensitivity and 97.0% specificity in this cohort. We also tested buccal swab DNA from a group of 19 females without TS and 69 females with TS. In this group, TS was identified with 97.1% sensitivity and 84.2% specificity.

Conclusions.—These results demonstrate the validity of a high-throughput, pyrosequencing based test for the accurate detection of TS, providing a potential alternative to karyotype testing.

▶ A highly accurate and noninvasive methodology for detecting sex chromosome aneuploidy would represent a significant addition to the diagnostic armamentarium of pediatricians and pediatric subspecialists. The implication that the test could be performed on buccal smears conveys an attractive element of symmetry because the initial diagnosis of Turner syndrome (TS) relied on quantification of Barr bodies in buccal smears. As the authors imply, this system of high throughput and pyrosequencing could easily be applied to multiple settings, including newborn screening programs, primary care, and subspecialty clinics. A few specific aspects of the study are worth noting. One of these is that a level of mosaicism so low that it would be missed on karyotype analysis could potentially be picked up by this method. Although it may initially be used as a screening test, it is intriguing that in some ways the high-throughput method could be more sensitive than the definitive confirmation by karyotype currently being recommended. Another issue worth considering is the authors' contention that adoption of this assay would result in earlier detection of TS. This does not logically follow, as it is usually a failure to consider the possibility of TS rather than the deterrent of venipuncture or cost (of chromosomal analysis) that lies at the root of delayed diagnosis. Regardless, the potential alternative of the high-throughput test is intuitively attractive and will certainly be met by enthusiasm on the part of physicians and their patients. It remains to be seen if and how this exciting new development will enter the arena of clinical care.

E. Eugster, MD

Maternal Thyroid Function during Early Pregnancy and Cognitive Functioning in Early Childhood: The Generation R Study

Henrichs J, Bongers-Schokking JJ, Schenk JJ, et al (Erasmus Med Univ Ctr, Rotterdam, The Netherlands; Erasmus Med Ctr—Sophia Children's Hosp, Rotterdam, the Netherlands; Erasmus Univ, Rotterdam, The Netherlands)
J Clin Endocrinol Metab 95:2010 [Epub ahead of print]

Context.—Thyroid hormones are essential for neurodevelopment from early pregnancy onward. Yet population-based data on the association between maternal thyroid function in early pregnancy and children's cognitive development are sparse.

Objective.—Our objective was to study associations of maternal hypothyroxinemia and of early pregnancy maternal TSH and free T_4 (FT_4) levels across the entire range with cognitive functioning in early childhood.

Design and Setting.—We conducted a population-based cohort in The Netherlands.

Participants.—Participants included 3659 children and their mothers.

Main Measures.—In pregnant women with normal TSH levels at 13 wk gestation (SD = 1.7), mild and severe maternal hypothyroxinemia were defined as FT_4 concentrations below the 10th and 5th percentile, respectively. Children's expressive vocabulary at 18 months was reported by mothers using the MacArthur Communicative Development Inventory. At 30 months, mothers completed the Language Development Survey and the Parent Report of Children's Abilities measuring verbal and nonverbal cognitive functioning.

Results.—Maternal TSH was not related to the cognitive outcomes. An increase in maternal FT_4 predicted a lower risk of expressive language delay at 30 months only. However, both mild and severe maternal hypothyroxinemia was associated with a higher risk of expressive language delay across all ages [odds ratio (OR) = 1.44; 95%confidence interval (CI) = 1.09–1.91; $P = 0.010$ and OR = 1.80; 95% CI = 1.24–2.61; $P = 0.002$, respectively]. Severe maternal hypothyroxinemia also predicted a higher risk of nonverbal cognitive delay (OR = 2.03; 95% CI = 1.22–3.39; $P = 0.007$).

Conclusions.—Maternal hypothyroxinemia is a risk factor for cognitive delay in early childhood.

▶ This study will undoubtedly add to the debate about whether routine prenatal screening of maternal thyroid function should be undertaken. Unlike a previous report of an adverse effect of mild maternal primary hypothyroidism on neuropsychological status in children at age 7 to 9,[1] this study included only mothers whose thyroid-stimulating hormone (TSH) was normal but whose free thyroxine (FT4) concentrations were low. The findings of an association between low FT4 and higher risk of expressive language delay (in both mild and severe hypothyroxinemia) and nonverbal cognitive delay (in severe maternal hypothyroxinemia) is troubling, especially as it is unclear whether these mothers had a true underlying thyroid condition and if so, what it was.

Unfortunately, no information about prepregnancy thyroid levels or iodine status is provided. Additionally, the possibility that some of these women had central hypothyroidism is not discussed. However, the authors make the excellent point that association does not prove causality and that their findings could be the result of other variables linking thyroid function and early childhood cognitive development. Regardless, this is an important study to be aware of. Particular strengths include the large sample size, cognitive assessments at 2 critical time points, and inclusion of neonatal thyroid status in a subset of children. Randomized prospective studies to examine the effect of thyroxine supplementation on the offspring's cognitive function in maternal hypothyroxinemia are clearly needed.

E. Eugster, MD

Reference

1. Haddow JE, Palomaki GE, Allan WC, et al. Maternal thyroid deficiency during pregnancy and subsequent neuropsychological development of the child. *N Engl J Med.* 1999;341:549-555.

Article Index

Chapter 1: Diabetes

Chapter 2: Lipoproteins and Atherosclerosis

Chapter 3: Obesity

Chapter 4: Thyroid

Chapter 5: Calcium and Bone Metabolism

Chapter 6: Adrenal Cortex

Chapter 7: Reproductive Endocrinology

Chapter 8: Neuroendocrinology

Chapter 9: Pediatric Endocrinology

Author Index

Printed and bound by CPI Group (UK) Ltd, Croydon, CR0 4YY

08/05/2025

01864677-0013